DRUG DESIGN

By

Dr. V. M. KULKARNI
Professor of Medicinal Chemistry,
Head of Pharmaceutical Division,
Department of Chemical Technology,
Matunga, Mumbai – 400 019.

Dr. K. G. BOTHARA
M. Pharm., Ph. D.
Principal and Professor
Sinhgad Institute of Pharmacy,
Narhe, Pune - 411 041.

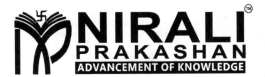

N1262

DRUG DESIGN

ISBN: 978-81-85790-11-4

Sixth Edition	:	**November 2014**
©	:	**Dr. K. G. Bothara**

The text of this publication, or any part thereof, should not be reproduced or transmitted in any form or stored in any computer storage system or device for distribution including photocopy, recording, taping or information retrieval system or reproduced on any disc, tape, perforated media or other information storage device etc., without the written permission of Dr. K. G. Bothara with whom the rights are reserved. Breach of this condition is liable for legal action.

Every effort has been made to avoid errors or omissions in this publication. In spite of this, errors may have crept in. Any mistake, error or discrepancy so noted and shall be brought to our notice shall be taken care of in the next edition. It is notified that neither the publisher nor the Dr. K. G. Bothara or seller shall be responsible for any damage or loss of action to any one, of any kind, in any manner, therefrom.

Published By:

NIRALI PRAKASHAN
Abhyudaya Pragati, 1312, Shivaji Nagar,
Off J.M. Road, PUNE – 411005
Tel - (020) 25512336/37/39, Fax - (020) 25511379
Email : niralipune@pragationline.com

Printed By:

REPRO INDIA LTD.
50/2 TTC MIDC Industrial Area,
MAHAPE
Navi Mumbai

DISTRIBUTION CENTRES

PUNE

Nirali Prakashan
119, Budhwar Peth, Jogeshwari Mandir Lane
Pune 411002, Maharashtra
Tel : (020) 2445 2044, 66022708
Fax : (020) 2445 1538
Email : bookorder@pragationline.com

MUMBAI

Nirali Prakashan
385, S.V.P. Road, Rasdhara Co-op. Hsg. Society Ltd.,
Girgaum, Mumbai 400004, Maharashtra
Tel : (022) 2385 6339 / 2386 9976,
Fax : (022) 2386 9976
Email : niralimumbai@pragationline.com

DISTRIBUTION BRANCHES

NAGPUR

Pratibha Book Distributors
Above Maratha Mandir, Shop No. 3, First Floor,
Rani Jhanshi Square, Sitabuldi, Nagpur 440012,
Maharashtra, Tel : (0712) 254 7129

HYDERABAD

Nirali Book House
22, Shyam Enclave, 4-5-947, Badi Chowdi
Hyderabad 500095, Andhra Pradesh
Tel : (040) 6554 5313, Mob : 94400 30608
Email: niralibooks@yahoo.com

CHENNAI

Pragati Books
9/1, Montieth Road, Behind Taas Mahal, Egmore,
Chennai 600008 Tamil Nadu, Tel : (044) 6518 3535,
Mob : 94440 01782 / 98450 21552 / 98805 82331
Email : bharatsavla@yahoo.com

JALGAON

Nirali Prakashan
34, V. V. Golani Market, Navi Peth, Jalgaon 425001,
Maharashtra, Tel : (0257) 222 0395
Mob : 94234 91860

KOLHAPUR

Nirali Prakashan
New Mahadvar Road,
Kedar Plaza, 1st Floor Opp. IDBI Bank
Kolhapur 416 012, Maharashtra. Mob : 9855046155

BENGALURU

Pragati Book House
House No. 1,Sanjeevappa Lane, Avenue Road Cross,
Opp. Rice Church, Bengaluru – 560002.
Tel : (080) 64513344, 64513355,
Mob : 9880582331, 9845021552
Email:bharatsavla@yahoo.com

RETAIL OUTLETS
PUNE

Pragati Book Centre
157, Budhwar Peth, Opp. Ratan Talkies,
Pune 411002, Maharashtra
Tel : (020) 2445 8887 / 6602 2707, Fax : (020) 2445 8887

Pragati Book Centre
Amber Chamber, 28/A, Budhwar Peth,
Appa Balwant Chowk, Pune : 411002, Maharashtra,
Tel : (020) 20240335 / 66281669
Email : pbcpune@pragationline.com

Pragati Book Centre
676/B, Budhwar Peth, Opp. Jogeshwari Mandir,
Pune 411002, Maharashtra
Tel : (020) 6601 7784 / 6602 0855
Email : pbcpune@pragationline.com

Pragati Book Centre
917/22, Sai Complex, F.C. Road, Opp. Hotel Roopali,
Shivajinagar, Pune 411004, Maharashtra
Tel : (020) 2566 3372 / 6602 2728

PBC Book Sellers & Stationers
152, Budhwar Peth, Pune 411002, Maharashtra
Tel : (020) 2445 2254 / 6609 2463

MUMBAI

Pragati Book Corner
Indira Niwas, 111 - A, Bhavani Shankar Road, Dadar (W), Mumbai 400028, Maharashtra
Tel : (022) 2422 3526 / 6662 5254
Email : pbcmumbai@pragationline.com

www.pragationline.com

info@pragationline.com

PREFACE

The chemical and physical properties of any molecule are governed by its structural features and biological activity does not stand exception to this. Inspite of the early recognition of this principle by Crum-Brown and Fraser, the quantitative relationship between the structure and properties of a molecule could not be established on a firm basis for almost a century. However, during last three decades, different approaches were designed to utilise the structural information coded in these physico-chemical properties as a quantitative descriptors of biological activity.

These approaches may be used effectively in drug design depending upon the institution, experience and general scientific awareness of the reader.

This text is an outgrowth of the medicinal chemistry courses taught at various Universities in India. In this book we have tried to provide a coherent and rational account of the principles underlying every aspect of drug design. Special chapters are devoted on Enzyme Inhibitors and Anti-Aids Agents to explain the strategy of the discovery and development of drugs. Since the basic principles of drug design remain sufficiently immutable, separate chapters were included to elaborate advances in the field of CVS - drugs and drugs affecting functioning of various neurotransmitter systems.

We wish to place on record our sincere thanks to our publisher Mr. D. K. Furia for his kind co-operation. Authors are greatly indebted to their colleagues for their generous help and criticism. They also wish to acknowledge indebtedness to all who have assisted with the completion of the book.

Suggestions from all corners of the profession are welcome. Authors are responsible for any deficiencies or errors that remained and would be grateful if readers would call them to our attention.

Pune   **Authors**

CONTENTS

1. Drug Design	1.1 – 1.30
2. Enzyme Inhibitors	2.1 – 2.19
3. Anti-Aids Agents	3.1 – 3.23
4. Microbial Bioconversions in Steroids	4.1 – 4.47
5. (a) Microbial Bioconversions in Prostaglandins	5.1 – 5.19
(b) Microbial Bioconversions in Antibiotics	5.20 – 5.27
6. Neurotransmitters	6.1 – 6.23
7. Drugs Acting on Cardiovascular System	7.1 – 7.29
8. Quantitative Structure Activity Relationship (QSAR)	8.1 – 8.72
9. Proteomics and Homology Modelling	9.1 – 9.8

1

DRUG DESIGN

1.1 INTRODUCTION

Drug design is an integrated developing discipline which portends an era of 'tailored drug'. It involves the study of effects of biologically active compounds on the basis of molecular interactions in terms of molecular structures or its physico-chemical properties involved. It studies the processes by which the drugs produce their effects, how they react with the protoplasm to elicit a particular pharmacological effect or response, how they are modified or detoxified, metabolised or eliminated by the organism.

Disposition of drugs in individual regions of biosystems is one of the main factors determining the place, mode and intensity of their action. The biological activity may be "positive" as in drug design or "negative" as in toxicology. Thus, drug design involves either total innovation of lead or an optimization of already available lead. These concepts are the building stones upon which the edifice of drug design is built up.

The current trend in the drug design is to develop new clinically effective agents through the structural modification of a lead nucleus. The lead is a prototype compound that has the desired biological or pharmacological activity but may have many undesirable characteristics, like high toxicity, other biological activity, insolubility or metabolism problems. Such organic leads once identified, are easy to exploit. This process is rather straight forward. The real test resides with the identification of such lead compounds and the optimum bioactive positions on the basic skeleton of such leads.

The examples of drug discovery without a lead are quite few in number. The most prominent examples include penicillium and librium. In 1928, Alexander Fleming noticed a green mold growing in a culture of *Staphylococcus aureus,* and where the two had converged, the bacteria were lysed. This led to the accidental discovery of penicillin, which was produced by the mold. Dr. Ronald Hare, colleague of Dr. Fleming, found that very special conditions were required to produce the phenomenon initially observed by Fleming. Another extraordinary circumstance was that the particular strain of the mold on Fleming culture was a relatively good penicillin producer, although most strains of that mold (Penicillium) produce no penicillin at all. The mold presumably came from the laboratory just below Fleming's laboratory where research on molds was going on. Thus, the discovery of penicillin could be possible because a combination of all unlikely events took place simultaneously.

The full extent of the value of penicillin was not revealed until late 1940s because of emergence of the sulphonamide antibacterials in 1935 and the outbreak of World War II. Thereafter the original mold (Penicillium notatum) was replaced by Penicillium chrysogenum because of relatively low yield of penicillin from the former. The correct structure of penicillin was reported in 1943 by Sir Robert Robinson (Oxford) and Karl Folkers (Merck). Once the structure was known, penicillin became lead nucleus for future analogs.

Yet another example of drug discovered without a lead is librium, the first benzodiazepine tranquilizer. A series of quinazoline-3-oxides (1) was synthesized by

Dr. Leo Sternbach at Roche in a program to develop a new class of tranquilizer drugs. Since, none of these compounds was found to be active, the scheme was terminated in 1955. However, a vial from the above scheme which remained untested was found in 1957 during a general laboratory cleanup.

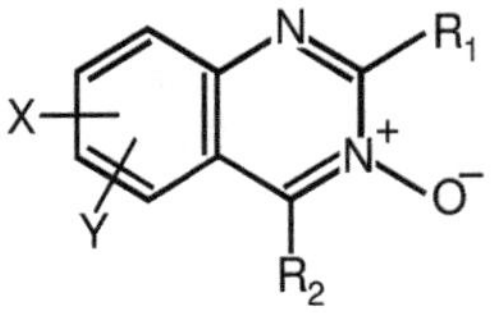

(1)

The compound (2) present in it, was submitted for pharmacological testing to complete official formalities. Surprisingly, it gave very promising results during preliminary screening for tranquilizing activity. It was found to be benzodiazepine-4-oxide, presumably produced in an unexpected reaction of the corresponding chloromethyl quinazoline-3-oxide with methylamine.

If that vial had not been found in the laboratory cleanup, the benzodiazepines may not have been discovered for many years to come. Thus, librium once identified as a lead, was then became exploited to develop future analogs like diazepam. The latter is about 10 times more potent than the lead.

The alkylating agents stood as the first systematic approach to cancer chemotherapy, especially in leukaemia where leukocytes multiply in an uncontrolled fashion. They were developed to lower down high toxicity of mustard gas whose anti-leucocytic action was evidenced when a ship loaded with mustard gas was bombed in an Italian harbour. The military personnel who came in contact with this gas showed an unusually low white blood cell count.

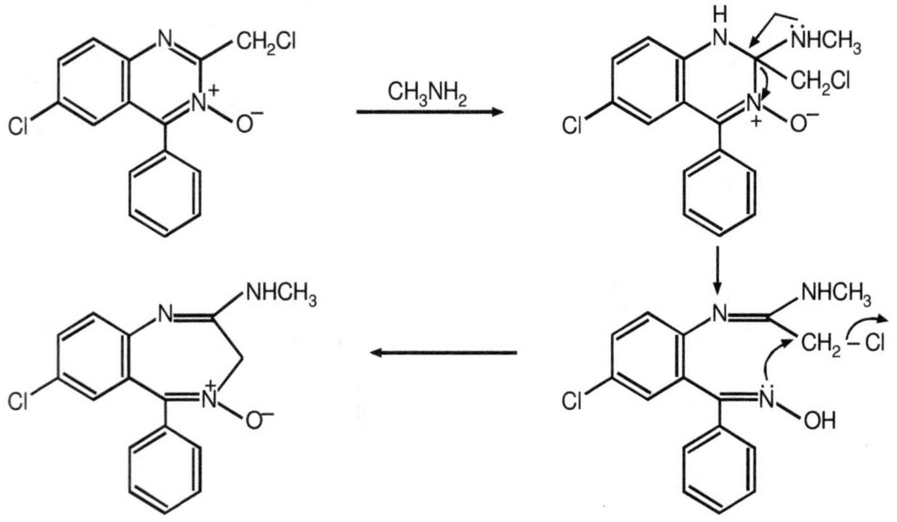

(2) Librium

1.2 METHODS OF LEAD DISCOVERY

There are several approaches which can be employed for lead identification. In order to identify a lead nucleus in a given series, the whole series should be analysed for a particular biological activity. Once the lead is identified, it can be structurally modified to improve the potency. There is a difference between the terms, activity and potency. Activity is the particular pharmacological activity while potency is the strength of that effect. Following are some of the important methods which can be used for lead identification.

(a) Random screening :

In this method, all compounds (including synthetic chemicals and natural products of plant, marine and microbial origin) from a given series are tested. Inspite of budgetary and manpower overuse, this method may be used to discover drugs or leads that have unexpected activities. Antibiotics like, streptomycin and tetracyclines were found out by this method.

A successful random search for antibacterial action was conducted by several pharmaceutical companies in the 1950s. They tested soil samples from all over the world, which resulted in the discovery of many novel structures and some spectacularly useful groups of antibiotics, notably the tetracyclines.

Recently, the large scale automated testing of microbial mutants has been done in combination with recombinant DNA techniques to speed up the efficient discovery and production of new antibiotics.

(b) Non-random screening :

It is a modified form of random screening which was developed because of budgetary and manpower restrictions. In this method, only such compounds having similar structural skeletons with that of lead, are tested.

(c) Drug metabolism studies :

Metabolism of drug occurs as an attempt by metabolizing enzymes to cut short the period of stay of the drug in the body. Structural modifications (i.e. metabolic biotransformation) are done in drug molecule by the enzymes to increase its polarity. It is brought about regardless of whether the resulting drug metabolite possesses more activity or toxicity. The discovery of sulfanilamide is reported through the metabolic studies of prontosil.

The antipyretic action of acetanilide was discovered by chance when a nurse by mistake dispensed acetanilide to a patient. Due to its toxicities, acetanilide could not stand in the market. Metabolic studies showed that the toxicities are due to its in vivo metabolite, p-aminophenol. These observations led to development of phenacetin and paracetamol.

(d) Clinical observations :

Many times the drug possesses more than one pharmacological activities. The main activity is called as therapeutic effect while rest of the actions are known as side-effects of the drug. Such drug may be used as lead compound for structural modifications to improve the potency of secondary effects.

Sulphonamide oral hypoglycemics arose directly from the clinical observation, in 1942, that a sulphathiazole derivative, which was being used specifically for treating typhoid, lowered the blood sugar drastically. The pronounced hypoglycemia exerted by

5 - isopropyl - 2 sulphanilamido - 1, 3, 4-thiadiazole indicated that an arylsulponyl thiourea moiety ($ArSO_2 - NH - C (= N) - S$) present in thiadiazoles is responsible for their blood glucose lowering effect. This observation led to the development of carbutamide by Franke and Fuchs through opening of thiazole ring to give a thiourea moiety in which = S was then replaced by = O.

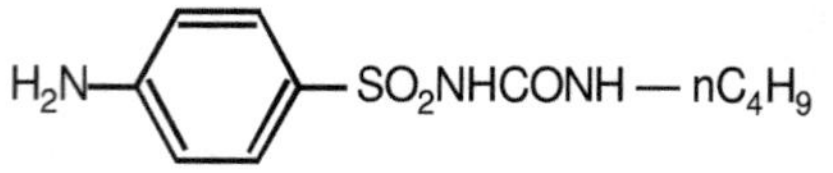

$$H_2N--SO_2NHCONH - nC_4H_9$$

Tolbutamide

In order to nullify the toxicity and antibacterial activity of the 4-amino group, it was replaced by other substituents resulting into tolbutamide, chlorpropamide and tolazamide.

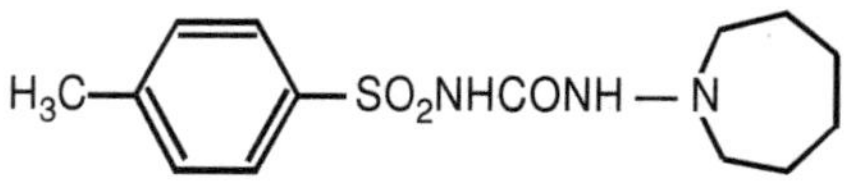

$$H_3C--SO_2NHCONH - N$$

Tolazamide

Using 4-methylhistamine as a lead, Ganellin and his colleagues developed H_2 - receptor antagonists with a side-chain terminating in a thiourea group. Because of severe side-effects seen in these thiourea derivatives, thiourea group was bioisosterically replaced by guanidine. Cyanoguanidine when introduced into the side-chain, resulted into cimetidine.

A series of aminoalkyl derivatives of iminodibenzyl was synthesized as analgesics, sedative and anti-histaminics by Hafliger and Schindler in 1951. Imipramine, one of the compounds, appeared to be potential anti-depressant during clinical studies by Kuhn in 1957. Many tricyclic anti-depressants, therefore were synthesized.

Similarly, due to the antifolate activity shown by chlorguanide, various diamino-pyrimidines were synthesized. Pyrimethamine was designed by deleting the bridging between two rings.

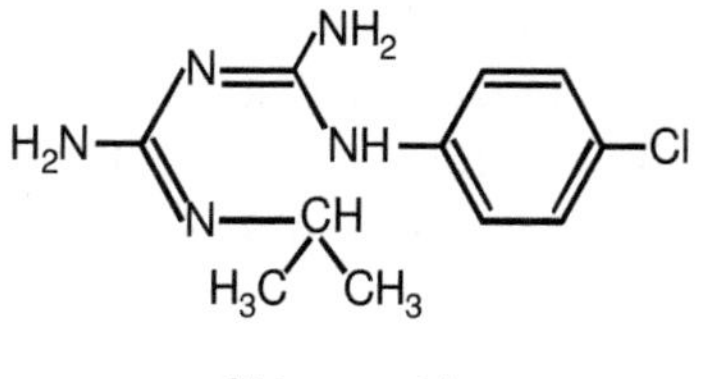

Chlorguanide

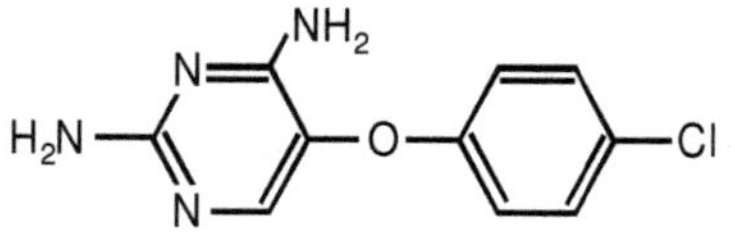

Diaminopyrimidine

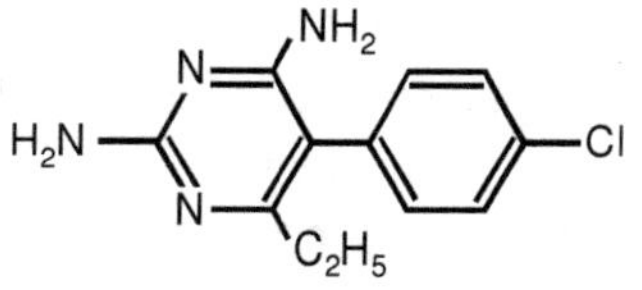

Pyrimethamine

With the knowledge of antimalarial activity of sulfapyrimidines at hand, British medicinal chemists F.L. Rose and F.H.S. Curd

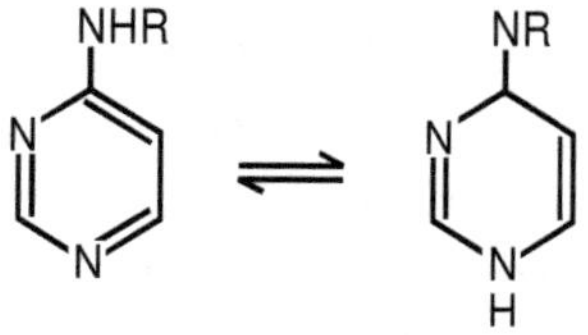

Proton tautomerism in aminopyrimidines

spotted a tautomeric proton shift in aminopyrimidines which was supposed to be an essential prerequisite for potent antimalarial activity as per Schonhofer's hypothesis proposed for amino-quinolines. Less toxicity may be expected from pyrimidine series when compared with quinolines/acridines, as the former are components of nucleotides.

*(e) **Rational approaches to lead discovery :***

The knowledge about the receptors and their mode of interaction with drug molecules plays an important role in drug design. This knowledge may be used to develop conformationally bioactive skeletons having exact three-dimensional complementarity to a receptor. Greater potency, higher selectivity and less adverse effects are expected by reducing the flexibility of the drug structure. For example, replacement of a terminal N, N-diethylamino group by piperidino exploits the decreasing valency angle at the tertiary nitrogen of the latter so that access of the basic group to anionic sites might be improved. This modification leads to the development of major tranquilizers, local anaesthetics, antihistaminics and spasmolytics. Incorporating a rigid ring leads to altered pharmacokinetic and pharmacodynamic features due to altered pKa of the amine and lipophilicity of the molecule.

This approach is of greater importance in identification of lead nucleus. It involves the use of signs and symptoms of the disease. Most diseases, atleast in part, arise from an imbalance of particular endogenous bioactive substances in the body. These imbalances may be corrected by agonism or antagonism of a receptor or by inhibition of a particular enzyme. Once the real site of such imbalance is identified, the natural enzyme substrate or endogenous substance may be used as a lead nucleus. For example, endogenous hormones, progesterone and 17 β-estradiol were used for developing oral contraceptives. The development of an anti-inflammatory drug, indomethacin from the lead nucleus, serotonin resulted at Merck with a belief that serotonin is a possible mediator of inflammation.

Medicinal chemistry has many examples of the development of successful therapeutics based on an exploration of endogenous compounds. The treatment of diabetes mellitus, for example, is based upon the administration of insulin, the hormone that is functionally deficient in this disease. The current treatment of Parkinson's disease is based upon the observation that the symptoms of Parkinson's disease arise from a deficiency of dopamine, an endogenous molecule within the human brain. Since, dopamine cannot be given as a drug, since it fails to cross the blood-brain barrier and enter the brain, its biosynthetic precursor, L-DOPA, has been successfully developed as an anti-Parkinson's drug.

Analogously, the symptoms of Alzheimer's disease arise from a relative deficiency of acetylcholine within the brain. Current therapies for Alzheimer's-type dementia are based upon the administration of cholinesterase enzyme inhibitors that prolong the effective half-life of remaining acetylcholine molecules within the brain.

Paul A. J. Janseen developed meperidine derivatives by replacing methyl group on piperidine nitrogen by alkyl aryl keto groups. While searching for a better substituent to replace carbethoxy group, tertiary alcohol group was finally selected.

Substitution of the aryl nucleus by halogens and pseudohalogens (F_3C) demonstrated that fluorine para to the keto group was optimal for neuroleptic potency. Out of several hundreds of analogs, haloperidol was selected in 1958 finally for clinical trial. Haloperidol was subjected to various molecular modifications to enhance neuroleptic activity at the expense of analgetic properties. For example, tetrahydropyridyl and piperazinyl rings were used to replace piperidine ring.

Molindone

Since the aminobutyrophenones are δ–aminoketones, homologs were synthesized. Molindone, a Mannich base of pyrrole ketone, is used as an antipsychotic.

In rational drug design, this cycle of "design-test-redesign-retest" can go on for several iterations until the optimized molecule is achieved.

In a chance test, numbing on the tongue was exerted by 2-dimethylamino-2-aceto-toluidine, an intermediate in the synthesis of gramine. This led to the synthesis of various anilides to get local anaesthetics. The presence of two sterically hindering ortho methyl groups protect the anilide linkage from hydrolysis and increase the duration of action of lidocaine. This principle was extended further to develop mepivacaine and dimethisoquine.

In Postwar France, the Berthier Pharmaceutical Company in Grenoble began to pursue a sideline project of producing soothing liquid bismuth preparations for acute tonsillitis. Being dissatisfied with the commonly used oils, they elected to use the physiologically inert valproic acid as a solvent for their bismuth compounds. Valproic acid is now used in the treatment of epilepsy and (migraine).

In 1962, Pierre Eymard, a graduate student at the University of Lyon, synthesized a series of Khellin. Khellin is a biologically active substance that occurs in the fruit of the wild Arabian Khell plant and which has been used for centuries for the treatment of kidney stones. When attempts to produce a solution of these Khellin compounds failed, advice was sought from H. Meunier of the nearby Laboratory, Berthier. In the view of Berthier's recent interest in valproic acid as a non-toxic inert solvent, Eymard's Khellin derivatives were dissolved in valproic acid and they were studied for anticonvulsant activity. These preliminary studies revealed profound anticonvulsant activity. The antiepileptic action of valproic acid was thus discovered completely by accident, with the first successful clinical trial occuring in 1963.

Bromine was discovered in seawater in 1826. Recognizing its chemical similarity to iodine, French physicians immediately exploited it as an iodine alternative for the treatment of numerous conditions, including syphilis and thyroid goiter. Although no beneficial effects were reported for either bromine or its potassium salt, their widespread use eventually helped to recognize the depressant effect of potassium bromide on the nervous system.

In 1857, Sir Charles Locock, the physician, with the view that epilepsy arose from excessive sexuality, introduced bromide to suppress the supposed hypersexuality of epileptics. The bromide salts (e.g., potassium bromide, sodium bromide) were administered in substantial doses ranging from 0.3 g/day in children to a staggering 14 g/day in adults. Although side effects had been considerable (and included psychoses and serious skin rashes), bromides were successful in 13 of the 14 patients treated. On 11 may 1857, at a meeting of the Royal Medical Society, Lucock proudly reported his success in treating "hypersexual" epilepsies with bromides.

Bromides were a major step forward in the treatment of epilepsy and their use persisted until the introduction of Phenobarbital in 1912.

Hypoglycemic Agents :

(a) Insulin analogues :

Attempts were made to synthesize various insulin analogues by specific amino acid substitutions of the β-chain of insulin molecule using recombinant DNA techniques. These analogues have different pharmacokinetic properties than the clinically used insulin. The monomeric insulin analogues appeared to be less immunogenic and allergic than insulin.

(b) Somatostatin analogues :

Somatostatin, a tetradecapeptide is a inhibitor of growth hormone release. It may also improve glycaemic control by slowing down nutrient absorption from the gut. Several somatostatin analogues have been synthesized. However, the high cost of production of these peptides might have limited their clinical utility.

(c) Fatty acid oxidation inhibitors :

In diabetic person, always an increased utilisation of fatty acids occurs. The fatty acid oxidation inhibitors exert hypoglycemic activity by promoting increased carbohydrate utilisation and inducing a reduction in fatty acid oxidation. These agents selectively block Carnitine Palmitoyl Transferase (CPT), a key enzyme in the oxidation of long-chain fatty acyl groups.

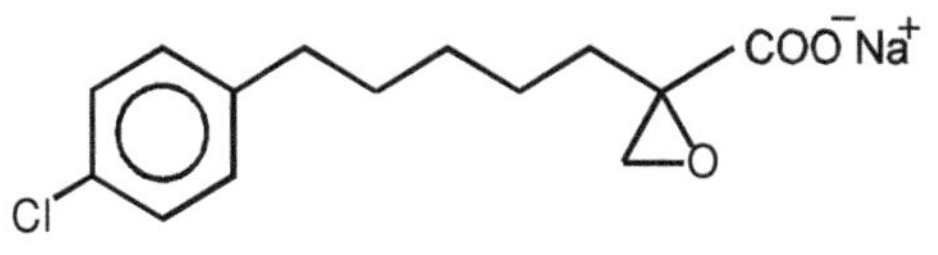

Chlorphenyl pentyloxirane carboxylate

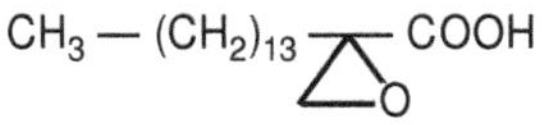

$$CH_3 - (CH_2)_{13} - COOH$$

2-tetradecylglycidate

$$(CH_3)_3\overset{+}{N} - CH_2 - \underset{\underset{NH_2}{|}}{CH} - CH_2 - COOH \quad Cl^-$$

2-(3-methyl cinnamyl hydrazone) propionate

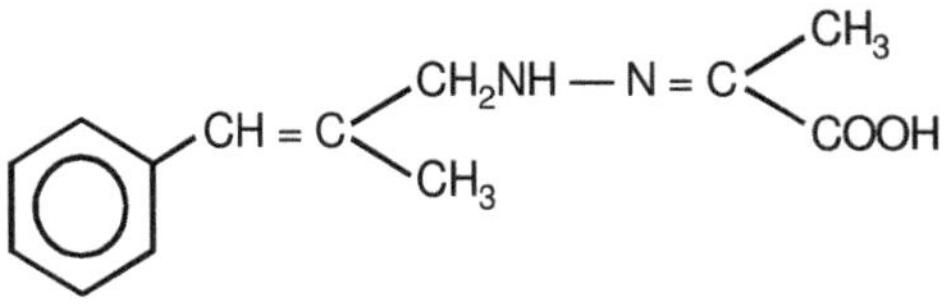

Aminocarnitine

(d) Anorectic agents :

Weight loss is an effective means to achieve improved glycaemic control in the treatment of obese non-insulin dependent diabetes millitus. A variety of anorectic agents which may be used for short-term therapy, include

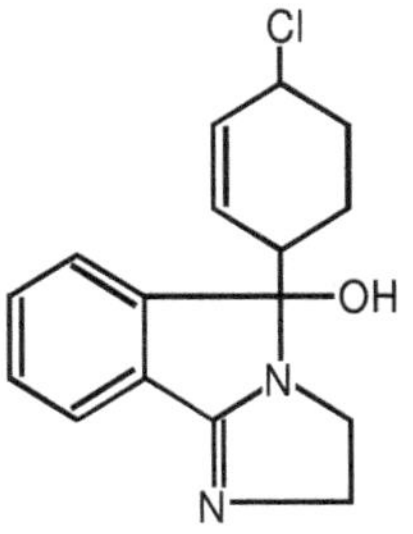

Mazindol 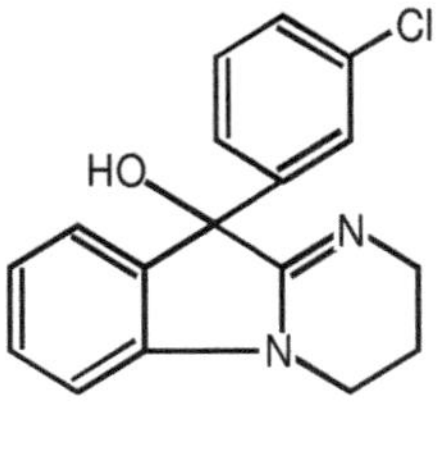   Ciclazindol

(e) Inhibitors of carbohydrate absorption :

The intestinal carbohydrate digestion can be delayed by inhibiting the enzymes which cleave the terminal glucose. Carbose is a clinically used example.

(f) Aldose reductase inhibitors :

Glucose is mainly metabolised in body by two pathways (i) glycolytic pathway involving an initial phosphorylation by the enzyme, hexokinase and (ii) polyol pathway by the enzyme, aldose reductase which reduces glucose to fructose via sorbitol.

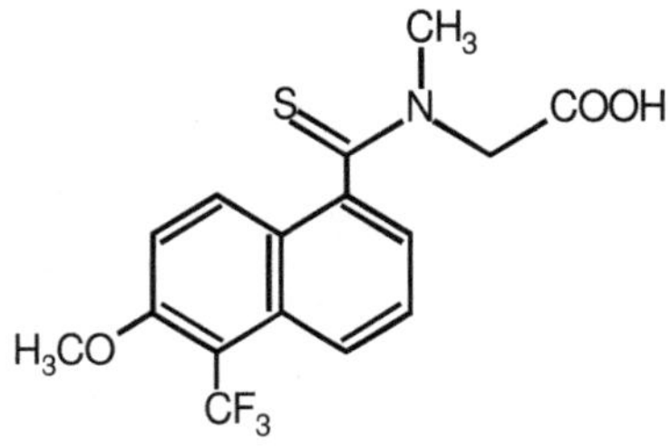

Tolrestat

Glucose is preferentially metabolised by glycolytic pathway in normal person. In diabetic patient, the high glucose concentration leads to saturation of glycolytic pathway. Excess glucose is then metabolised by polyol pathway resulting into production of sorbitol and fructose. Since, the rate of formation of sorbitol is higher than its rate of conversion to fructose, sorbitol selectively accumulates and causes complications of chronic diabetes like, cataract, neuropathy and retinopathy.

Tolrestat is an example of clinically used agent useful in the prophylaxis of diabetic neuropathy, retinopathy and cataract.

Antimalarials :

The planar conformation of the acridine ring is optimal for antimicrobial activity. However separation of individual phenyl ring from the whole tricyclic skeleton does not affect activity. This observation led the synthesis of 2-(p-chlorophenyl) amino-pyrimidines by Rose, thus retaining the overall flat area. Since, dialkylamino-alkylamino side chain was already present in some of the anti-malarials, it was attached to the skeleton. In order to simplify the structure, the pyrimidine ring was opened to get biguanides. However because of the increased basicity (due to diethylamino group and two basic guanidines), the terminal guanidino group was replaced by simple alkyl groups. This resulted into development of chlorguanide where the alkyl group is an isopropyl moiety.

Anticoagulants :

(1) **Heparinoids :** Heparinoids are the sulphuric acid esters of various polysaccharides. They were found to be more active than heparin in animals.

(2) In 1922, a disease characterized by internal bleeding was reported in cattle which was found to be due to the ingestion of sweet clover hay. Investigations of the later identified 3, 3 - methylenebis (4-hydroxycoumarin) as a causative agent.

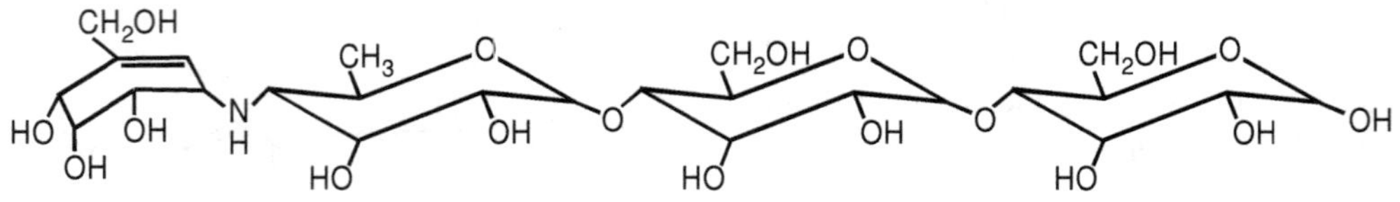

Acarbose

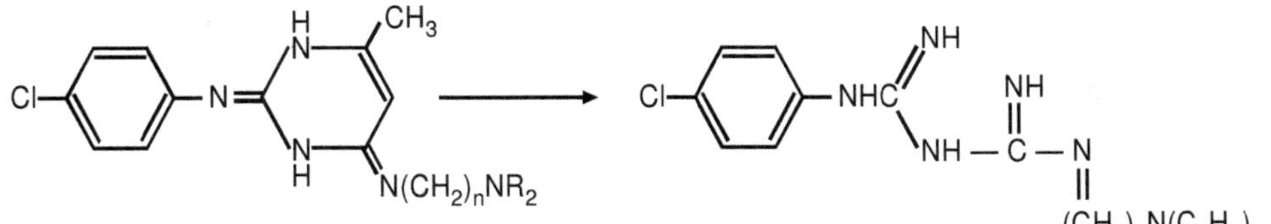

Biguanide

At the same time, warfarin, another coumarin derivative was routinely used as a haemorrhagic rat poison. Using both these leads, various synthetic compounds were prepared by molecular modifications.

(3) Indanedione, yet another lead was developed by ring contraction of coumarin. This resulted in the introduction of phenindione and diphenadione. They exert anticoagulant action by inhibiting prothrombin biosynthesis as well as the synthesis of factors VII, IX and X, through the formation of active cyclic ketals.

Since vitamin K may also generate a cyclic ketal-like structure, the oral anticoagulants may act by antagonising vitamin K competitively at the active sites :

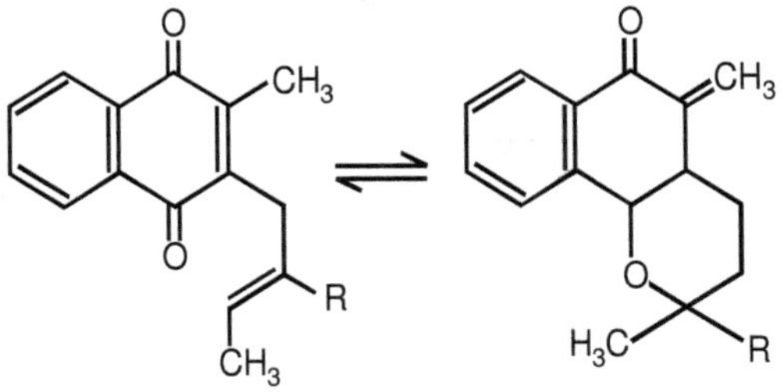

Postulated cyclization of vitamin K

1.3 OPTIMIZATION OF THE LEAD

Once the lead nucleus is identified, it is easy to exploit. This process is rather straight forward. Various approaches are employed in order to improve the desired pharmacological properties of the lead nucleus. Important amongst them are,

(a) Identification of the active part (the pharmacophore) :

Any drug molecule consists of both, essential and non-essential parts. Essential part is important in governing pharmacodynamic (drug-receptor interactions) property while non-essential part influences pharmacokinetic features. The relevant groups on a molecule that interact with a receptor are known as bioactive functional groups. They are responsible for the activity. The schematic representation of nature of such bioactive functional groups along with their interatomic distances is known as pharmacophore.

A **pharmacophore** was first defined by Paul Ehrlish in 1909, as "a molecular framework that carries the essential features responsible for a drug's biological activity". In 1977, this definition was updated by Peter Gund to "a set of structural features in a molecule that is recognized at a receptor site and is responsible for that molecule's biological activity". The IUPAC definition of pharmacophore is "an ensemble of steric and electronic features that is necessary to ensure the optimal supra molecular interactions with a specific biological target and to trigger (or block) its biological response".

In 1958, Daniel Koshland suggested a modification to the lock and key model. Since enzymes are rather flexible structures the active site is continually reshaped by interactions with the substrate as the substrate interacts with the enzyme. The active site continues to change until the substrate is completely bound, at which point the final shape and charge is determined.

The active site geometry of a protein complex depends heavily upon conformational changes induced by the bound ligand.

Once such pharmacophore is identified, structural modifications can be done to improve pharmacokinetic properties of the drug. For example, the presence of a phenyl ring, asymmetric carbon, ethylene bridge and tertiary nitrogen are found to be minimum structural requirement for a narcotic analgesic to become active. Similarly, the presence of two anionic sites and one cationic site must be present in cholinergic agent.

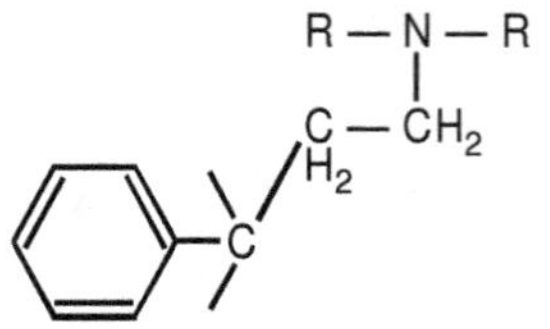

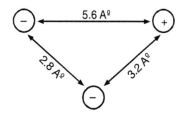

Fig. 1.1 : Pharmacophore for Narcotic Drug

Fig. 1.2 : Pharmacophore for Cholinergic Drug

Morphine, the prototype narcotic agent has a pentacyclic structure. The complexity of structure leads to appearance of several adverse effects. Hence, the pharmacophore of morphine has been recognized through molecular dissection and was used to develop still simpler and even acyclic analogs. For example, methadone is as potent as analgesic as morphine.

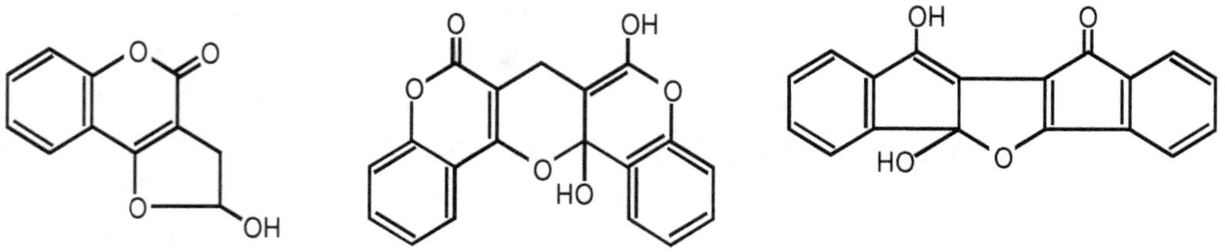

Potential cyclic ketal structures of oral anticoagulant

Methadone

Type - I : Histamine (4.55 Å)

Type - II : Histamine (3.60 Å)

Type - I : Antihistamine (4.80 ± 0.2 Å)

Type - II : Antihistamine (± 3.60 Å)

Fig. 1.3 : The Two Nearly Equally Preferred but Significantly Different Conformations for Histamine

Similarly, in estrogenic compounds two bioactive sites, having ability to undergo H-bonding, should be separated by a minimum distance of 8.5 A°.

In 17-β-estradiol, the distance is 10.9 A° while in diethyl stilbestrol it is 12.1 A°.

On the contrary, in certain cases, an increase in structural complexity (increased rigidity) is required for selectivity of action and to increase potency. For example, buprenorphine is about 10-12 times potent than morphine and has a very low level of dependence liability.

Buprenorphine

(b) Functional group optimization :

The activity of a drug can be correlated to its structure in terms of the contribution of its functional groups to the lipophilicity, electronic and steric features of the drug skeleton. Hence, by selecting proper functional group, one can govern the drug distribution pattern and can avoid the occurrence of side-effects. For example, the amino group of carbutamide (antibacterial agent) was replaced by a methyl group to give tolbutamide (antidiabetic agent).

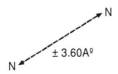

Carbutamide : R = NH_2
Tolbutamide : R = CH_3

Similarly, removal of sulfonamide side-chain of chlorothiazide (an antihypertensive drug with diuretic activity) helped to design diazoxide (an antihypertensive drug without diuretic activity).

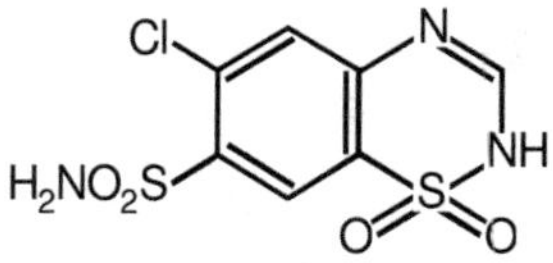

Chlorothiazide

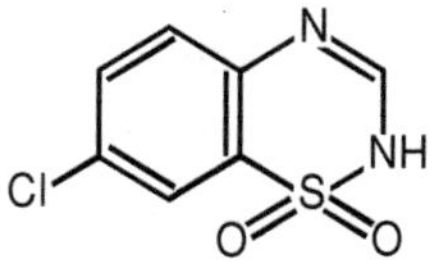

Diazoxide

Since a neuroleptic activity runs parallel with the α-adrenoceptor blocking activity, piperoxan, an alpha adrenoceptor blocking agent was chosen as a lead to get pentamoxane which showed high neuroleptic activity in animal studies.

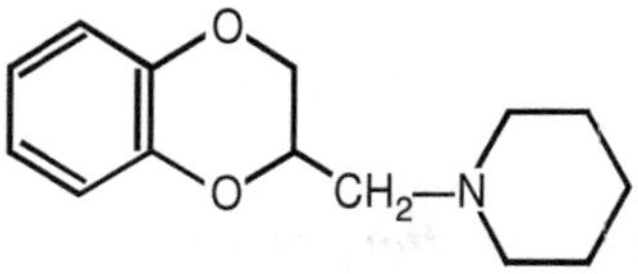

Piperoxan

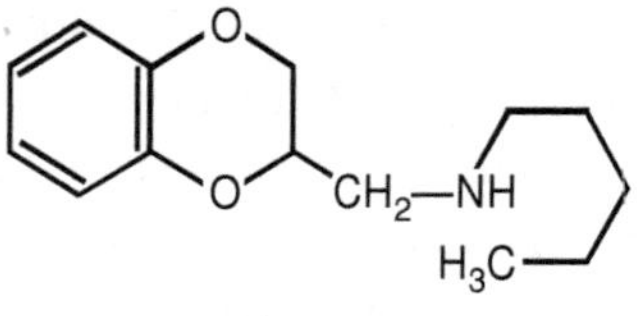

Pentamoxane

The replacement of –Cl by CF_3 in ring position 2 and the modification of the basic side-chain to include a piperazine moiety in chlorpromazine is thought to enhance neuroleptic potency by increasing lipophilicity so that CNS-entry of the drug is facilitated.

(c) Structure-activity relationship studies :

The physiological action of a molecule is a function of its chemical constitution. This observation is the basis of SAR studies.

SAR studies usually involve the interpretation of activity in terms of the structural features of a drug molecule. Generalised conclusions then can be made after examining a sufficient number of drug analogs. For example, sulphonamides are found to be associated with diuretic and antidiabetic activities in addition to their antibacterial activity. The generalised structures needed for individual activity are represented below.

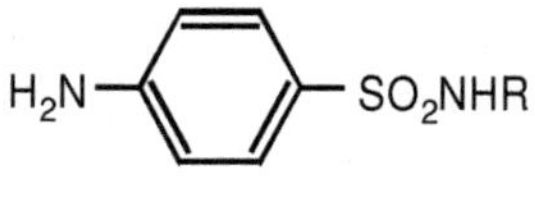

Antibacterial sulphonamide

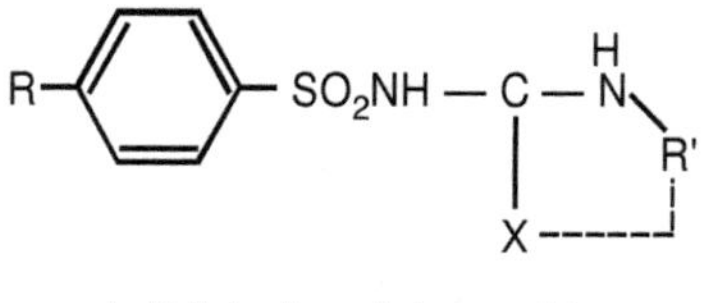

Antidiabetic sulphonamide

(X = O, S or N)

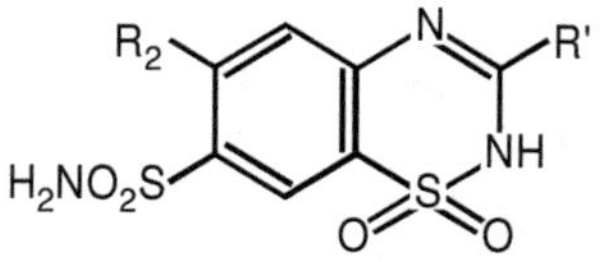

Diuretic sulphonamide

Because of hepatotoxic side-effects of hydrazines and hydrazides, structurally diversified compounds were synthesized resulting into the introduction of pargyline and tranylcypromine. Tranylcypromine was developed as a structural analog of amphetamine and is used as an anti-depressant agent. Due to pronounced effect on blood pressure, the former was used as an antihypertensive agent. Further structural modification of pargyline skeleton resulted into cyclogyline.

Pargyline

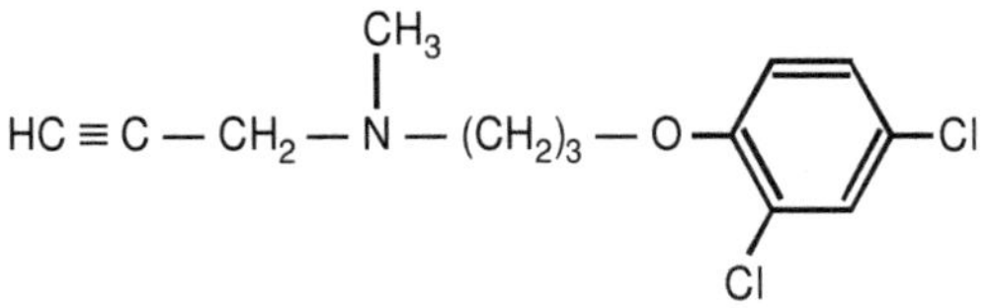

$$HC \equiv C - CH_2 - \underset{\underset{CH_3}{|}}{N} - (CH_2)_3 - O - \text{(ring)} - Cl$$

Clorgyline

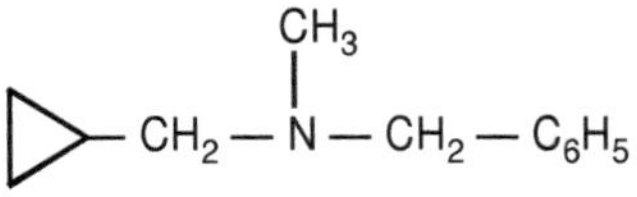

$$\text{(cyclopropyl)} - CH_2 - \underset{\underset{CH_3}{|}}{N} - CH_2 - C_6H_5$$

Cyclogyline

(d) Homologation :

The variation in the substituent can be used to increase or decrease the polarity, alter the pKa, and change the electronic properties of a molecule. Exploration of homologous series is one of the most often used method to induce these changes in a very gradual manner. A homologous series is a group of compounds that differ by a constant unit, generally a CH_2 group. Usually, increasing the length of a saturated carbon side-chain from one (CH_3) to 5 to 9 atoms (pentyl to nonyl) produces an increase in pharmacological effects. Further increase results in a decrease in the activity. This is probably either due to increase in lipophilicity beyond optimum value (hence decreased absorption and distribution) or

decrease in concentration of free drug (i.e., micelle formation). For example, maximum hypnotic activity is seen from 1-hexanol to 1-octanol. Thereafter activity decreases for higher homologs. Similarly, in a series of 4-alkyl substituted resorcinol derivatives, 4-n-hexyl resorcinol (clinically used topical anaesthetic in throat lozenges) was found to possess maximum antibacterial activity. While in a series of mandelate esters, n-nonyl ester has maximum anti-spasmodic activity. In the same series, branching leads to decrease in the activity, probably due to interference with receptor binding. For example, primaquine (an antimalarial agent) is much more potent than its secondary or tertiary homologs.

(e) Cyclization of the side-chain :

Change in the potency or change in the activity spectra can be brought about by transformation of alkyl side-chain into cyclic analogs. For example, chlorpromazine (i) has more neuroleptic activity than its cyclic analog (ii). Similarly the compound (iii) has anti-depressant (imipramine like) activity than neuroleptic activity. While in compound (iv) the antiemetic activity is greatly enhanced.

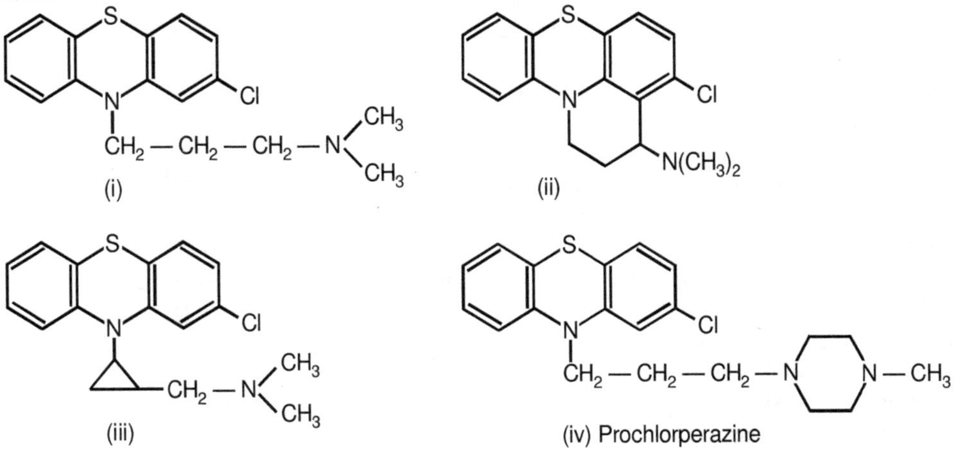

Cyclization of the side chain

Sometimes bridging of two carbon atoms (secondary cyclization) also leads to an increase in potency or change in activity spectrum. Examples include thebaine (oripavine) derivatives, atropine, bridged piperazine derivatives of phenothiazines etc.

(f) Bioisosterism :

The purpose of molecular modification is usually to improve potency, selectivity, duration of action and reduce toxicity. The physicist Langmuir introduced the term, isosterism in 1919. The term, bioisosterism, introduced by friedmen in 1951. Bioisosters are substituents or groups that have similar physical or chemical properties and hence similar biological activity pattern. Isosteric groups, according to Erlenmeyer's definition are isoelectronic in their outermost electron shell. Bioisosteric replacement may help to decrease toxicity or to change activity spectra. It may also alter the metabolic pattern of the drug. The parameters being changed are molecular size, steric shape (bond angles, hybridization), electron distribution, lipid solubility, water solubility, the pKa, the chemical reactivity to cell components, and the capacity to undergo H-bonding (receptor interaction). Even if the bioisosteric replacement is relatively minor (Cl for CH_3 or vice versa). Cl may block metabolic hydroxylation, whereas CH_3 may be bio-oxidized and the compound may have shorter half-life. For example, tolbutamide (R=CH_3) has shorter half-life than chlorpropamide (R=Cl). Erlenmeyer defined isosters as atoms, ions or functional groups in which the peripheral layers of electrons can be considered to be identical. These are known as classical bioisosters. While non-classical bioisosters do not have the same number of atoms and do not fit the steric and electronic rules of classical isosters, but they do produce a similarity in biological activity. More recently Burger subdivided bioisosters as :

(1) Classical bioisosters :

(a) Univalent atoms and groups :

Such groups include

(i) – Cl, – Br, – I

(ii) – CH_3, – NH_2, – OH and – SH

(b) Bivalent atoms and groups :

(i) R-O-R ; R-NH-R; R-CH_2-R; R-S-R; R-Se-R

(ii) –$COCH_2$R; –CONHR; –CO_2R; –COSR

(c) Trivalent atoms and groups :

(i) –CH = ; –N =

(ii) –P = ; –As =

(d) Tetravalent atoms :

(i) =C= ; =N=; =P=
$$\overset{\oplus}{} \quad \overset{\oplus}{}$$

(ii) $-\overset{|}{\underset{|}{C}}-$; $-\overset{|}{\underset{|}{Si}}-$

(e) Ring equivalents :

(i) –CH = CH– ; –S– (e.g., benzene, thiophene)

(ii) –CH= ; –N= (e.g., benzene, pyridine)

(iii) –O– ; –S– ; –CH_2 ; –NH–

(e.g., tetrahydrofuran, tetrahydrothiophene, cyclopentane, pyrrolidine).

The size, shape, electronic distribution, lipid solubility, water solubility, pKa, chemical reactivity, and hydrogen bonding are the parameters that influence the potency, selectivity and duration of action of the drug. Bioisosterism becomes effective because it affects all the above parameters to less or more extent. In the design of bioisosters, the biochemical mode of action may play an important role e.g., aspirin acts by acetylating cyclo-oxygenase enzyme. Isosters of aspirin are inactive because they cannot release the acetyl group at all (X=CH_2) or at an adequate rate (X=S, NH).

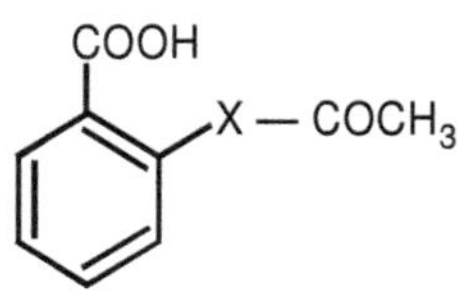

(2) Non-classical Bioisosters :

(a) Halogens : Cl, F, Br, CF, CN

(b) Ethers : —S—; —O—; CN-N ; (CN)₂C(CH₃)₂

(c) Carbonyl group : ketone; C(CN)₂; S=O; SO₂

(d) Carboxylic acid group : —C(=O)OH ; —SO₂OH ; —P(=O)(OH)(NH₂)

(e) Hydroxy group : —OH; —NH—C(=O)—R; —NHSO₂R; —CH₂OH; —NH—C(=O)—NH₂

(f) Catechol : catechol ; benzimidazole ; 3-hydroxy-4-pyridinone ; 1-hydroxy-2-pyridinone

(g) Thiourea : —NH—C(=S)—NH₂ ; —NH—C(=N—CN)—NH₂ ; —NH—C(=CH—NO₂)—NH₂

(h) Spacer group : —(CH₂)₃—; cyclohexyl ; phenyl

(i) Ionizing analogues : Ar—OH⁺ ; Ar N⁺H SO₂CH₃ ; Ar N⁺H HCN

(j) Ring Bioisosters :

1. Indole ↔ Indazole ↔ 3,4-dimethoxy phenyl ↔ Furopyridine
   ↕
   Thienopyrrole

2. Hydroxamic acid ↔ Acyl cyanamide ↔ Acyl sulphonamides

1.4 APPLICATION OF BIOISOSTERISM IN DRUG-DESIGN

(a) An important compound from catecholamine series is phenylephrine in which phenolic hydroxyl group takes part in H-bonding with bioactive site on the receptor. The hydroxyl group can be replaced by other group having ability to undergo H-bonding. Hence, alkylsulphonamido derivative of phenylephrine was found to retain activity.

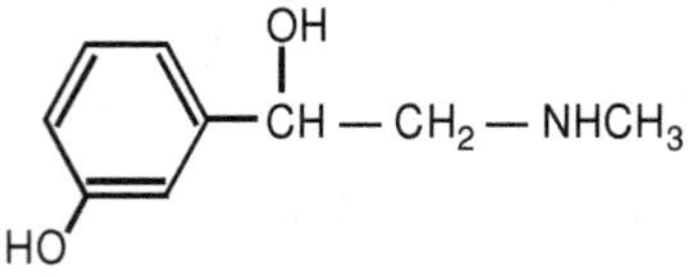

Phenylephrine

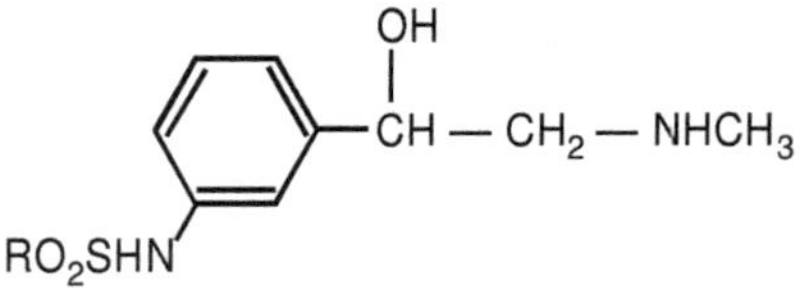

Alkylsulphonamido derivative

(b) A classic example of ring versus non-cyclic structure is diethylstilbestrol and 17 β-estradiol.

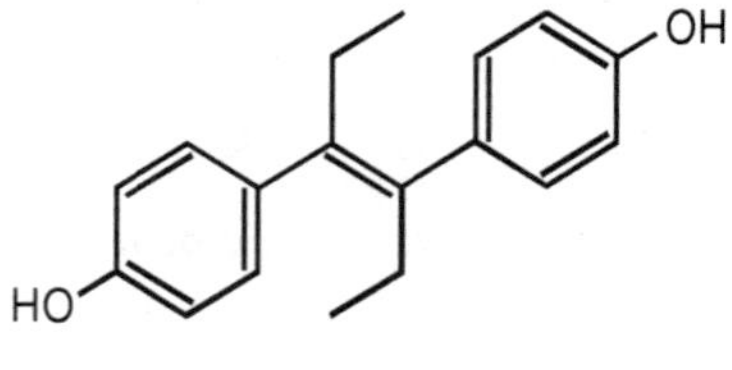

Trans-Diethyl stilbestrol

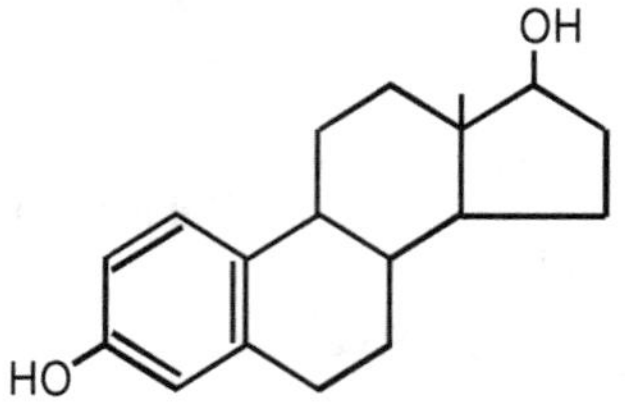

17-β-estradiol

Diethylstilbestrol has about the same potency as that of naturally occurring estradiol. The central double bond of diethyl stilbestrol is highly important for the correct orientation of the phenolic and ethyl groups (trans) at the receptor site.

(c) Bioisosteric analogs in neuroleptic category include

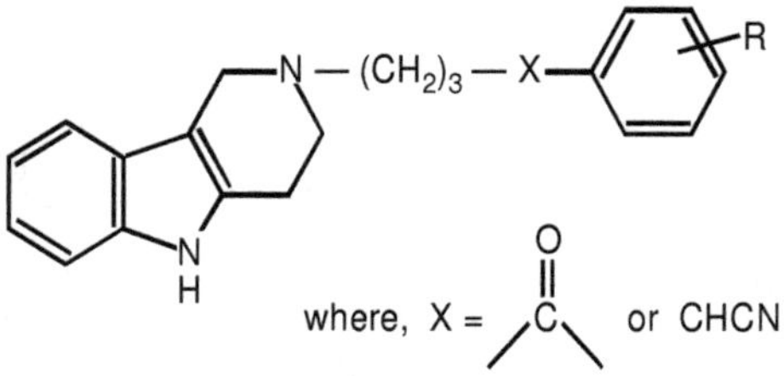

where, X = $\overset{O}{\underset{}{C}}$ or CHCN

(d) Bioisosteric analogs in anti-inflammatory category include

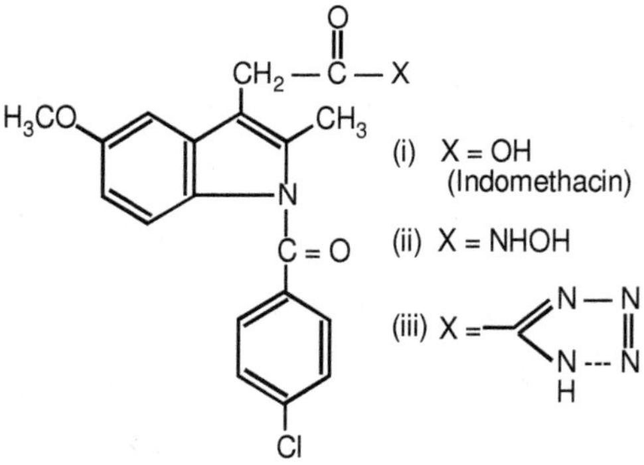

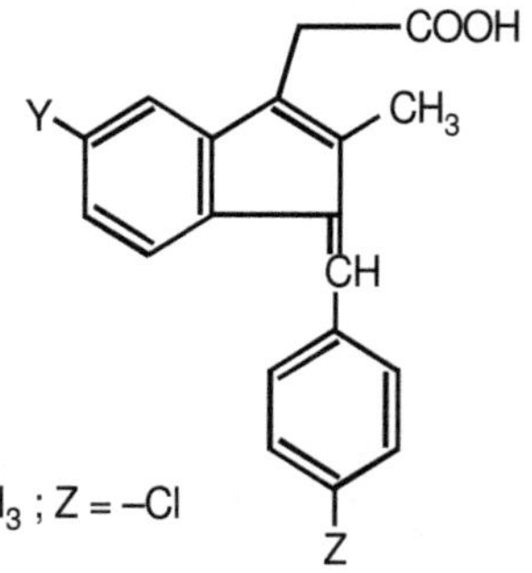

(i) X = OH (Indomethacin)

(ii) X = NHOH

(iii) X = tetrazole

(i) Y = –OCH$_3$; Z = –Cl

(ii) Y = –F;
      Z = –S –CH$_3$ (Sulindac)

(e) Bioisosterism in anti-histaminic agents

$$R - X - (CH_2)_n - Y \; ; \; X = NH, O, CH_2$$

(i) $Y = N(CH_3)_2$ (n = 2)

(ii) $Y =$ (imidazoline ring) (n = 1)

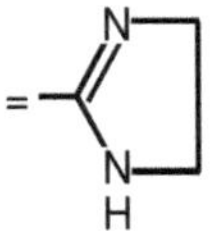

(iii) $Y =$ (imidazole ring) (n = 1, 2)

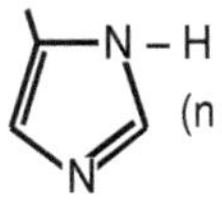

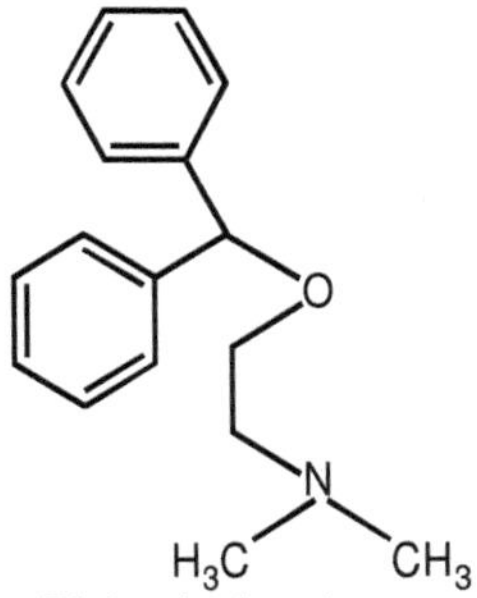

Diphenhydramine

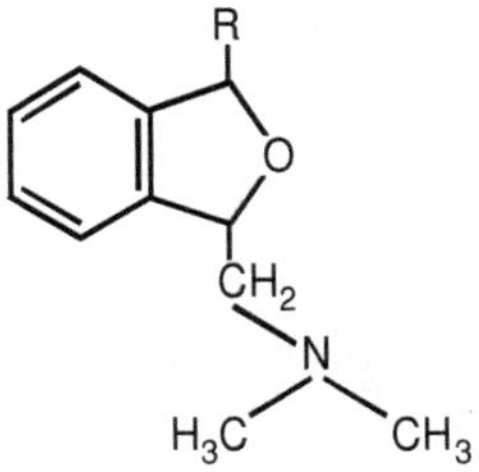

Bioisoster (Isobenzofurans)

(f) The non-thiazide category of diuretic agents has been developed by replacing ring SO_2 by carbonyl group. e.g., Quinazolinone derivatives.

(g) Metoclopramide shares features of both anticholinergic (–O– is bioisosterically replaced by –NH–) and antidopaminergic (antiemetic) agents. It is in fact used as antiulcer agent.

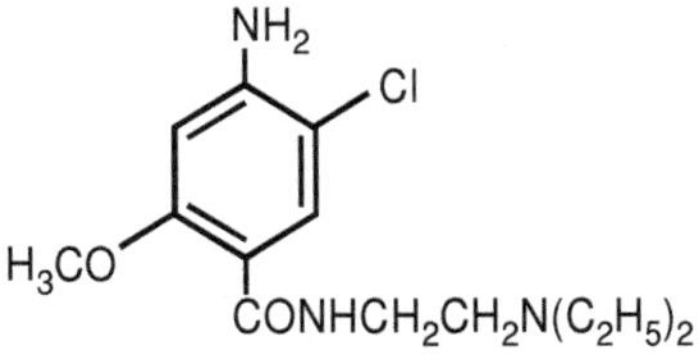

Metoclopramide

(h) Pirenzepine, an antimuscarinic agent, possesses structural similarity with tricyclic antidepressant agents. However, it lacks antidepressant activity due to its poor penetration ability in the CNS. Hence, other tricyclic antidepressant agents (e.g., doxepin and trimipramine) are undergoing clinical investigations for antiulcer activity.

Table 1.1

Parent compound	Bioisosters	Activity of parent compound
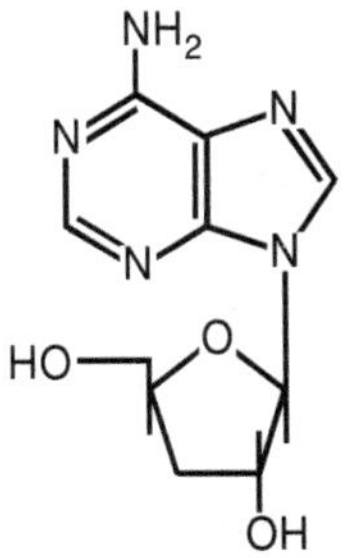 (adenosine structure)	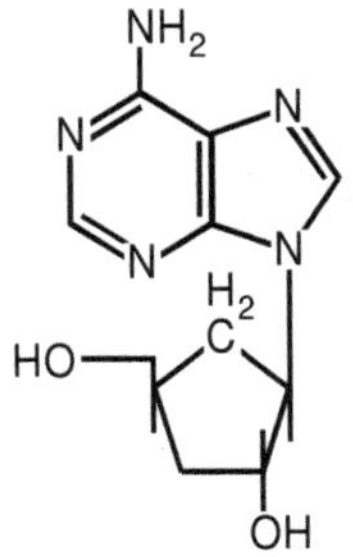 (adenosine bioisoster structure)	Adenosine deaminase activity (−)

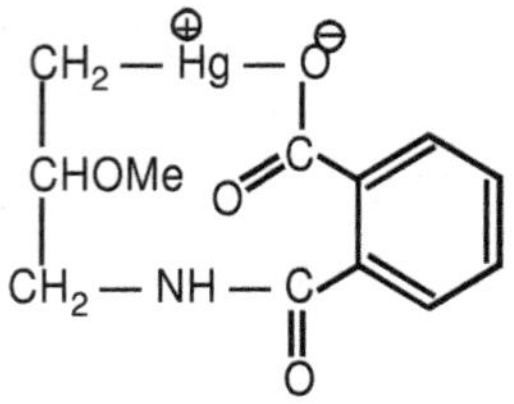	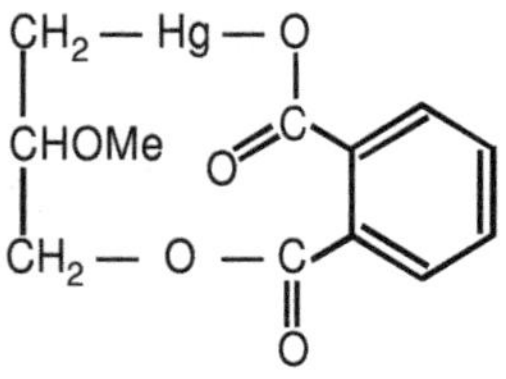	Diuretic (+)
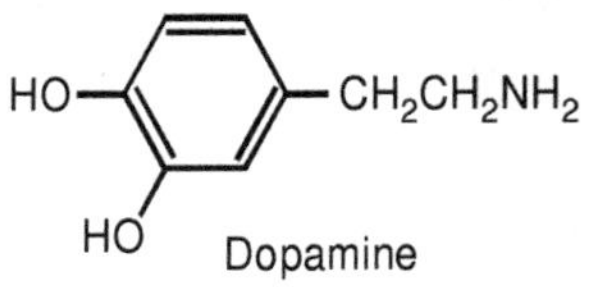 Dopamine	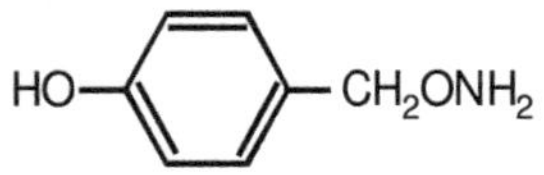	Increases inhibition

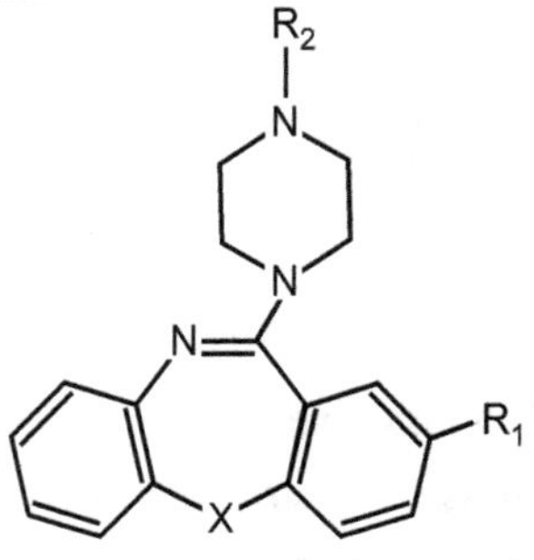

X	R_1	R_2	Compound
S	Cl	CH_3	Clotiapine
O	Cl	CH_3	Loxapine
O	Cl	H	Amoxapine
CH_3	H	CH_3	Periapine

Isosteric replacement in clozapine analogues

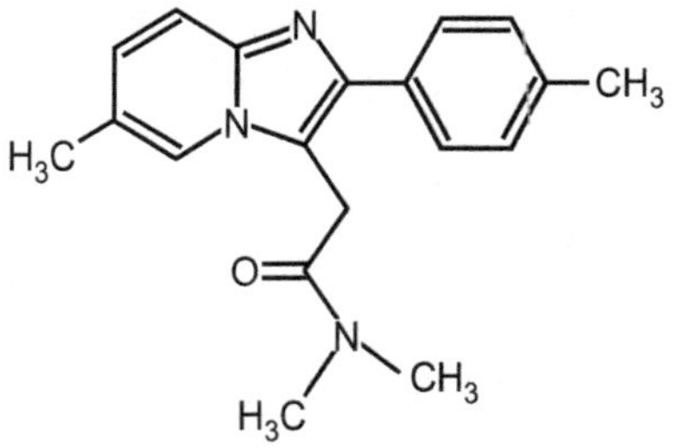

Zolpidem

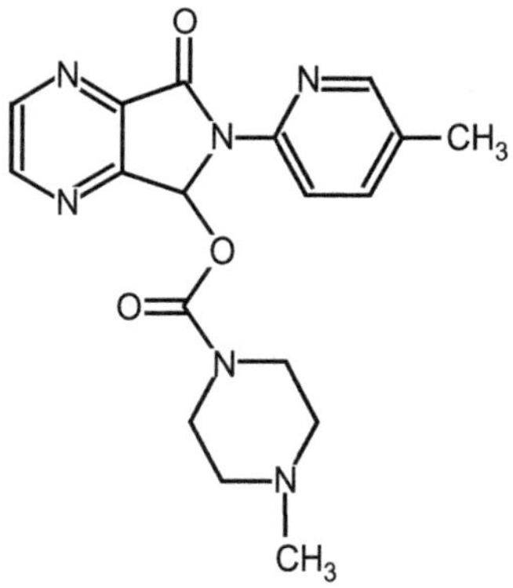

Zopiclone

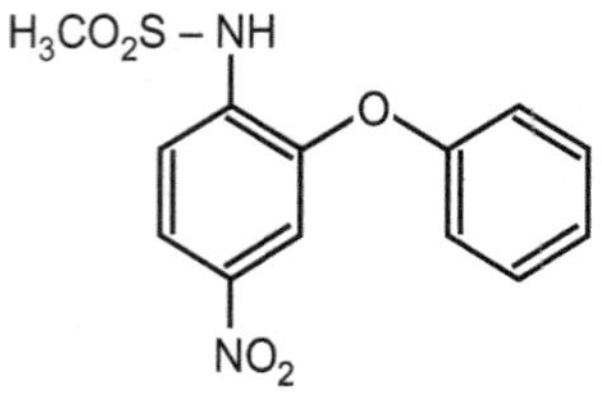

Nimesulide

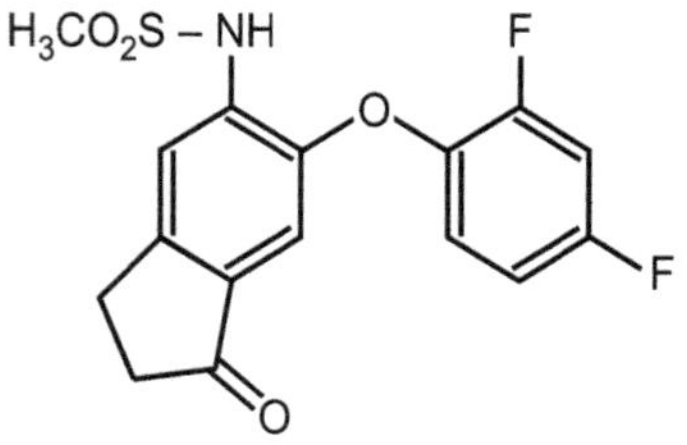

Flosulide

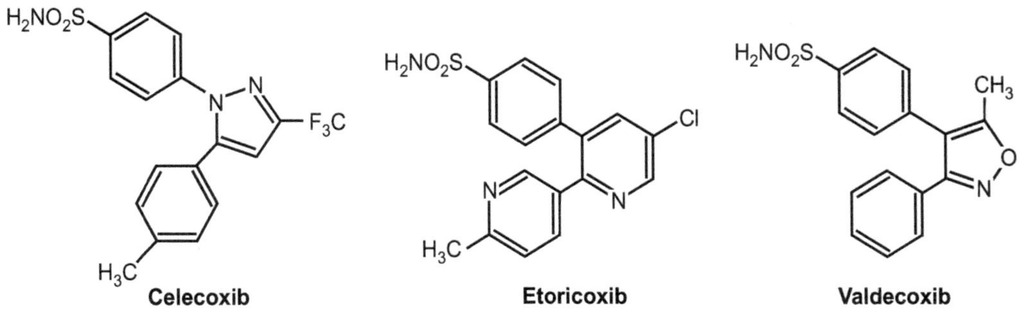

Celecoxib

Etoricoxib

Valdecoxib

Application of bio-isosterism in selective COX$_2$-inhibitors.

Table 1.1 contains a variety of bioisosters (including classic and non-classic bioisosters) which are either clinically used or used as investigational compounds. If a particular substituent does not change the activity of the original compound, it does not necessarily follow that the groups substituted are bioisosteric. It may simply be that substitution at this site plays little role in the interaction of the molecule with its site of action. Accordingly, groups can only be accepted to be truely bioisosteric when they can be replaced in a number of drug series.

Inspite of the great success of the classical methods of drug design, their unpredictability and the tremendous amount of wasted effort expended, have necessitated the development of more rational methods with a much higher predictive capability, in an effort to project drug design as a science rather than an art. The approach involving selection of lead nucleus remains unchanged, the organic chemistry used in the design of its analogs was still there; however ways to select substituents for structural modification were changed and models based on multiple regression analysis and pattern recognition methods, using computer techniques are employed as aids.

The knowledge of drug metabolism in vivo can be utilized to improve a wide variety of drug characteristics. Using this knowledge, an active drug is not modified irreversibly, but in such a way that it will be regenerated by metabolic processes. Such temporarily modified structure usually inactive in nature is called as prodrug.

The search for a new drug became a risky affair due to the monetary cost, the time involved (from 7 to 10 years) and high rate of failures. These factors have compelled the medicinal chemists to find out new ways of putting the existing drugs to better use. Two major objectives that stand behind the optimization of the lead nucleus :

(a) to maximize the drug's desired activity and

(b) to minimize the intensity and frequency of side effects associated with the drug. Drugs usually have multiple pharmacological effects and the drug designer tries to improve selectivity of action. The aim of a medicinal chemist should be to optimize and not only to maximize the activity, to provide better affinity to the target sites.

One of the ways is to improve the intensity of beneficial side effect associated with the drug. An effect considered as a side effect today, may be appreciated as a therapeutic effect tomorrow. This will be possible only if both these components of action are based on different mechanisms of action at essentially different sites of action.

Examples are anti-histamines with a strong sedative action (e.g., chlorpromazine) as a side-effects were latter developed as neuroleptics and tranquilizing agents. The tranquilizing properties (strong sedation, state of indifferent and disinterest without effecting sleep) of chlorpromazine were observed during its clinical evaluation as an anti-histamines.

Sulphonamides, used as antibacterial agents exhibited acidosis as a side-effect due to its inhibition of renal carbonic anhydrase. This observation led to the development of the diuretic, acetazolamide and subsequently the chlorthiazide group of diuretics. Since, guanidine was found to lower blood sugar level, polymethylene diguanides were synthesized. To improve hypoglycemic action and to decrease toxicity of these synthalins, biguanides (e.g., phenformin) were prepared.

1.5 PRODRUG DESIGNING

Prodrug is a chemically modified form of a drug which has a superior delivery properties. The term prodrug was coined by Albert.

In 1958, another similar term 'drug latentiation' proposed by Harper (1959) is defined as the chemical modification of a biologically active compound to form a new compound which, upon in vivo enzymatic attack, will liberate the parent compound. It refers to a pharmacologically inactive compound that is converted to an active drug by a metabolic biotransformation at appropriate time and place in the body without substantial direct elimination or untoward metabolism. This activation may occur at any time during absorption, distribution or metabolism. For instance, castor oil is a laxative because it is hydrolyzed intenstinally to the active, ricinoleic acid. Another classical example is conversion of prontosil to sulfanilamide.

Prodrug thus may be considered as drug containing specialized non-toxic protective group utilized in a transient manner to alter or eliminate undesirable properties in the parent drug.

Prodrug designing is required to overcome many formulation, pharmacokinetic or pharmacodynamic drawbacks. The prominent drawbacks include.

(i) unpleasant taste or odour (gastric irritation),

(ii) a wide range of adverse effects,

(iii) shorter duration of action,

(iv) instability.

(v) site non-specificity,

(vi) poor absorption or distribution,

(vii) poor water solubility,

(viii) some compounds are more active but unable to reach the site of action (e.g., GABA).

1.6 TYPES OF PRODRUG

(a) Non-intentional prodrug :

Sometimes, after administration of the drug the metabolic studies indicate the prodrug nature of drug. It becomes accidentally evident that the activity of a drug is because of its metabolite and not because of the parent drug. Example includes the anti-inflammatory agent, sulindac.

(b) Carrier-linked prodrug :

It is a compound that contains an active drug linked to a carrier group that can be removed enzymatically, such as an ester which is hydrolysed to an active carboxylic acid containing drug. The carrier group must be non-toxic and biologically inactive when detatched from the drug. It should be removed easily to allow the active drug to be released efficiently in vivo. The most common reaction for activation of carrier-linked prodrugs is hydrolysis.

A simple hydrolysis reaction cleaves the transport moiety at the adequate rate (e.g., progabide, bacampicillin).

Targetting of Drugs : The side effects associated with a drug are the outcome of non-specific distribution of the drug administered. Targetted drug delivery not only decreases the side effects but also helps to lower down the therapeutic dose of the drug by enhancing the selectivity of attack. This can be achieved by selecting pharmacologically inert, ready to degrade and non-immunogenic carriers to convey the drug molecules selectively towards their target cells. The link between the drug and its carrier should remain inert and stable in the blood stream and extracellular spaces but should be sensitive to the enzymes present in or around the target sites. Nanoparticles, microspheres, lisosomes, glycolipids, antibodies and peptide hormones are being evaluated as carriers for a variety of medicinally active agents. At present targetted drug delivery systems have been utilized for the chemotherapy of cancer and protozoal diseases. It may also be extended in the chemotherapy of intracellular infections such as those caused by protozoa and viruses.

(c) Bioprecursor :

The bioprecursor does not contain a temporary linkage between the active drug and a carrier moiety, but designed from a molecular modification of the active principle itself.

It is a compound that is converted to active drug through metabolic biotransformation. For example, if the drug contains a carboxylic acid group, the bioprecursor may be a primary amine which is metabolized by oxidation to the aldehyde which is further metabolized to the carboxylic acid drug. e.g. fenbufen, phenyl-butazone / oxyphenbutazone, acetanilide (Paracetamol), imipiramine (demethyl-imipramine).

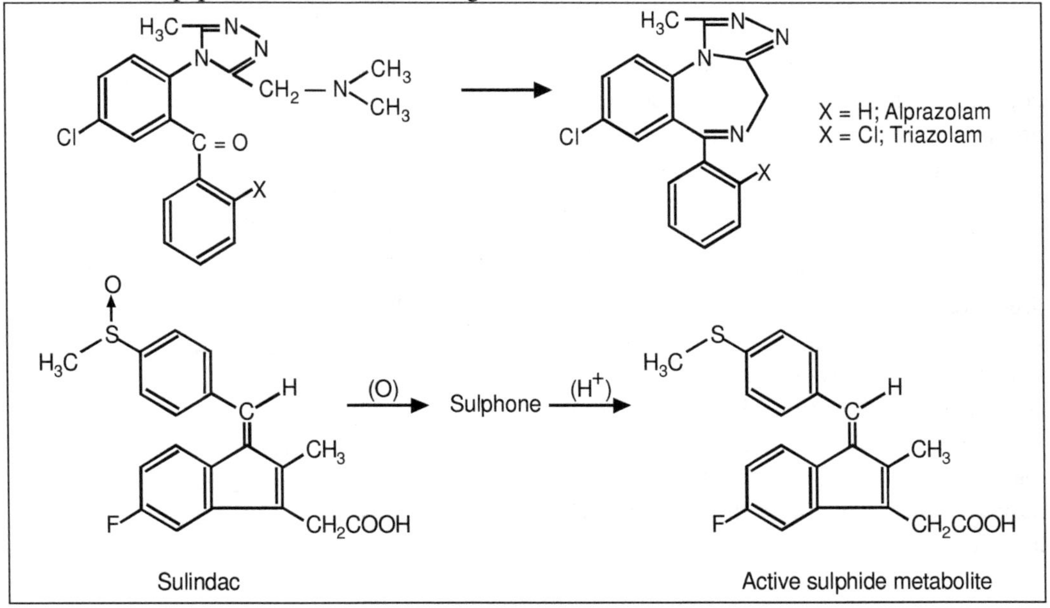

X = H; Alprazolam
X = Cl; Triazolam

Sulindac   →(O)→ Sulphone →(H+)→   Active sulphide metabolite

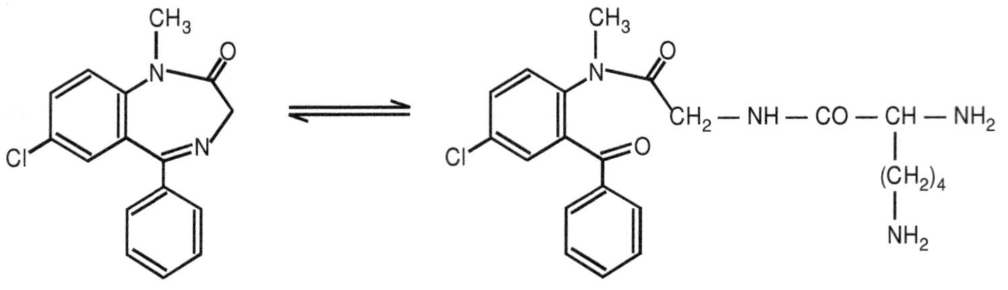

Fig. 1.4 : In-vivo Conversion of Diazepam Prodrug to Diazepam

Similarly, pyrrolines are the bioprecursors of GABA and its analogs. N-alkylaminobenzophenones were designed to get in-vivo benzodiazepines by N-dealkylation of tertiary amine and ring closure. The linkage between the drug substance and the transport moiety is usually a covalent bond.

Sulindac, a non-steroidal anti-inflammatory bioprecursor, gets converted to the sulphide metabolite (active drug) via sulphone.

1.7 CARRIER-LINKED PRODRUGS

Alcohol-containing drugs can be acylated with aliphatic or aromatic carboxylic acids to decrease water-solubility (increase lipophilicity) or with carboxylic acids containing amino or additional carboxylate group to increase water solubility. Conversion to phosphate or sulphate esters also increase water solubility. Thus, by changing the degree of water-solubility, we can impart desirable absorption and distribution properties to the drug molecule. Succinate esters can be used to accelerate the rate of hydrolysis by intramolecular catalysis. If a hydrolysis is too slow, addition of electron withdrawing groups on the alcohol part of the ester can increase the rate. If a slower rate of ester hydrolysis is desired, long-chain aliphatic or sterically hindered esters can be used.

Activated amides, generally of low basicity amines or amides of amino acids are more susceptible to enzymatic cleavage. Phenyl carbamates ($R\ NHCO_2Ph$) can also be used as prodrugs because of their susceptibility to the attack of plasma enzymes.

The anticonvulsant agent progabide is a prodrug form of γ-aminobutyric acid, an important inhibitory neurotransmitter. Its lipophilicity helps it to cross blood-brain-barrier. Once it enters the CNS, it is hydrolyzed to GABA.

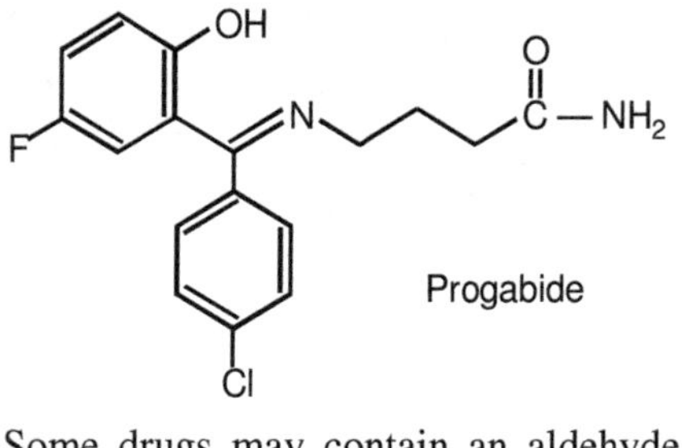

Progabide

Some drugs may contain an aldehyde or ketone functional group. The carbonyl group may be converted to Schiff base, oxime, acetal (ketal), enol ester, oxazolidine or thiazolidine.

(a) Prodrugs for increased water solubility :

The hydrophilic characteristic of a drug can be improved by formation of hemisuccinates, hemiglutarates, hemiphthalates or metasulphobenzoates which then serve as a site of formation of water soluble sodium, potassium or amine salts. Phosphates have been used to prepare the hydrophilic carrier prodrugs in the fields of steroids and vitamins. Water solubility of 1, 4-benzodiazepines may be elevated by the formation of a peptide bond between the drug and L-lysine.

Similarly, β-glycosidation helps to get a non-irritating water-soluble derivative of menthol.

Prednisolone and methylprednisolone are poorly water soluble cortico steroid drugs. Prednisolone phosphate (PO_3Na_2) is a water soluble prodrug for prednisolone that is activated in-vivo by phosphatases. Methylprednisolone sodium succinate is a water soluble prodrug of methylprednisolone. Since, amidase catalyzed hydrolysis occurs rapidly in human serum, water soluble amide prodrug forms of benzocaine can be prepared with various amino acids.

(b) Prodrugs for improved absorption and distribution :

Drugs applied to the skin are poorly absorbed. Corticosteroids for the topical treatment of inflammatory, allergic and pruritic skin conditions can be made more suitable for topical absorption by esterification or acetonidation. Once absorbed through the skin, an esterase can release the drug.

Examples include fluocinolone acetonide and fluocinonide. Dipivaloylepinephrine (dipivefrin), a prodrug for epinephrine, has better cornea penetration rate than epinephrine and is used in the treatment of glaucoma. Similarly, estradiol-3-benzoate-17-cyclooctenyl ether was designed for a sustained release formulation of oestradiol.

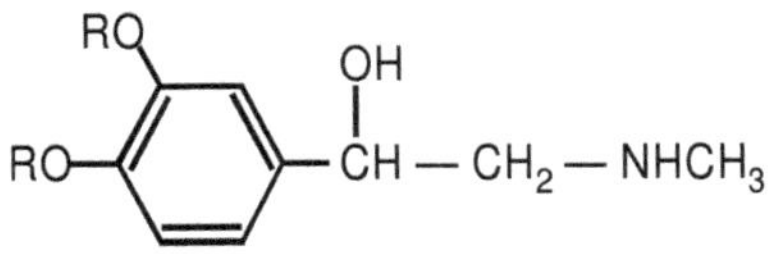

(i) Epinephrine : R = H

(ii) Dipivefrin : R = $(CH_3)_3$ CCO

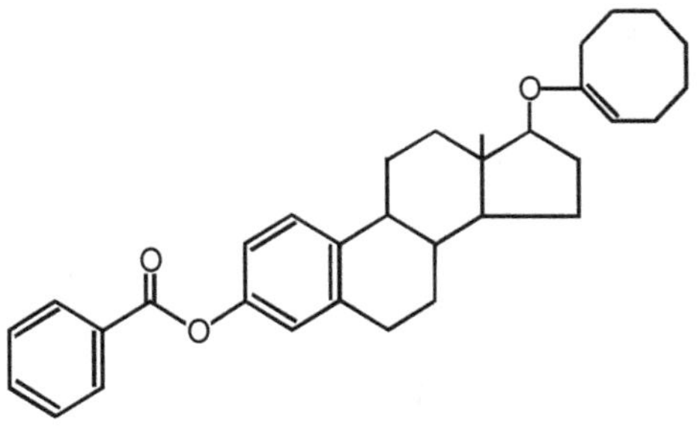

Estradiol-3-benzoate-17-cyclooctenyl ether

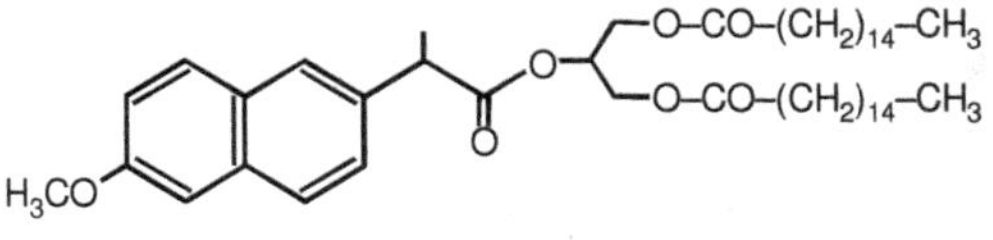

Naproxen - 2- glyceride
(less gastric irritation and higher plasma level)

Fig. 1.5 : Lipophilic Carrier Prodrugs

Similarly ampicillin, when administered orally only about 40% of dose is absorbed. Hence, ampicillin, when presented in the form of its esters, has increased oral absorption, e.g., bacampicillin, pivampicillin.

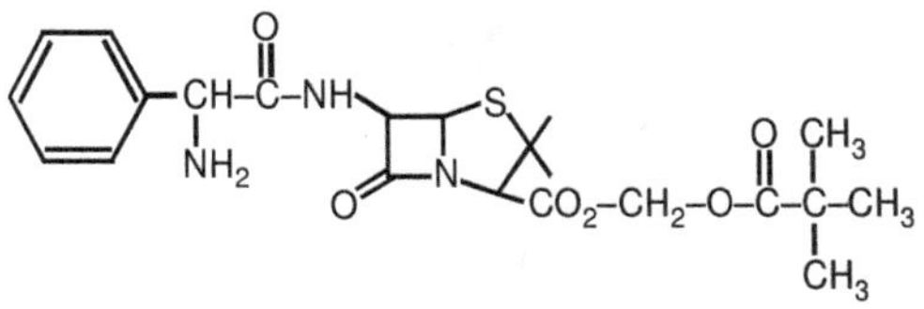

Pivampicilline

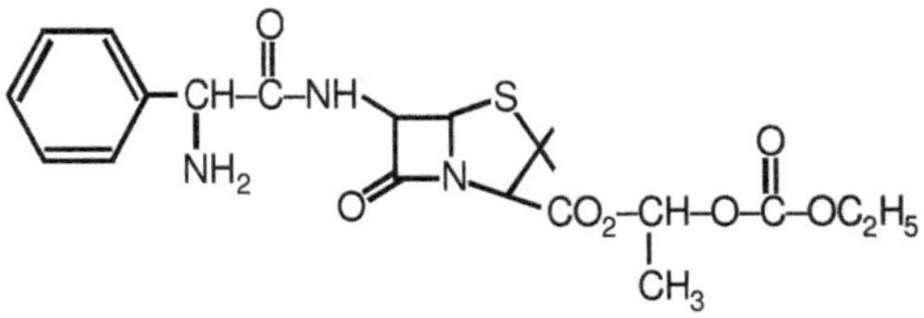

Bacampicilline

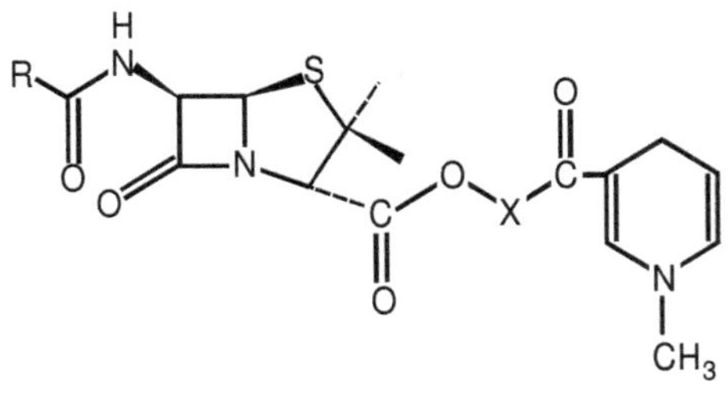

(c) Prodrugs for site specificity :

The designing of centrally acting drugs need ability to cross the blood-brain-barrier. The approach is based on attaching a lipophilic carrier to the hydrophilic drug in a loosely bound form. The complex releases hydrophilic drug in the CNS.

For example, β-lactam antibiotics may be used in the treatment of bacterial meningitis. Since, the β-lactam antibiotics are hydrophilic, they enter the brain very slowly, but they are actively transported back into the blood. Bodor and co-workers have synthesized dihydropyridine-penicillin prodrugs that deliver β-lactam antibiotic in high concentrations into the brain.

The phosphoamidases are abundant in neoplastic cells than in normal cells and hence, cyclophosphamide is developed by phosphorylating the nitrogen mustard. The drug might be hydrolysed in tumour cells by the enzyme phosphoamidases.

Another example is progabide which is a prodrug of an inhibitory neurotransmitter, GABA. Oxyphenisatin (R = H) is a bowel sterilant that is active only when rectally given. An orally active prodrug can be designed (R = CH_3CO) which releases an active drug, oxyphenisatin, in the intestine through hydrolysis.

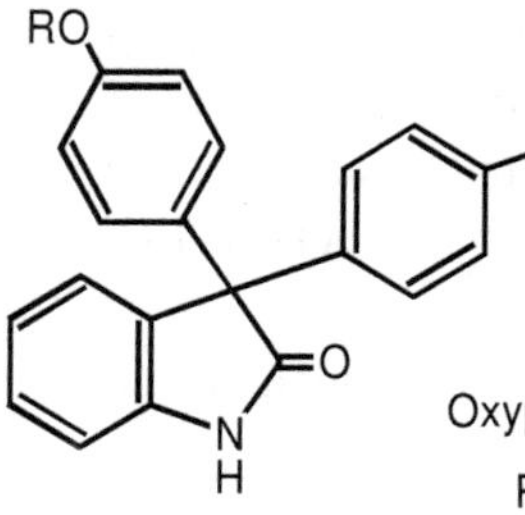

Oxyphenisatin
R = –H

Another approach for site specific drug delivery is to design a prodrug that requires activation by an enzyme found predominantly at the desired site of action. Diethylstilbestrol diphosphate (R = PO_3^{--}) was designed for site-specific delivery of diethylstilbestrol to prostatic carcinoma tissues, since tumour cells were found to have higher concentration of phosphatases and amidases than the normal cells.

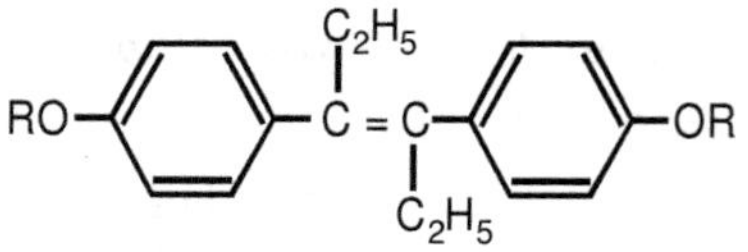

Yet another example of site-specific delivery prodrug design is the conversion of dopamine to L-dopa and preparation of aliphatic and steroidal esters of GABA.

The high concentration of two enzymes, γ-glutamyl transpeptidase and L-aromatic amino acid (DOPA) decarboxylase present in the kidneys leads to the development of γ-glutamyl-DOPA as a selective renal vasodilator.

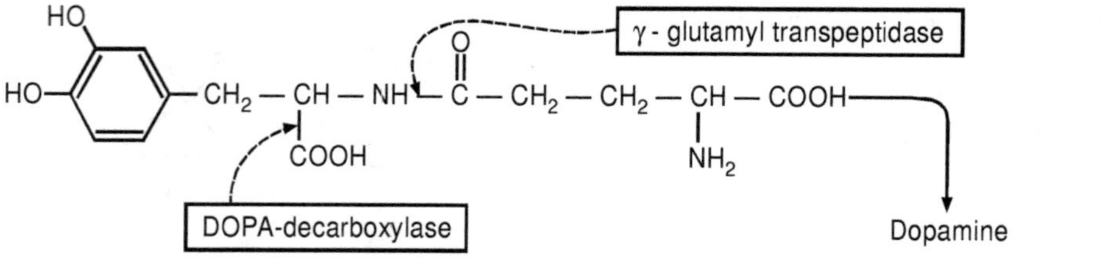

(d) Prodrugs for stability :

Extensive first-pass metabolism in liver is the most important cause that restricts oral effectiveness of many drugs. Metabolic studies of drugs provide such clues as how to make the drug resistant to first-pass metabolism and to increase oral effectiveness. For example,

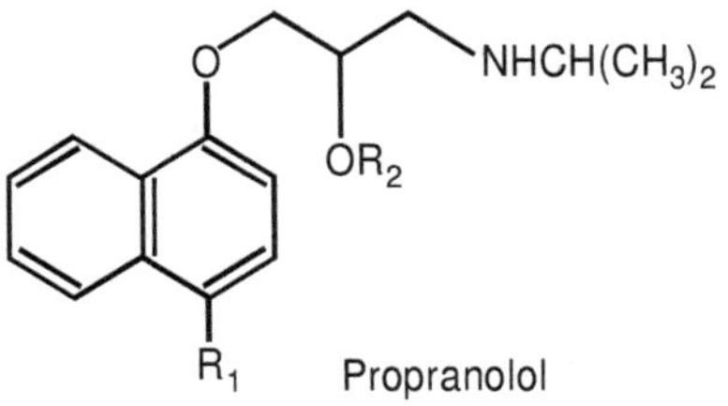

Propranolol
$R_1 = R_2 = H$

the major metabolites of propranolol were found to be propranolol -o-glucuronide ($R_1 = -H$, $OR_2 = $ glucuronide), p- hydroxypropranolol ($R_1 = -OH$, $R_2 = -H$) and its o-glucuronide ($R_1 = -OH$; $OR_2 = $ glucuronide). Hence, oral administration of propranolol hemisuccinate ($R_1 = H$, $R_2 = COCH_2 CH_2 COOH$) elevates plasma levels of propranolol about 8 times.

Similarly, naltrexone (R = H), undergoes extensive first-pass metabolism. When its ester analogs, namely anthranilate (R = CO -o-NO_2Ph) and the acetylsalicylate (R = CO -o-ACOPh) used, the bioavailability of naltrexone was found to be increased to 45 and 28-times respectively.

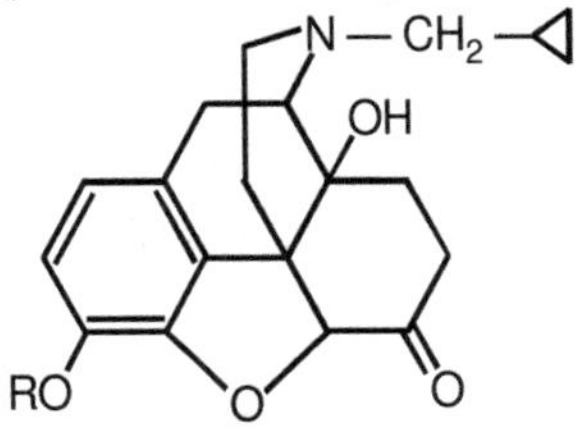

(e) Prodrugs for slow and prolonged release :

It can best be achieved by making a long chain aliphatic ester because these esters hydrolyze slowly. This principle has been well

elaborated in the drug designing of sex hormone derivatives e.g.; progestins or androgens. Examples include haloperidol decanoate [R = $CO(CH_2)_8CH_3$] which when injected intramuscularly as a solution in sesame oil, its activity lasts for about one month in comparison to haloperidol (R = H) as such (2-6 hrs). Similarly, another antipsychotic agent, fluphenazine enanthate [R = $CO(CH_2)_5CH_3$] and decanoate [R = $CO(CH_2)_8-CH_3$] have duration of action of about a month in comparison to plain fluphenazine (6-8 hrs).

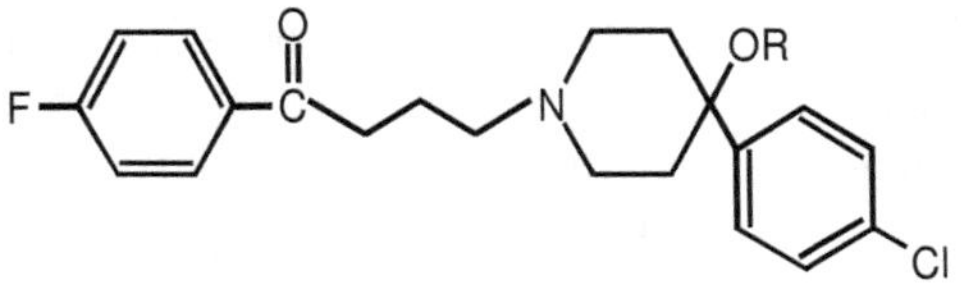

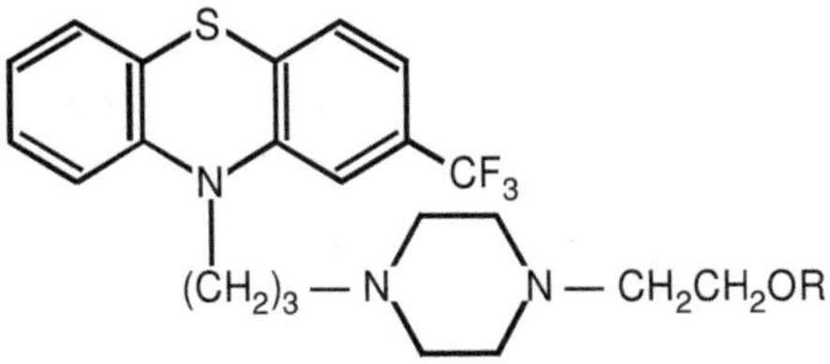

When a glycine conjugate (R = NH CH_2COOH) of anti-arthritis drug, tolmetin sodium (R = O – Na^+) is used, both potency and duration of action are prolonged because of the slow hydrolysis of the prodrug amide linkage. Among local anaesthetics, procaine is an ester, and is therefore easily hydrolyzed by esterases. By conversion of the ester into an amide (lidocaine), the duration of action is increased by several folds.

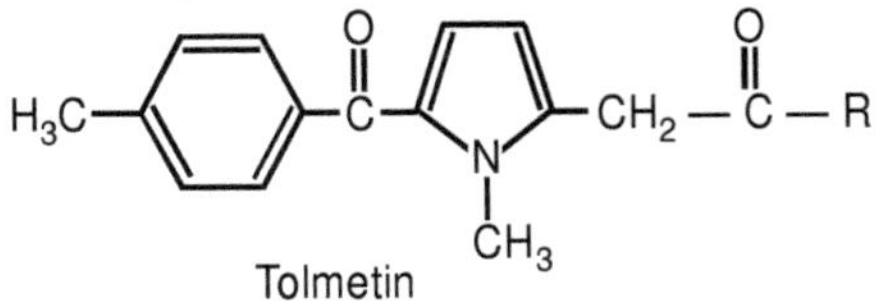

Tolmetin

(f) Prodrugs to lower toxicity profile :

Examples include the use of prodrug dipivaloylepinephrine (R = Me_3CCO) instead of epinephrine (R = H) in the treatment of glaucoma. Similarly, the side effects associated with the use of aspirin are gastric irritation and bleeding. Esterification of aspirin (R = alkyl) greatly suppresses gastric ulcerogenic activity.

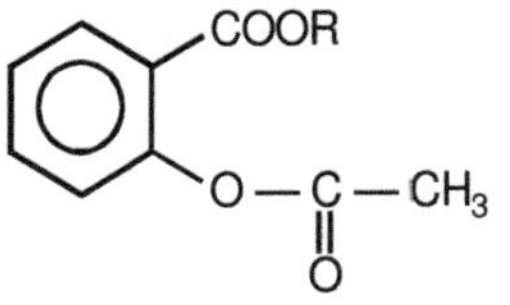

Aspirin (R = H)

(g) Prodrugs to improve patient acceptance :

Clindamycin (R = H) has a bitter taste, so it is not well accepted by children. It was found that by increasing the chain-length of 2-acyl esters of clindamycin, the taste improved from bitter (acetate ester) to a non-bitter taste (palmitate ester). Bitter taste results from a compound dissolving in the saliva and interacting with a bitter taste receptor in the tongue. Esterification with long-chain fatty acids makes the drug less water-soluble, resulting into non-bitter taste. Yet another example from this category is chloramphenicol palmitate.

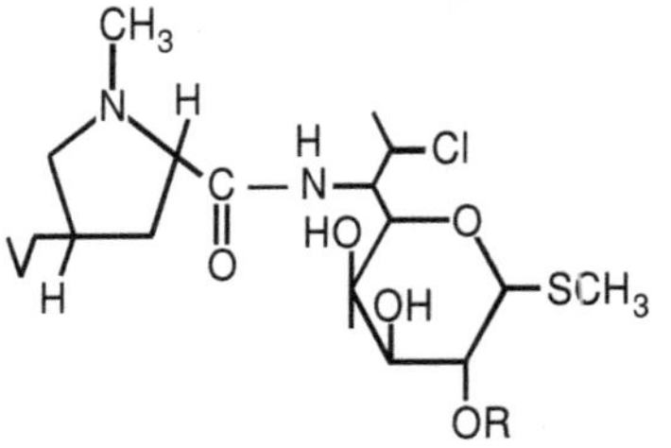

Clindamysin; R = H

Thus in summary, prodrug concept may be utilized to improve the undesirable properties of the drug. Such undesirable properties may include,

(a) Physico-chemical properties : e.g. poor solubility, instability, unpleasant taste or odour.

(b) Pharmacokinetic properties : e.g. poor bioavailability due to incomplete absorption or shorter duration of action due to high rate of metabolism.

(c) Toxicities or side-effects : e.g. gastric irritation. Sometimes drug may be more active but unable to reach its site of action. In other cases, due to large volume of distribution, drug may get distributed to other sites alongwith its site of action. This leads to appearance of side-effects, because of drug concentration of unintended sites. In all such cases prodrug concept can be applied. However toxicity testing of prodrug is also necessary.

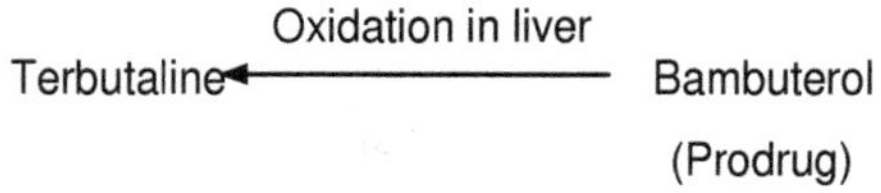

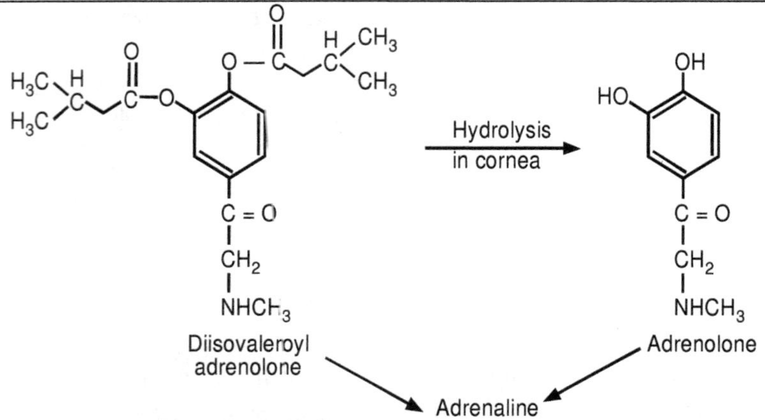

Terbutaline ← —————— Bambuterol
          Oxidation in liver   (Prodrug)

Fig. 1.6 : Ophthalmic Delivery of Drugs (Adrenaline Diesters)

Table 1.2 : Clinically used Prodrugs

Prodrug	Active form	Prodrug	Active form
Levodopa	Dopamine	Proguanil	Proguanil triazine
Enalapril	Enalaprilat	Prednisone	Prednisolone
Alpha methyl dopa	Alpha methylnorepinephrine	Bacampicillin	Ampicillin
Dipivefrine	Epinephrin	Sulfasalazine	5-ASA
Sulindac	Sulfide metabolite	Cyclophosphamide	Aldophosphamide, Phosphoramide mustard, Acrolein
Hydrazide (MAO inhibitor)	Hydrazide derivative	Primidone, phenobarbitone	Phenobarbitol
Mercaptopurine	Methylmercaptopurine ribonucleotide	Bambuterol	Terbutaline
Valaciclovir	Aciclovir	Dipyridamole	Adenosine
Psilocybin	Psilocin	Fosphenytoin	Phenytoin
Heroin	Morphine	Midodrine	Desglymidodrine
Nabumetone	6-MNA	Melagatran	Ximelagatran
Lovastatin and simvastatin	Active-hydroxyl derivatives	Alatrovafloxacin	Travafloxacin
Phenacetin	Acetaminophen	Famciclovir	6-deoxypenciclovir
Chloramphenicol palmitate	Chloramphenicol	Tenofovir disoproxilfumarate	Tenofovir
Azathioprine	Mercaptopurine	Dipivefrin	Epinephrine
Bacampicillin	Ampicillin	Enalapril	Enalaprilat
Benonrylate	Aspirin + Paracetamol	Levodopa	Dopamine
Cortisone	Hydrocortisone	Proguanil	Proguanil triazine
Cyclophosphamide	Aldophosphamide	Sulindac	Sulfide metabolite
Sulfasalazine	5 Aminosalicylic acid	Zidovudine	Zidovudine triphosphate

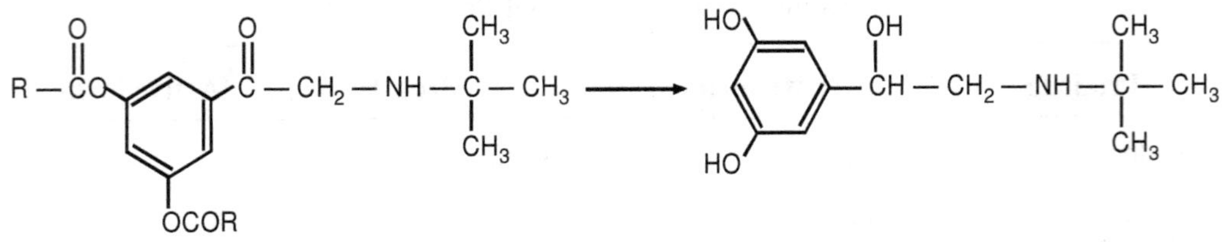

Ketone-diester of t-butaline

t-butaline

Applications of Prodrug Concept :

(a) Increasing absorption of drugs :
  e.g. ampicillin esters.

(b) Improve site specific drug delivery;
  e.g. epinephrine.

(c) Prolongation of drug action :
  e.g. testosterone.

(d) Decrease side-effects and toxicity :
  e.g. NSAID.

(e) Improve taste and odour :
  e.g. chloramphenicol palmitate.

(f) Delivery to brain : e.g. dopamine to L-dopa. L-dopa to its methyl ester

GABA to its aliphatic and steroid esters.

1.8 DRAWBACKS OF PRODRUG APPROACH

The prodrug concept may become a potential source of toxicities if,

(a) the prodrug generates toxic metabolites which are not generated by the parent drug;

(b) increased consumption of glutathione during the conversion of prodrug to active metabolite may leave vital cell constituents unprotected;

(c) the inert carrier moiety could not remain inert and leads to formation of toxic metabolites.

(d) the prodrug or/and carrier moiety generate such metabolites which alter the pharmacokinetic features of the parent drug by either inducing metabolic enzymes or by competing the active drug for binding with plasma-proteins.

1.9 SOFT DRUG CONCEPT

Prodrugs are designed in such a way that the active drug is generated by the major metabolic pathway. Prodrugs might effectively eliminate some toxicities by protecting the drug from unwanted degradations, particularly those occurring in GIT prior to and during absorption or possibly during the first passage through the liver. The application of the concept of 'soft drugs' is necessary to overcome and to improve (a) pharmacokinetic insufficiencies, (b) transportability, and (c) site specificity. The soft drugs are defined as therapeutically beneficial agents characterized by a predictable and controllable in-vivo metabolism to non-toxic moieties, after they achieve their therapeutic role. The site-specific delivery via chemical modifications involves the design of a soft drug from an inactive metabolite. The designed drug is then transformed by facile and predicted routes of metabolism ultimately resulting in the delivery of the active drug at the expected sites of action. The concept was successfully applied to local delivery of steroids, drugs acting on specific areas in the eye, brain and testes. If it is possible to deliver potent drugs exactly at the site of action, very less dose will be required, which will not cause unexpected toxicities.

For example, increased separation of activity from toxicity (i.e. improved selectivity) may be achieved by using 3-spirothiazolidine derivative of hydrocortisone. Unlike hydrocortisone, it lacks specific hydrocortisone binding and affinity properties, even if it is absorbed systemically during topical administration.

This is because, the 4, 5-unsaturated 3-ketone group is absent in this derivative which is slowly generated in dermal cells by stepwise hydrolysis of thiazolidine ring to deliver the active 3-keto compound. Using similar approach, an antiacne topical progesterone preparation was developed containing the cystein 3,20-bisthiazolidine derivative of progesterone.

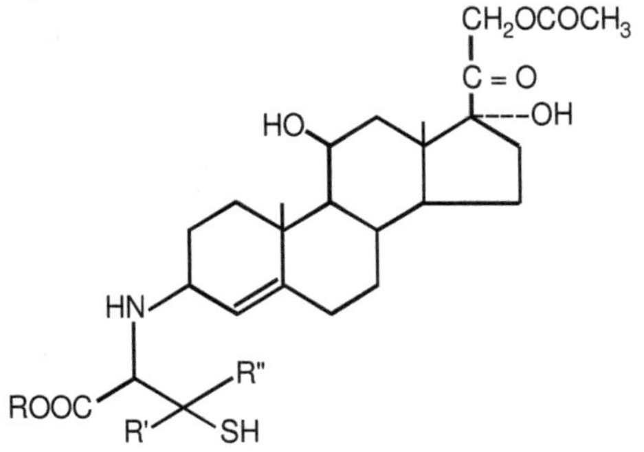

The concept of 'soft drug' may also be applied to develop selective and safer ocular drug delivery systems for the treatment of glaucoma, ocular inflammations and infections. It was found by Bodor et al. in 1978 that diester derivatives of adrenolone have a high level of ocular sympathomimetic activity due to the conversion of former to adrenaline via a combined reduction-hydrolysis process in the eyes.

Using same approach, tertbutaline was generated selectively in the iris-ciliary tissues by the action of reductases and esterases on ketone-diester precursors of tertbutaline.

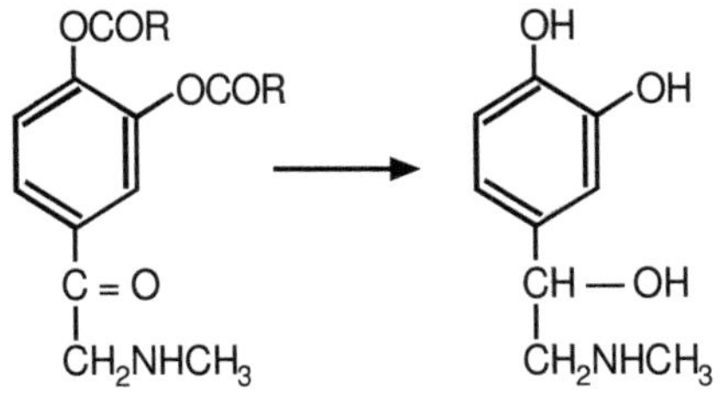

Diester of adrenolone

Adrenaline

Similarly propranolol is generated at the iris-ciliary body by the action of esterases and reductases on the topically applied keto-oxime derivative of propranolol.

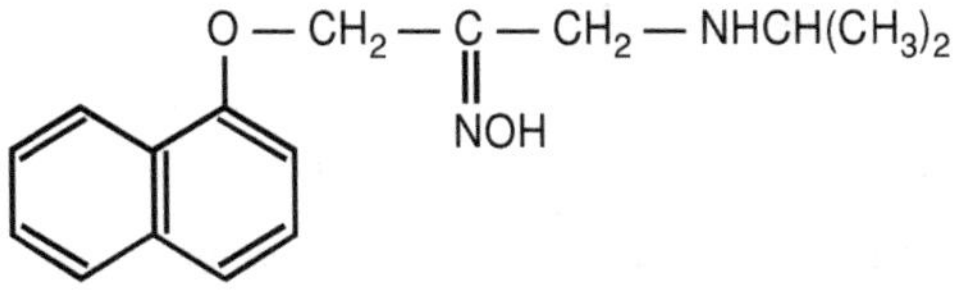

The 'soft drug' concept was utilized to develop loteprednol etabonate, a topical anti-inflammatory and anti-allergic agent.

It is locally potent but systemically safe.

1.10 HIGH THROUGHPUT ASSAY

A variety of high throughput assays have been developed and perfected over the past 10-20 years. These include the following basic types of assay.

1. Microplate activity assays : This assay is carried out in solution in a well; the result of the assay, such as enzyme inhibition, is linked to some observable event, such as color change to enable identification of bioactivity.

2. Gel diffusion assays : In such assay, the biological target is mixed in soft agar and spread as a thin film; the compound library is spread on the surface of the film; after allowing for compound diffusion, an appropriate developing agent is sprayed on the agar surface and areas in which bioactivity has occurred will show up as distinct zones.

3. Affinity selection assays : The compound library is applied to a protein target receptor; all compounds that do not bind are removed; compounds that do bind are then identified.

Of course, microplate assays are probably the most widely used. Screening combinatorial libraries in 96- or even 384-well microplates is time and cost efficient. Using modern robotic techniques, it is possible to perform more than 100,000 bioassays per week in a microplate system (permitting the 200,000 compound library to be screened in two weeks, rather than over a century).

In addition to selecting an appropriate assay, it is also necessary to have a pooling strategy. It is more efficient to test many compounds per well on the microplate, rather than one. If one could test 100 compounds per well, then the standard 96-well plate would enable almost 10,000 compounds to be evaluated in one experiment.

Currently, multiwell plates containing more than 96 wells are routinely being used. To facilitate effective pooling, the library of compounds is usually divided into a number of nor-overlapping subsets. The synthetic strategy employed during the combinatorial synthesis can be used to assist in determining these pooling strategies. In random incorporation synthesis, a single bead could contain millions of different molecular species. In mix and split synthesis (also called pool and divide synthesis or one bead-one compound synthesis) only one compound is attached to any given solid-phase synthetic bead.

1.11 PHARMACOGENOMICS AND FUTURE OF LEAD COMPOUND DISCOVERY

Conventional drug design attempts to discover drugs to treat particular diseases; pharmacogenomics attempts to design individualized drugs to treat particular people with particular diseases. Traditionally, drug design has developed, drugs for "everyone" with a given disease; pharmacogenomics will enable the tailor-made design of chemotherapies for specific populations or individuals with diseases.

Pharmacogenomics will rely upon genetic data such as single nucleotide polymorphism maps. The assembly of a Single Nucleotide Polymorphism (SNP) map for the genome will represent a set of characterized biomarkers spread throughout the human genome; this SNP map will highlight individual variations within particular genes, some of which may be associated with particular diseases, thus identifying the genetic variability inherent in human populations that is crucial to the task of individualized drug design.

2

ENZYME INHIBITORS

2.1 INTRODUCTION

Enzymes are the specialized proteins which catalyze various biochemical reactions. The status of mental and physical health of a person depends on the rates of no-going biochemical reactions. The concept of enzyme inhibition is routinely utilized to affect biosynthesis and metabolic pattern of various hormones, autacoids and neurotransmitters because of extraordinary specificity and catalytic power of the enzymes. Urease was the first enzyme isolated in pure crystalline form in 1926 by J. B. Sumner. Thousands of enzymes are found to be present in the human body. On the recommendation of an International Enzyme Commission, a scheme of classification of enzymes has been proposed. Each enzyme is assigned a recommended name for everyday use, a systematic name to identify the reaction which it catalyses and the classification number which may be used where an accurate and unambiguous identification of an enzyme is required.

International Classification of Enzymes :

1.   Oxido-reductases : These enzymes act on

$$\ce{>C=O, >CH-OH, >C=CH-, >CH-NH_2, >CH-NH-}$$

functional groups.

2.   Transferases : These enzymes catalyse the transfer for one carbon units to acyl group, aldehydic or ketonic group, glycosyl group, phosphate group or sulfur containing moieties.

3.   Hydrolases : These enzymes have the ability to induce hydrolysis of esters, acid anhydrides, glycosidic bonds, peptide bonds and other C-N bonds.

4.   Lyases : These enzymes catalyze such reactions characterized by addition to double bonds in molecules containing

$$\ce{>C=C<, >C=O} \text{ and } \ce{>C=N} \text{ linkages.}$$

5.   Isomerases : These enzymes catalyze recemization or isomerization reactions.

6.   Ligases : These enzymes catalyze the formation of bonds with ATP cleavage in molecules containing C–O, C–S, C–N, C–C linkages.

Coenzymes usually function as intermediate carriers of functional groups that are transferred in the overall enzymatic reactions. The coenzyme is called as a prosthetic group when it is very tightly bound to the enzyme molecule.

2.2 ENZYME INHIBITION

Enzymes often are the targets of drug action; drugs, however, may be and often are targets for enzymes as well. Inhibition of a biochemical pathway will be most effective if the drug acts on the rate limiting step. For example, the conversion of tyrosine to dopa is a rate limiting step in the biosynthesis of norepinephrine. However, it may not be always possible to block the rate limiting step in a biochemical pathway. In such cases, if one of the other remaining steps is blocked, the quantity of end-product formed will be greatly reduce. This minimizes the feed-back inhibition exerted by the end-product on all previous steps. This results into an increase in the turnover in the sequence of steps located before the enzyme blocked. The net outcome is an accumulation of the intermediate product which normally is the substrate for the enzyme so blocked. As the consequence, the inhibitor will be displaced from the enzyme surface by the substrate thus accumulated.

Also the accumulation of intermediate products as such may lead to complications. The situation may become serious especially if no or only a limited capacity for the elimination of the intermediate product is available.

2.3 CLASSIFICATION OF ENZYME INHIBITORS

A number of drugs in clinical use exert their action by inhibiting a specific enzyme, the target enzyme, present either in the tissues of the individual under treatment or in those of an invading organism. The inhibition of a suitably selected target enzyme leads to build-up in concentration of substrate(s) and a corresponding decrease in the concentration of the metabolite(s), one of which leads to a useful clinical response.

Type of inhibitor selected for a particular target enzyme plays an important role in producing a useful clinical effect. Various parameters may be given due consideration in selecting an enzyme inhibitor. Important amongst them are :

(a) biochemical environment of the target enzyme,

(b) specificity of action not associated with toxic or undesirable side-effects.

The time-period for which an enzyme is blocked becomes the basis of the classification of enzyme inhibitors. Various clinically used enzyme inhibitors may be broadly categorised into :

(a) Reversible enzyme inhibitors, and

(b) Irreversible enzyme inhibitors.

The inhibitor may temporarily block the enzyme. The enzyme inhibited by this way gets readily reactivated back. Such types of agents are called reversible enzyme inhibitors. Some enzymes undergo irreversible inactivation when they are treated with agents capable of reacting covalently and permanently modifying a functional group required for catalysis making the enzyme molecule inactive.

(a) Reversible enzyme inhibitors :

Reversible enzyme :

Inhibitors may further be categorised into competitive, uncompetitive and non-competitive enzyme inhibitors. In competitive inhibition, the inhibitor reacts reversibly with an enzyme to form an enzyme inhibitor complex, analogous to enzyme substrate complex.

$$E + I \rightleftharpoons EI$$

The inhibitor must possess structural similarity with the natural substrate to act as competitive enzyme inhibitor.

In competitive inhibition, an inhibitor can combine with the free enzyme in such a way that it competes with the normal substrate for binding at the active site. Though the inhibitor is structurally related to the natural substrate, the inhibitor molecule is not chemically altered by the enzyme.

In uncompetitive inhibition, the inhibitor combines with enzyme substrate complex rather than with the free enzyme to give inactive enzyme inhibitor complex.

$$E + S \rightleftharpoons ES$$
$$ES + I \rightleftharpoons ESI$$

A non-competitive inhibitor can combine with either the free enzyme or the enzyme-substrate complex, interferring with the action of both. A non-competitive inhibitor deforms the shape of enzyme instead of binding with the active site of an enzyme. The altered shape and conformation of the enzyme slow down both, the rates of formation and dissociation of enzyme-substrate complexes. These effects are reversed by increasing the substrate concentration.

The majority of reversible enzyme inhibitors act through competitive antagonism pathway. However in many cases, potent in vitro enzyme inhibitors lose their potency when tested in vivo. Various mechanisms have been proposed to explain this loss in potency. Important among them include,

(i) Because of in-vivo metabolism, the lipophilicity required to penetrate the desired cellular membranes before reaching the target enzyme can not be maintained.

(ii) The rate-controlling step in the metabolic chain need not to be always catalysed by the target enzyme. Moreover the drug operates well below its maximum efficiency so that inhibition has little effect on the overall pathway.

(iii) Similarly to exert competitive inhibition, a required concentration of the drug does not always built up at target sites.

Table 2.1 : Some Clinically used Reversible Enzyme Inhibitors

Drug	Enzyme inhibited	Clinical use
Allopurinol	Xanthine oxidase	Treatment of gout
Acetazolamide, Dichlorophenamide	Carbonic anhydrase	Diuretic
Trimethoprim, Pyrimethamine, Methotrexate	Dihydrofolate reductase	Antibacterial, Antimalarial, Anticancer agent
Aspirin	Prostaglandin synthetase	Anti-inflammatory
Cardiac glycosides	Na^+, K^+–ATPase	Cardiotonic
Amphenone, Metyrapone	11β-Hydroxylase	Test for pituitary function
6-Mercaptopurine, Azathioprine	Riboxyl amidotransferase	Anticancer agent
5-Fluorouracil, Floxuridine	Thymidylate synthetase	Anticancer agent
Captopril	Angiotensin-converting enzyme	Hypotensive agent
Sulthiame	Carbonic anhydrase	Treatment of epilepsy
Sodium valproate	GABA transaminase	Treatment of epilepsy
Idoxuridine	Thymidine kinase and thymidylate kinase	Antiviral agent

contd...

Drug	Enzyme inhibited	Clinical use
Cytosine arabinoside (Ara-C)	DNA and RNA polymerases	Antiviral and anticancer agents
Aminoglutethimide	Aromatase	Oestrogen-mediated breast cancer
ε-aminocaproic acid	Plasmin	Antifibrinolytic agent
Nitrefazole	Aldehyde dehydrogenase	Alcoholism
Sorbinil	Aldose reductase	Diabetes mellitus complications

Table 2.2 : Some Clinically used Irreversible Enzyme Inhibitors

Drug	Enzyme	Clinical use
α-Mono(di)fluoromctltyldopa	Dopa decarboxylase (peripheral)	Hypotensive
Sulphonamides	Dihydropteroate synthetase	Antibacterial
Neostigmine, pyridostigmine	Acetycholinesterase	Glaucoma, Myasthenia gravis
lproniazid, phenelzine	Mono amino-oxidase	Antidepressant
Azaserine	Formylglycinamide ribotide amido transferase	Anticancer agent
Penicillins, cephalosporins	Transpeptidase	Antibiotics
Clavulanic acid	β-lactamase	Adjuvant to penicillin antibiotics
Organo-arsenical	Pyruvate dehydrogenase	Anti-protozoal agent
5-Fluorouracil	Thymidylate synthetase	Anti-inflammatory agent
Serazide, carbidopa	Dopa decarboxylase	In conjunction with L-Dopa in Parkinsonism disease.
Acetohydroxamic acid	Bacterial urease	Urinary infection
D-cycloserine	Alanine racemase	Antibiotic
γ-Vinyl GABA	GABA transaminase	Antiepileptic

2.4 MECHANISMS OF ENZYME INHIBITION

A number of drugs in clinical use exert their action by inhibiting a specific target enzyme. The different ways of enzyme inhibition are as follows :

(a) In a very simplified process, the blockade of an enzyme, catalysing a particular biochemical reaction leads to accumulation of the substrate. This results into a desired biological response. Sometimes undesired biochemical effects (i.e., disease) appear due to excessive production of the metabolite from the substrate. By inhibiting this conversion, these undesirable effects may be lowered down.

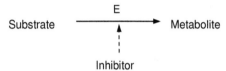

(b) In a multistep biochemical pathway, the rate limiting step governs the rate of production of the final product which may be essential for a particular biochemical function. The inhibition of an enzyme that catalyses the rate-limiting step decreases the production of a metabolite which may be responsible for clinically undesired effects or for bacterial or cancerous growth.

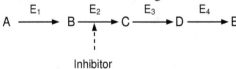

(c) Most of the enzymes need co-factors to catalyse the biochemical pathway. Inhibitors can be developed selectively for the co-factor involved. The inhibitor leaves the co-factor either a non-usable or a non-replaceable form.

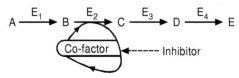

(d) A single inhibitor with a single site of action could cause multiple effects when it acts on an enzyme that is a member of a regulated steady-state system. To minimize the toxicities and the risk of development of resistant strains of bacteria, two inhibitors may be employed simultaneously to achieve a greater therapeutic effects. For example, co-trimoxazole contains a combination of trimethoprim and sulphamethoxazole.

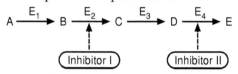

(e) In a variety of biochemical pathways, the rate of production of end-product is governed by feed-back mechanisms. If the metabolism of the end-product is minimised, the accumulated end-product decreases the activity of an enzyme on its substrate. Hence, a useful clinical effect may be achieved by inhibiting the disposal of the end-product.

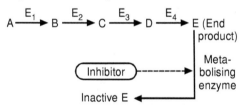

(f) The drug-metabolising enzymes cut short the duration of stay of drug molecule in the body. Inhibition of metabolizing target enzyme permits higher plasma levels of administered drug to persist which lead to an increase in the plasma half-life of the drug.

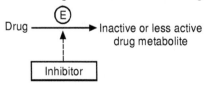

For example, clavulanic acid inhibits β-lactamase enzymes which are responsible for inactivation of β-lactam antibiotics. Hence, clavulanic acid is used as an adjuvant to penicillin therapy.

(g) Multisubstrate analogues : When a substrate interacts with an enzyme, the concentration and orientation of substrate at the active site of the enzyme govern the catalytic efficiency of an enzyme. A multisubstrate compound consists the features of binding sites of two or more different substrates in the same molecule. The binding ability of a multisubstrate analog may exceed the combined affinities of individual substrates towards the concerned enzymes. For example, pyridoxyl alanine (multisubstrate analog) has more binding ability towards pyruvate transaminase than pyridoxal and alanine. Phosphonoacetyl - L - aspartate (multisubstrate analog) has a greater binding ability to aspartate transcarbomoylase than phophonoacetic acid and diethyl aspartate. Similarly, the binding affinity of coenzyme A towards acetyl transferase enzyme may be increased by alkylating coenzyme A with bromoacetic acid.

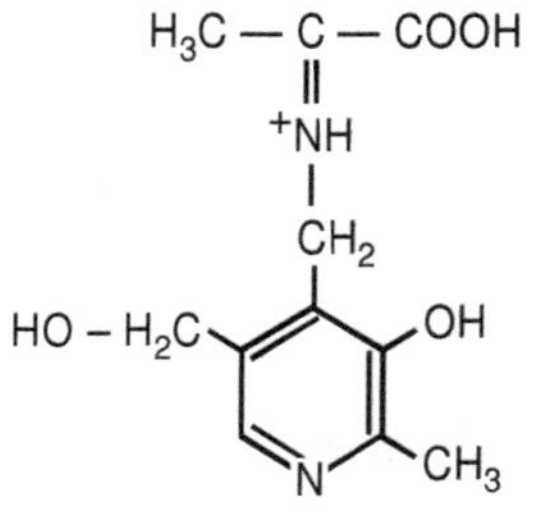

Pyridoxal alanine

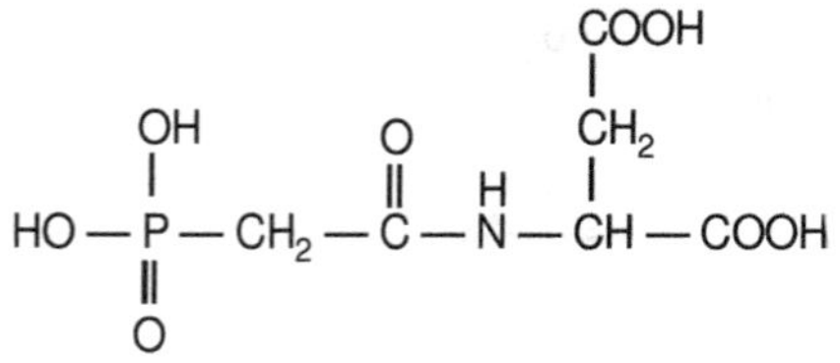

Phosphonoacetyl-L-aspartate

(h) Transition state analogues : An enzyme interacts with a substrate to form enzyme substrate complex through a tetrahedral transition state.

Transition state

Enzyme-substrate complex

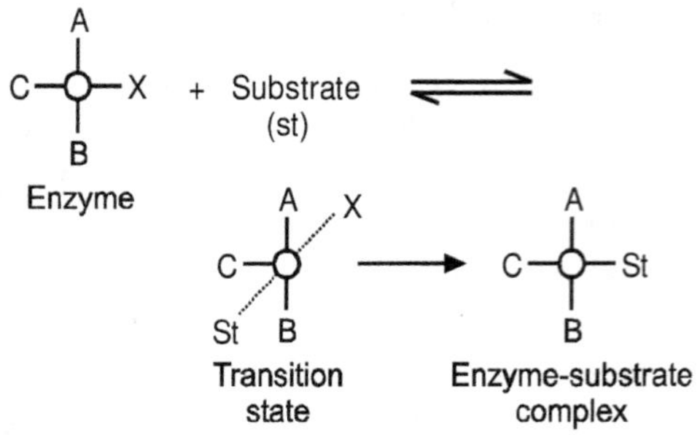

A stable compound that resembles the intermediate is expected to bind strongly to enzyme and acts as an inhibitor. Such compounds are called as transition state analogues. Since, the transition state is unique characteristic of any enzyme reaction, an enzyme will bind the transition state of the reaction which it catalyses many orders of magnitude more tightly than it will bind the substrate. A transition state analog binds more tightly to an enzyme than it does its substrate. The transition state analogues are the examples of potent reversible inhibitors which are highly specific in their action. In order to design such as analog, the mechanism of the enzymatic reaction must be thoroughly understood.

For example, a tetrahedral transition state is proposed in the acetylation of serine residue in cholinesterase during hydrolysis of acetylcholine. The boronic acid analog of acetylcholine acts as potential transition state analogs for acetylcholinesterase. Under ideal conditions (pH 7.5 and $25^\circ C$), the boronic acid analog binds about four orders of magnitude more tightly to cholinesterase compared with acetylcholine. Penicillin is another example of a transition state analog which bind to the peptidoglycan transpeptidase, an enzyme involved in cross-linking of preformed peptidoglycan stands in bacterial cell wall synthesis.

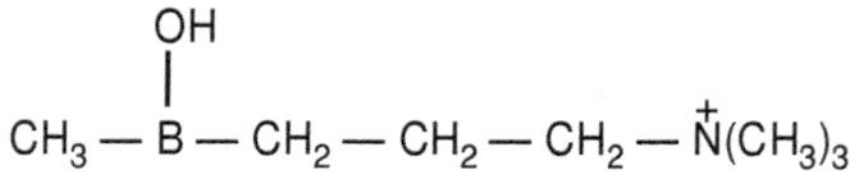

Boronic acid analog of acetylcholine

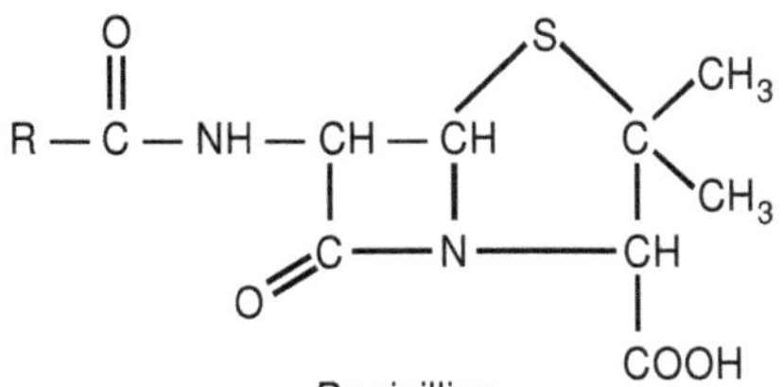

Penicillins

(i) Suicide Enzyme Inhibitors (Kcat inhibitors) : This is a category of irreversible enzyme inhibitor which utilises highly electrophilic species such as α-halogenated carbonyl compounds or other strongly alkylating agents which in turn irreversibly react with a nucleophilic group on the enzyme. Such inhibitors are expected to bind tightly to the enzyme through covalent bonding and can not be washed out readily. The enzyme is thereby inhibited permanently and is regenerated slowly by biosynthesis.

Suicide enzyme inhibitors are the compounds that possess latent reactive functional groups which are unmasked by the catalytic action of the enzyme. These unmasked reactive functional groups will then inhibit the enzyme function in irreversible way. Thus the enzyme gets inactivated by its own mechanism of action. The design of suicide enzyme inhibition utilizes the knowledge of chemical bond making and breaking, mechanism used by the enzyme to catalyze the reaction, and binding energy of the non-reacting parts of the substrate and enzyme. Examples include inhibition of aldehyde dehydrogenase by cyclopropanone, a metabolite of coprine. The irreversible enzyme inhibition occurs by the formation of a stable thiohemiketal bond with the thiol group of the enzyme.

Another example of suicidal enzyme inhibitor is tranylcypromine which inhibits monoamine oxidase enzyme by following mechanism.

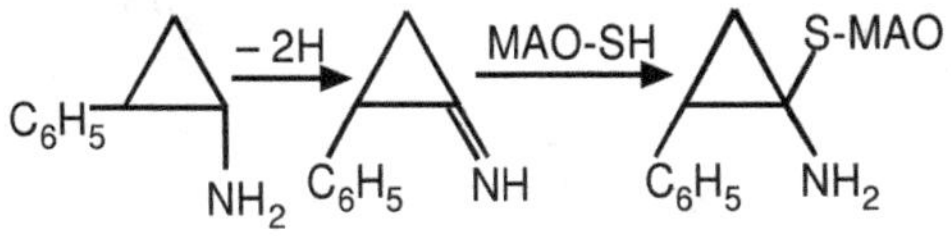

In pyridoxal phosphate dependent enzymes (i.e. decarboxylases or transaminases), the catalytic process begins with the formation of a schiff base. Hence, a suicidal enzyme inhibitor for pyridoxal phosphate dependent enzymes may be developed by incorporating a sufficiently reactive amino group which will help to form a schiff base with pyridoxal phosphate (Py-CHO).

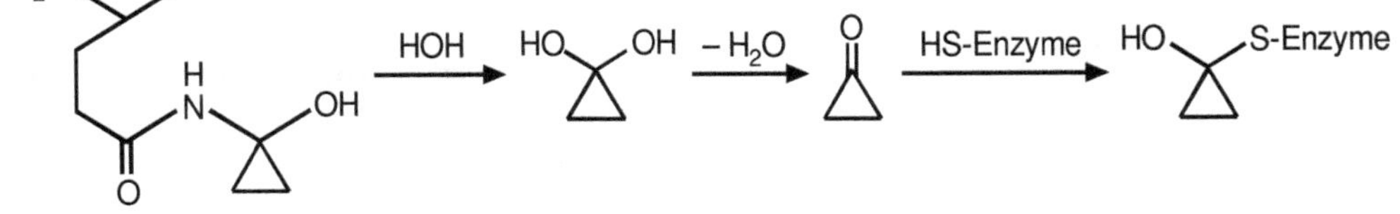

Coprine

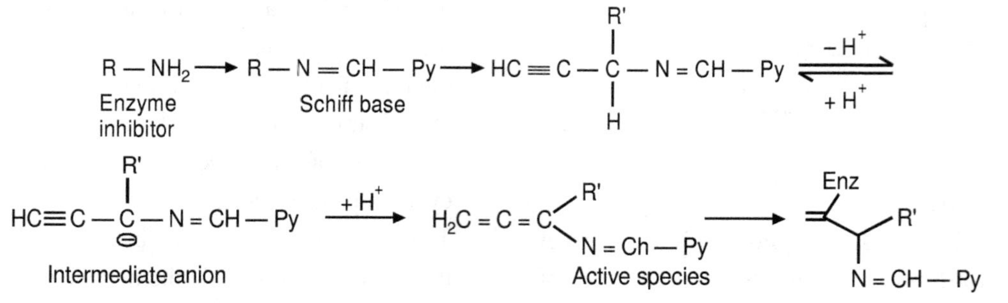

(j) Active site directed irreversible inhibitors : This category of inhibitors may be designed by two important aspects. In first approach, the inhibitor has some similarity with either a substrate or cofactor of the enzyme. Sometimes a section of the reactive part of the enzyme may be incorporated into the inhibitor to recognize and to direct the inhibitor molecule to the enzyme's active site. In another approach, a strong nucleophile is placed in the inhibitor molecule which is expected to interact with an electrophile moiety located near the active enzyme site with the formation of a firm covalent bond to the enzyme's peptide backbone or side-chains. The most prominent example of the approach is alkylating agents of whose leaving groups interact with electrophilic sites of the enzyme by way of carbonium ions, aziridinium ions and similar nucleophiles.

(k) Quinone inhibition of enzymes : The sulfhydryl groups of an enzyme are essential for its catalytic function. By virtue of their oxidising property, quinones can oxidise two SH-groups to form an S-S linkage

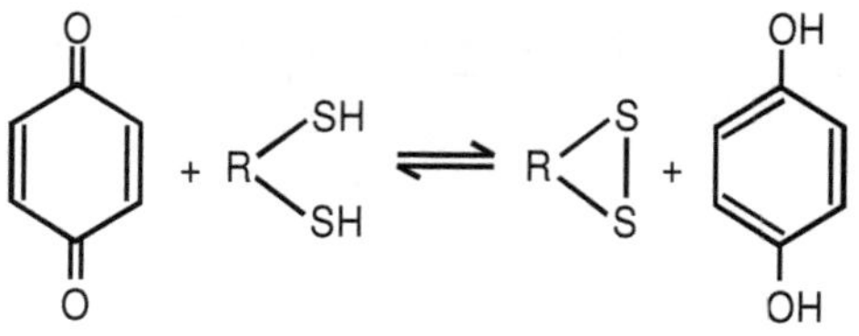

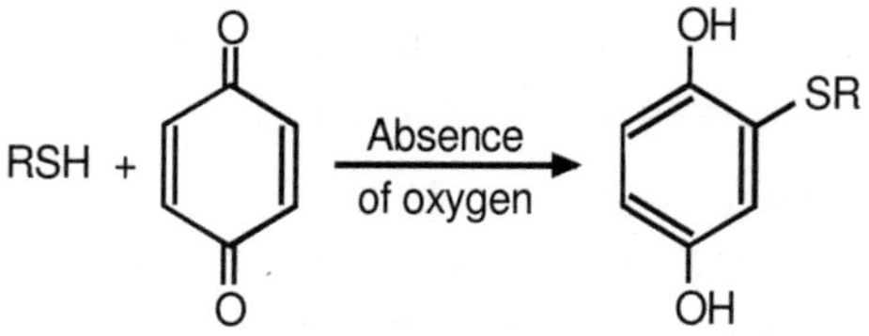

If the inhibitor contains a quinone moiety, the enzymes containing the sulfhydryl groups may be protected against the inhibitory action by the addition of other SH - containing substances like cysteine, glutathione, BAL (2,3 – dimercaptopropanol) and p-benzoquinone. Addition of such compounds may partially reverse and regenerate an already inhibited enzyme. The oxidising property of quinone can be nullified by 2, 3-dimercaptopropanol in the following way.

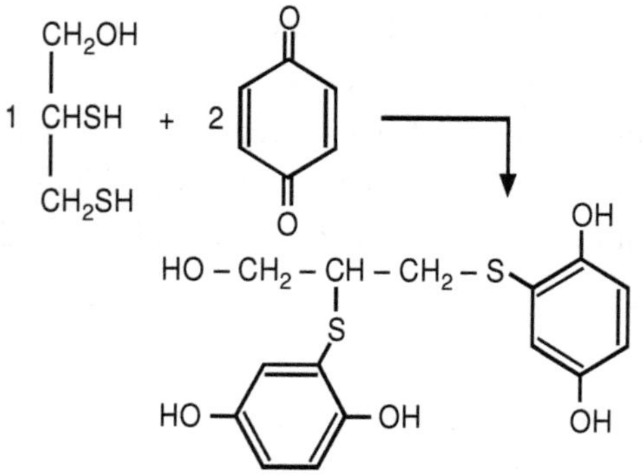

The mechanism of action of certain vitamins like vitamin K_1 and K_2 is based on the presence of a quinone ring in their structure. Quinone inhibition of non-oxidative sulfhydryl enzymes is the mechanism of quinone action on enzymic oxidoreduction processes.

Dicoumarol acts as a competitive inhibitor of phosphorylation where oxidation is not inhibited. Since, vitamin K may generate a cyclic ketal-like structure, the oral anticoagulants may act by antagonising vitamin K competitively at the active sites.

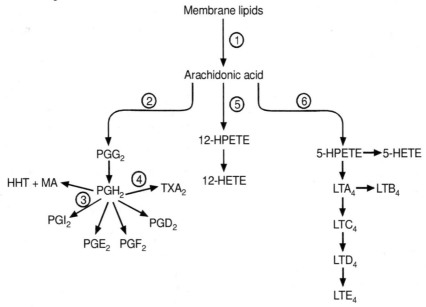

The overall sequence of reactions include

where,

HHT : 12-L-hydroxy-5, 8, 11 - heptadecatrienoic acid

MA : Malondialdehyde

HETE : 12-L-hydroxy-5, 8, 10, 14, - eicosatetraenoic acid

HPETE : 12-L-hydroperoxide analogue

Enzymes involved in the biosynthesis of prostaglandins :

(1) Phospholipases (acyl hydrolases)
(2) Cyclooxygenase (PG - endoperoxide synthetase)
(3) Prostacyclin synthetase
(4) PC-endo-thromboxane A isomerase (thromboxane A_2 synthetase)
(5) 12-Lipooxygenase
(6) 5-Lipooxygenase

Fig. 2.1 : Biosynthetic Pathway for Various Prostaglandins

2.5 ENZYME INHIBITORS ACTING ON PROSTAGLANDIN BIOSYNTHETIC PATHWAY

Prostaglandins are known to be distributed widely in mammals. They have been extensively studied because of their profound effects on various physiological processes. Prostaglandins are synthesized enzymtatically from certain open chain C_{20}-unsaturated fatty acids which include.

(a) 8, 11, 14-eicosatrienoic acid (dihomo - 7 - linolenic acid)

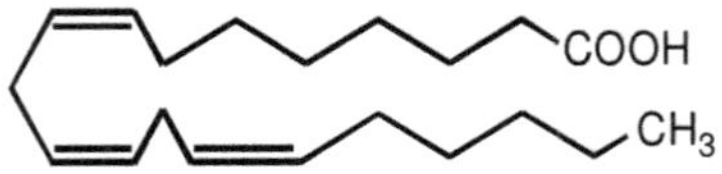

(b) 5, 8, 11. 14- eicosatetraenoic acid

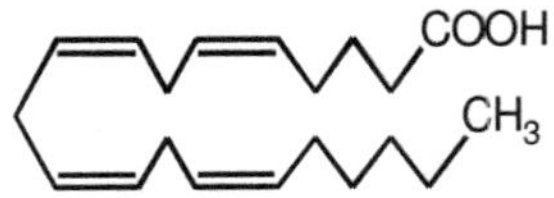

(c) 5, 8, 11, 14, 17 - eicosapentaenoic acid

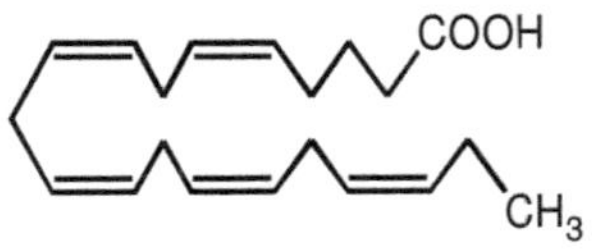

Hydroperoxyeicosatetraenoic acids (HPETEs) are obtained from arachidonic acid. HPETEs are unstable intermediates and are further metabolised by a variety of enzymes. All HPETEs may be converted to their corresponding hydroxy fatty acid (HETE) either by a peroxidase or non-enzymatically.

(a) Inhibitors of phospholipase enzyme :

The phospholipase enzyme causes the hydrolysis of arachidonyl phosphatidyl choline fraction of membrane lipids and releases free arachidonic acid. Various compounds like mepacrine, lipocortin, chloroquine, p-bromophenacyl bromide, were found to inhibit phaspholipase activity.

The steroidal anti-inflammatory agents like hydrocortisone and dexamethasone limit the availability of free arachidonic acid presumably by affecting the activity of phospholipase enzyme.

(b) Inhibitors of cyclooxygenase enzyme :

Aspirin and related analgesic – anti-inflammatory agents block the synthesis of prostacyclin, TxA_2, PGE_2 and other products of cyclooxygenase pathway while the metabolites derived from arachidonic acid via lipooxygenase pathway remain unaffected. Aspirin exerts irreversible inhibition by acetylating serine residue at the active site of cyclooxygenase. These drugs inhibit other enzymes including phosphodiesterase, PLA_2 and 15-hydroxyprostaglandin dehydrogenase.

(c) Inhibitors of lipooxygenase enzyme :

Arachidonic acid is partly utilised by lipooxygenase enzymes to form leukotrienes which are responsible for hypersensitivity reactions. Hence, when cyclooxygenase is blocked, the amount of arachidonic acid available for lipooxygenase pathway gets doubled resulting into more production of leukotrienes. This explains the occurrence of hypersensitivity reactions seen during the therapy of non-steroidal anti-inflammatory agents. This drawback can be overcomed by developing a selective inhibitor of 5-lipooxygenase (5-LO) or a dual inhibitor of both 5-LO and cyclooxygenase enzymes. Selective inhibitors of 5-LO include flavonoids, quercetin, esculetin, baicalein, benoxaprofen and cirsilol.

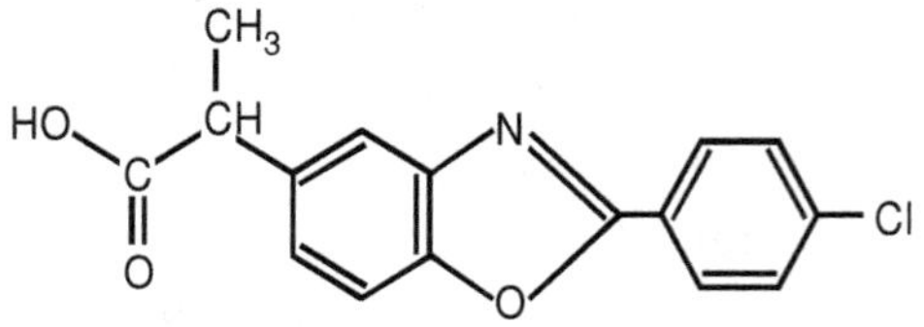

Benoxaprofen

Originally designed by BAYER to act as an antithrombotic agent, nafazatrom was found to act as a selective inhibitor of 5-LO. Since nafazatrom is believed to be a reducing co-factor for peroxidase, it acts by increasing 5-HETE synthesis which in turn may inhibit 5-LO through negative feed-back inhibitory mechanism.

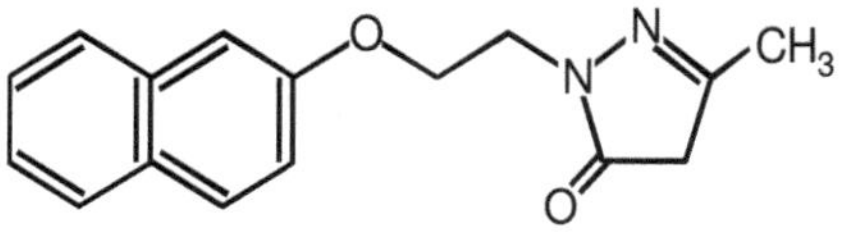

Nafazatrom

Other examples of selective inhibitor of 5-LO include piroprost and AA 861. These agents help to decrease the generation of leukotrienes in the prostaglandin biosynthetic pathway and may be useful to treat allergic broncho constriction.

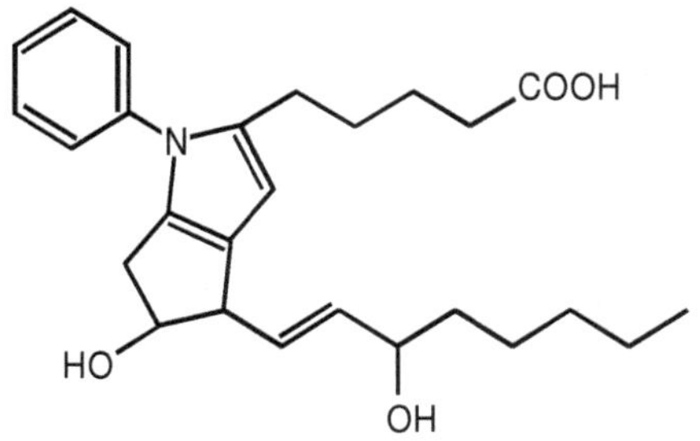

Piroprost

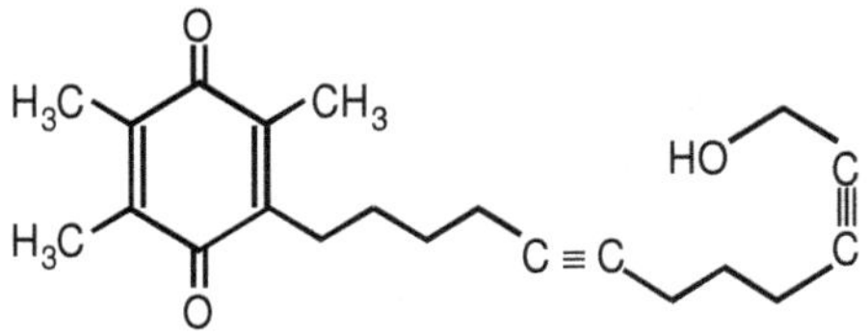

AA 861

(d) Inhibitors of thromboxane synthetase :

Thromboxane A_2 is a vasoconstrictor and inducer of platelet aggregation. By blocking the cyclooxygenase pathway, aspirin exerts anti-thrombotic action for which it may be used in the treatment of various CVS - disorders. However a selective inhibitor of thromboxane synthetase offers many advantages over aspirin in anti-thrombotic therapy. By blocking the formation of thromboxane A_2, it increases the availability of PGH_2 for the production of prostacyclin. The re-direction of prostaglandin endoperoxide metabolism to increased formation of anti-thrombotic prostacyclin (PGI_2) and PGD_2 helps to get selectivity of action. Examples of selective inhibitors of thromboxane synthetase includes.

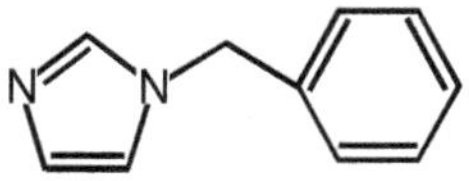

Benzyl imidazole

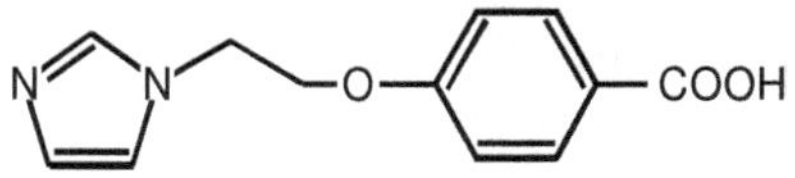

Dazoxiben (pfizer)

2.6 ENZYME INHIBITORS ACTING ON NOREPINEPHRINE BIOSYNTHESIS PATHWAY

The enzymes that participate in the biosynthesis of epinephrine are summerised below :

The key enzyme is tyrosine hydroxylase, which requires a tetrahydrofolate coenzyme, oxygen and Fe^{++} and is quite specific. Dopa-decarboxylase acts on all aromatic L-amino acids including histidine, tyrosine, tryptophan, 5-HT, phenylalanin and requires pyridoxal phosphate as a co-factor Dopamine β-hydroxylase, located in the membranes of storage vesicles, is a copper containing protein, a mixed function oxygenase that utilises oxygen and ascorbic acid. Dopamine β-hydroxylase dose not show a high degree of substrate specificity and acts in-vitro on a variety of substrates, oxidising almost any phenylethylamine to its corresponding phenyl-ethanolamine. Finally phenyl-ethanolamine-N- methyl transferase, located in the adrenal medulla and in the brain, uses S-adenosylmethionine as a methyl donar. The adrenal medullary enzyme shows poor substrate specificity on a variety of β-hydroxylated amines.

(a) Inhibitors of dopa decarboxylase :

Dopa decarboxylase catalyzes the conversion of dopa to dopamine. Alpha-methyl dopa and α-monofluoro methyl dopa are the examples of effective inhibitor of the enzyme. Since, the rate of decarboxylation of these compounds is considerably slower than that of dopa, they tie up the enzyme for a longer period of time. The α-monofluoro methyl dopa causes depletion of catecholamine levels in the brain, heart and kidneys. Phenylalanine and tyrosine are weak inhibitors of dopa decarboxylase but their keto acids and some cinnamic acid derivatives are effective inhibitors.

The aldehyde group of co-decarboxylase makes it susceptible to reaction with carbonyl-trapping agents such as hydroxylamine, hydrazine, semicarbazide etc.

(b) Inhibitors of dopamine-β-hydroxylase :

Inhibitors of dopamine β-hydroxylase (DBH) serve as potential lead for further antihypertensive agents. They inhibit the enzyme in competitive or non-competitive way. The former category includes analogues of phenylethylamine skeleton like picolinic acid, benzyloxyamine, aromatic thioureas and ascorbate-2-sulphate. Non-competitive inhibitors include histidine, hydralazine, prazosin and diethyldithio-carbamate. Many DBH inhibitors were found to act as metal-chelating agents. Other examples of effective inhibitors of dopamine-β-hydroxylase include 2-mercapto-l-methylimidazole, diethylpyro-carbonate, bleomycin and benzylhydrazine.

Dopamine-β-hydroxylase can be inhibited by a variety of compounds. The most effective are compounds which chelate copper : D-cysteine and L-cyteine, gluta-thione, mercaptoethanol and coenzyme A. The inhibition can be reversed by addition of the N-ethylmaleimide, which reacts with the sulfhydryl groups and interfers with the chelating properties of these substances. Copper chelating agents such as diethyldithiocarbamate (i.e., disulfiram) and [bis - (1 - methyl - 4 - homopiperazinyl-thiocarbonyl) - disulfide] have proved to be effective inhibitors both in-vivo and in-vitro.

(c) Inhibitors of L-tyrosine hydroxylase :

The enzyme L-tyrosine hydroxylase was identified by Udenfriend and colleagues in 1964. The enzyme is stereospecific and has a high degree of substrate specificity. It catalyzes the rate limiting step in catecholamine biosynthesis.

Effective inhibitors of this enzyme include α-methyl-p-tyrosine and its ester, α - methyl - 3 - iodotyrosine, 3-iodotyrosine, α - methyl - 5 - hydroxytryptophan, catechol derivatives, tropolones and selective iron chelators. A marked increase in activity in the case of the tyrosine analogues can also be produced by substituting a halogen at the 3-position of the benzene ring.

Inhibitors of dopa decarboxylase :

Carbidopa, a hydrazine analogue of α-methyldopa, is an important DOPA decarboxylase inhibitor. The exclusive peripheral mode of action of carbidopa in the therapy of parkinson's disease is due to its ionic character and inability to cross the blood-brain barrier.

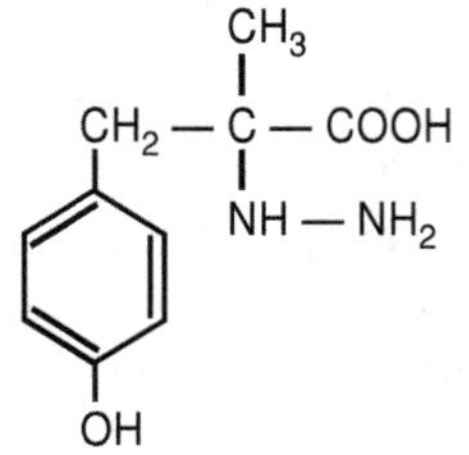

Carbidopa

Benserazide is another inhibitor having similar activity.

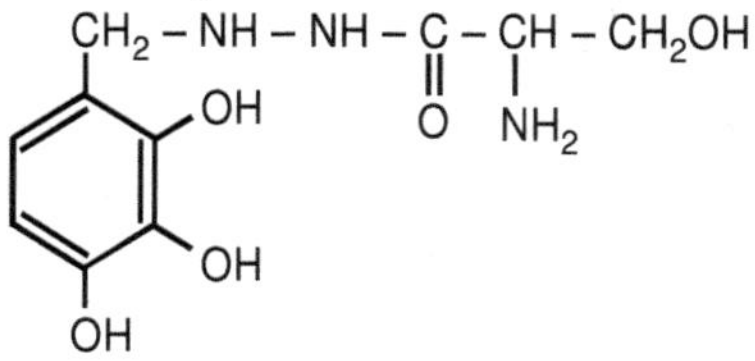

Benserazide (Roche)

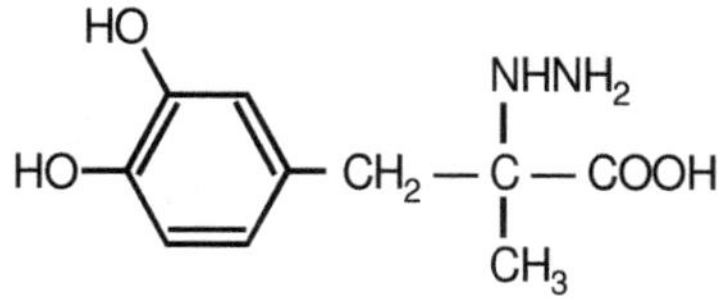

N-Amino methyl dopa (Merck)

Enzyme inhibitors of mono amino oxidase :

The non-hydrazine MAO-inhibitors (e.g., pargyline and tranylcypromine) are preferred in therapy due to the hepatotoxic side-effects of hydrazine-hydrazide MAO-inhibitors. Due to pronounced effect on blood pressure, pargyline is used as an antihypertensive agent while tranylcypromine was developed as a structural analog of amphetamine and is used as in anti-depressant agent. Further structural modifications of pargyline skeleton lead to clorgyline and cyclogyline.

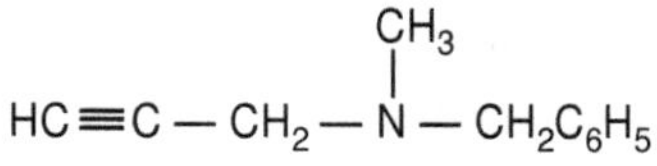

Pargyline

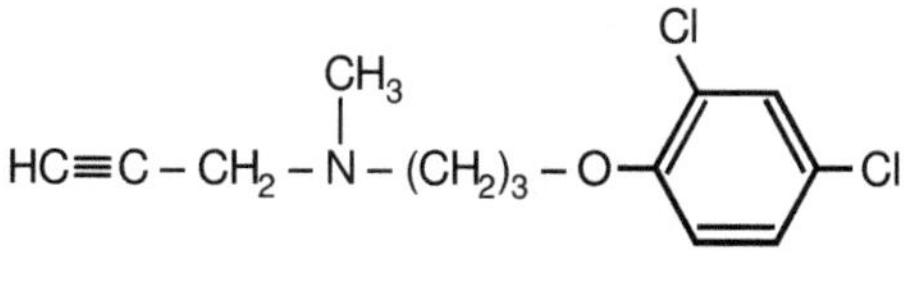

Clorgyline

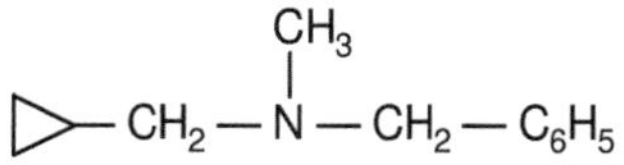

Cyclogyline

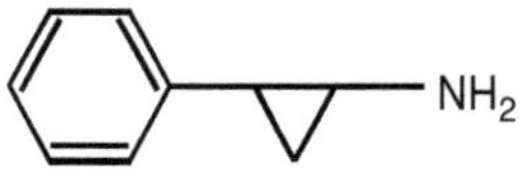

Tranylcypromine

Pargyline inactives the MAO by interacting with flavin co-enzyme across the 1, 4-additive system. The covalent adduct formed suggests an irreversible inhibition of MAO – enzyme.

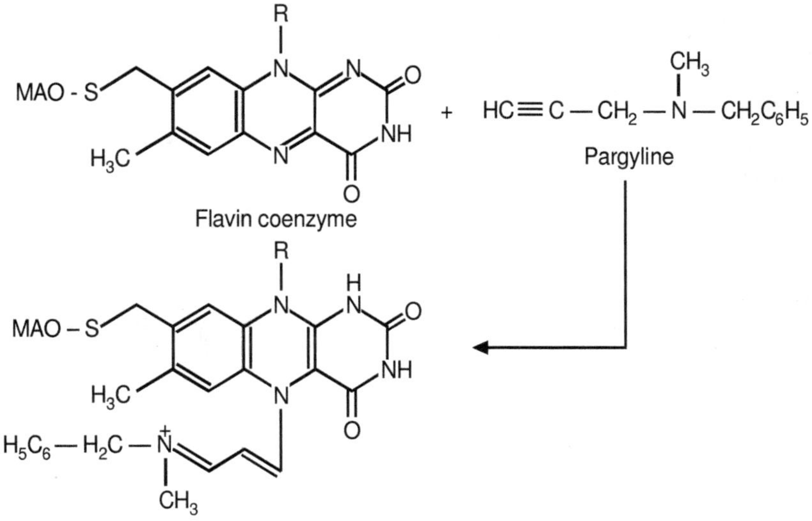

Flavin coenzyme

Pargyline

2.7 SEROTONIN SYNTHESIS INHIBITORS

Tryptophan hydroxylase catalyzes the first rate-determining step in serotonin synthesis P-Chlorophenylalanine is found to block tryptophan hydroxylase.

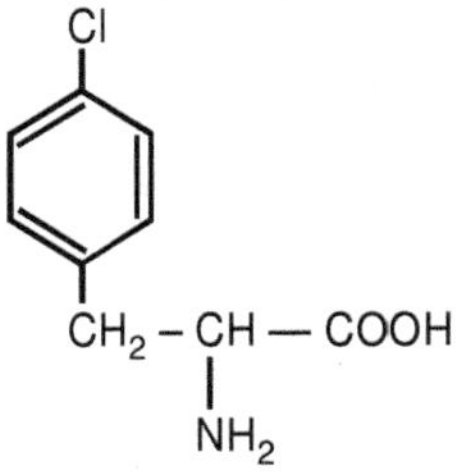

P-chlorophenylalanine

Dihydropteridine reductase :

During the hydroxylation of tyrosine to DOPA, the reduction of the quinonoid dihydropterin is catalysed by this enzyme. Since reduced pteridines are essential for tyrosine hydroxylation, any effect on the activity dihydropteridine reductase will influence the activity of tyrosine hydroxylase. Dihydropteridines with an amine substitution at positions 2 and 4 are found to be effective inhibitors of dihydropteridine reductase.

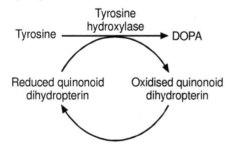

2.8 INHIBITORS OF MEMBRANE BOUND ATPase

The ATPase activity of a high molecular weight ATPase complex resides in its water soluble protein fraction (F_0) (F). Certain lipoidal agents dissolve in the biological membranes and deprive the ATP synthetase of its energy input. This results into inhibition of ATP synthesis. Such agents include, 2, 4-dinitrophenol, carbonylcyanide, m-chlorophenyl-hydrazone, trichlorosalicylamide, chlorhexidin, etc.

The inhibitors of water-insoluble protein fraction (F_0) of the membrane bound ATPase include oligomycin, rutamycin, leucinostatin, venturicidin, etc.

2.9 GABA-METABOLISM INHIBITORS

An inhibitory central neurotransmitter GABA, is found to play an etiological role in generation of epileptic seizures. An antiepileptic drug, sodium valproate, blocks succinic semialdehyde dehydrogenase, the enzyme oxidizing the semialdehyde.

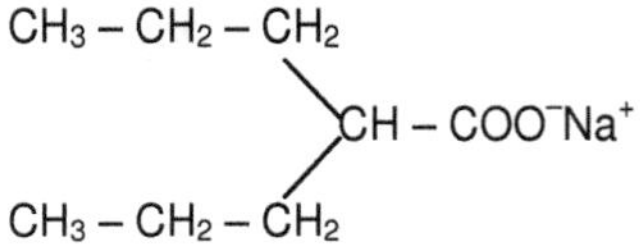

Sodium valproate

As this metabolite accumulates GABA - transaminase (GABA-T) activity is suppressed by end - product inhibition and the neurotransmitter concentration increases, thus inhibiting the seizures. The direct inhibitors of GABA-T enzyme include,

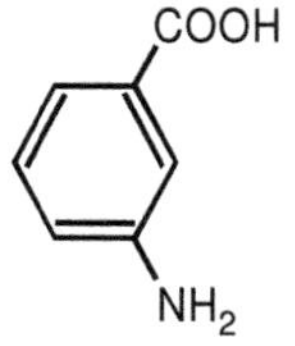

Gabaculine

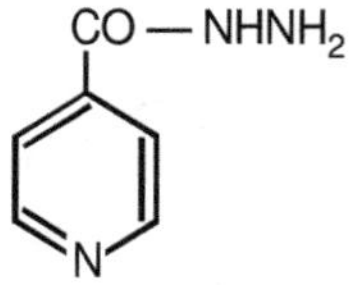

Isonicotinic acid hydrazide

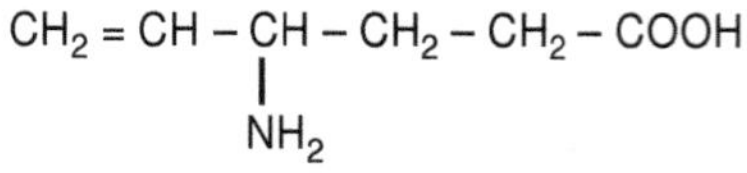

4-aminohex-5-enoic acid

2.10 INHIBITORS OF HIV-REVERSE TRANSCRIPTASE (HIV-RT)

The first clinically used anti-aids agent, azidothymidine (AZT) is found to act by inhibiting HIV-RT enzyme. The drug in its activated form (AZT-triphosphate) acts as a potent inhibitor of the virus reverse transcriptase. The virus enzyme becomes ineffective in elongating a primer terminated with AZT. The drug also inhibits cellular DNA polymerases at much high concentration level. AZT is an example of nucleoside RT-inhibitor.

Non-nucleoside RT-inhibitors have binding sites on reverse transcriptase which are distinct to that of nucleoside inhibitors. These agents include pyridinone, dipyrido-diazepinone. HEPT and TIBO.

2.11 HYPOGLYCEMIC AGENTS ACTING THROUGH ENZYME INHIBITION

(a) Inhibitors of carbohydrate absorption :

The intestinal carbohydrate digestion can be delayed by inhibiting the enzymes that cleave the terminal glucose. Acarbose is such a clinically used agent.

(b) Aldose reductase inhibitors :

The two major pathways by which glucose is metabolised in the body include glycolytic pathway and polyol pathway. The former pathway is preferred in normal person. In diabetic person the excess sugar left after saturation of glycolytic pathway is metabolised by polyol pathway. In polyol pathway, glucose is metabolised to fructose via sorbitol by aldose reductase enzyme.

Since the rate of formation of sorbitol is higher than its rate of conversion to fructose, the resulting accumulation of sorbitol is responsible for complications of chronic diabetes like cataract, neuropathy and retinopathy. Tolrestat acts by inhibiting aldose reductase enzyme and may be used in the prophylaxis of diabetic neuropathy, retinopathy and cataract.

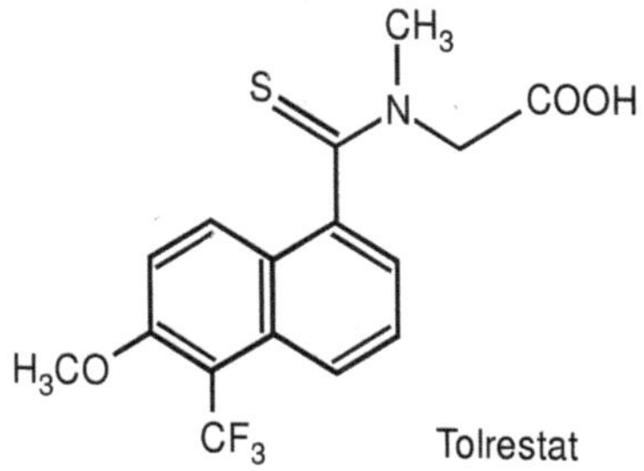

Tolrestat

2.12 CARBONIC ANHYDRASE INHIBITORS

Certain sulphonamides exert diuretic, anti-glaucoma and antiepileptic activities by inhibiting carbonic anhydrase enzyme. The interaction between the NH of sulphonamido group and the active site of enzyme is proposed to be hydrogen bonding. In comparison with most other carbonic anhydrase inhibitors, sulphonamides equilibrate rather slowly with the enzyme.

2.13 INHIBITORS OF XANTHINE OXIDASE

The oxidation of hypoxanthine and xanthine to uric acid is catalysed by xanthine oxidases.

Examples of xanthine oxidase inhibitors include purine analogs, pteridine, allopurinol, pterin-6-aldehyde, xanthopterin, isoxanthopterin, leucopterin, etc.

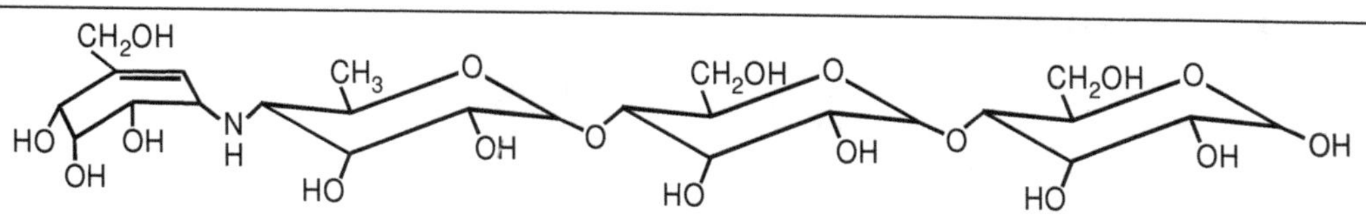

Acarbose

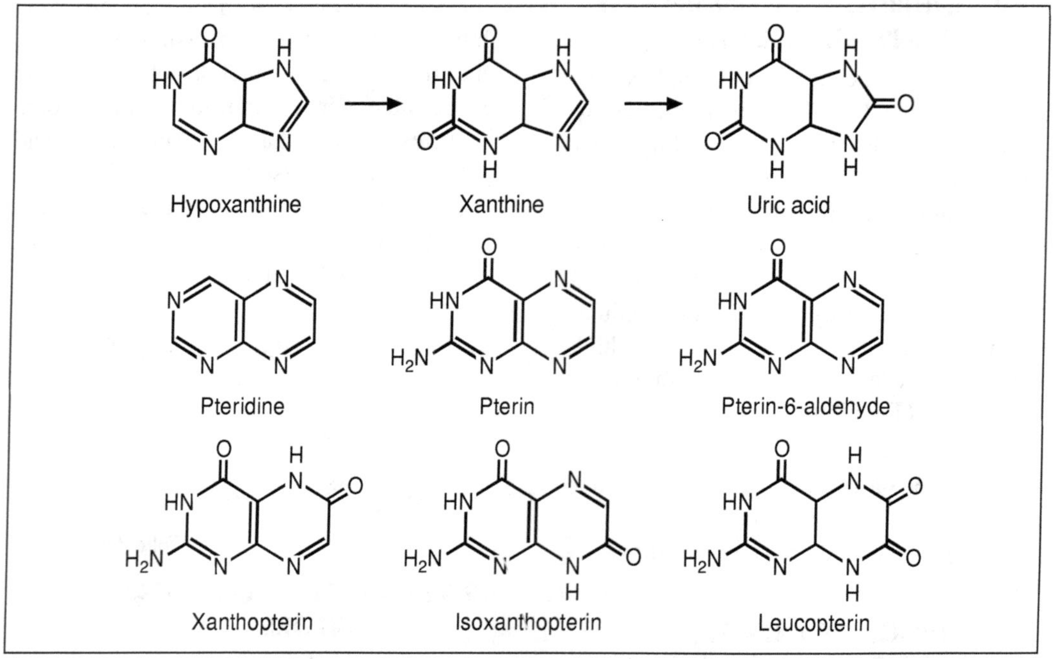

Hypoxanthine → Xanthine → Uric acid

Pteridine   Pterin   Pterin-6-aldehyde

Xanthopterin   Isoxanthopterin   Leucopterin

2.14 AROMATASE INHIBITORS

The ring A aromatization is an important step in the biosynthesis of estrogens. The aromatase inhibitors, therefore may find place in the therapy of metastatic hormone-dependent breast cancer. Aminoglutethimide, an aromatase inhibitor was found to be effective in many trials with postmenopausal women.

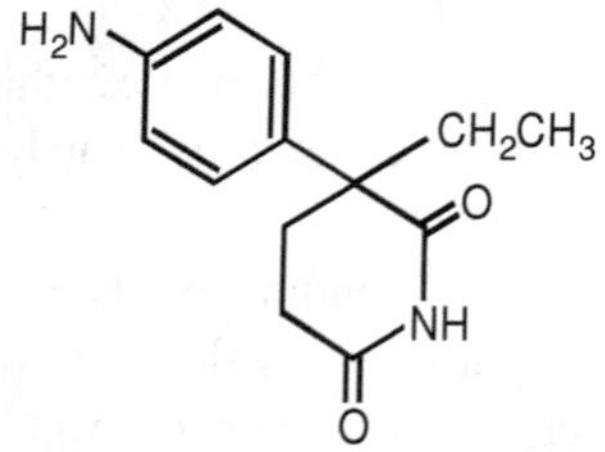

Aminoglutethimide

2.15 Na$^+$ – K$^+$ – ATPase INHIBITORS

Digitalis and related drugs reversibly inhibit Na$^+$ – K$^+$ – ATPase through allosteric binding. Besides them, many low molecular weight, non-steroidal inhibitors of diversified lead skeletons have been prepared and evaluated for inhibition of Na$^+$ – K$^+$ – ATPase pump.

2.16 RENIN INHIBITORS

Human renin is an aspartyl protease which is synthesized, stored and secreted into the renal arterial circulation by the granular juxlaglomendar cells. The active form of renin is a glycoprotein having 340 amino acids. It catalyses the generation of angiotensin I (decapcptide) from a plasma protein substrate, an -α_2-globulin known as angiotensinogen. Renin inhibition is one of the important targets considered in antihypertensive therapy. Following are the examples of renin inhibitors.

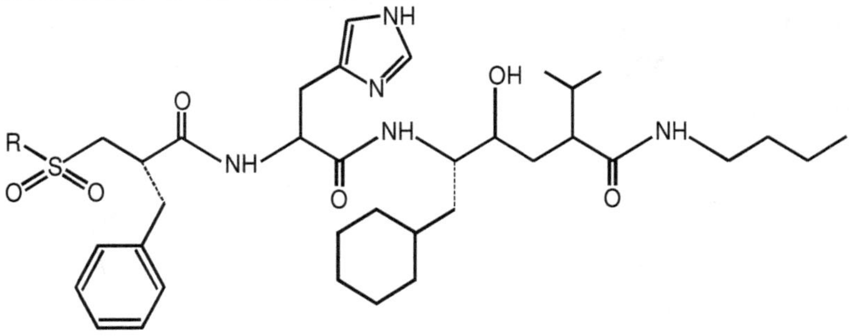

Drug Design   2.17   Enzyme Inhibitors

R = CH₃;   CGP - 38259
R = t-Bu;   CGP - 38560

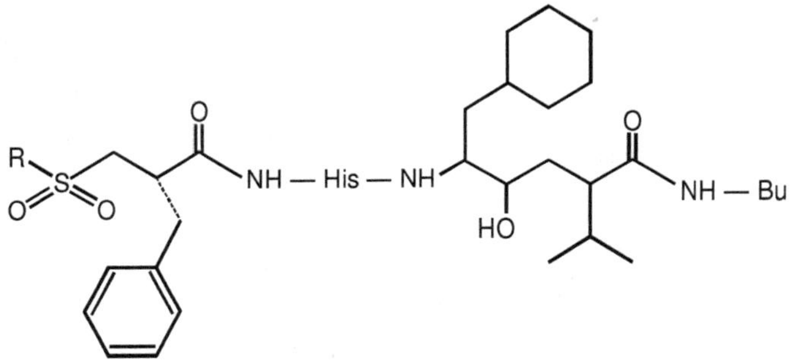

(Ciba Geigy; CGS - 38560)

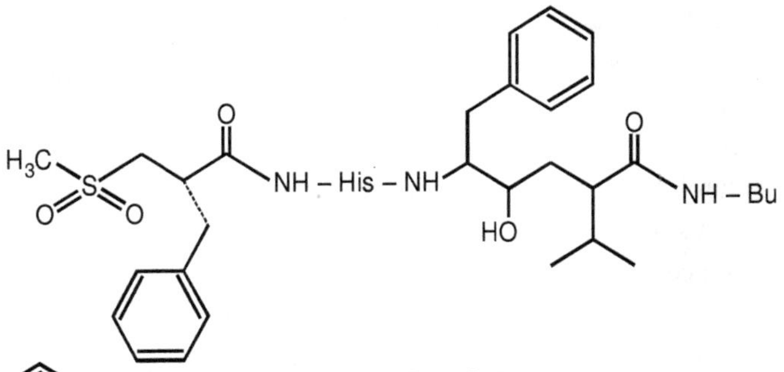

CGS - 38561 (Ciba Geigy)

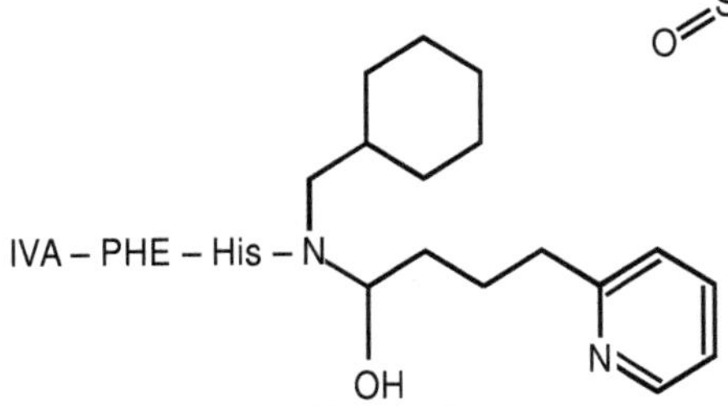

IVA – PHE – His – N

(Hoechst)

IVA – PHE – His – NH

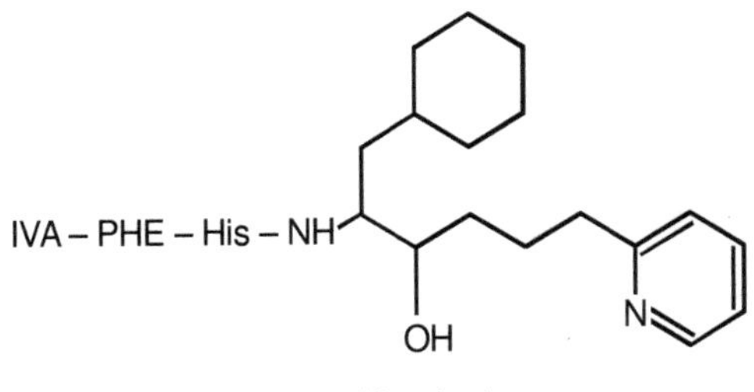

(Hoechst)

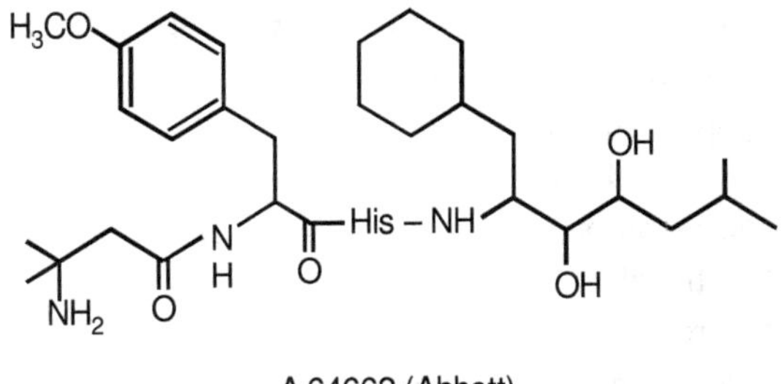

A 64662 (Abbott)

2.17 INHIBITORS OF ANGIOTENSIN CONVERTING ENZYME (ACE-INHIBITORS)

Human angiotensin converting enzyme (ACE) is a large protein containing 1278 amino acids. It catalyzes the conversion of angiotensin I (decapeptide) to angiotensin II (octapeptide), one of the most potent natural precursor substrates

H–Asp–Arg–Val–Tyr–Ile–His–Pro–Phe–His–Leu–OH

Angiotensin-I

ACE

H–Asp–Arg–Val–Tyr–Ile–His–Pro–Phe–OH

Angiotensin-II

Although a slow conversion of angiotensin-I to angiotensin-II occurs in the plasma, its rapid metabolism in-vivo is brought about by tissue-bound ACE. Zinc ions occur frequently at the active sites of ACE. Since carboxypeptidases and ACE are the examples of zinc hydrolases, the known structural features of carboxypeptidases were utilized to predict the structural features of ACE. The most important features of carboxypeptidases include the presence of a positive charge which may be expected to interact with the c-terminal carboxyl group of angiotensin I and a Zn^{++} ion that activates the carbonyl group of the scissile peptide bond. The activation is thought to be due to the ability of zinc to form stable mono or bidentate complexes with tetrahedral intermediates in substrate hydrolysis, thus favouring the attack of water. Taking these features into consideration, analogs incorporating functional groups that can form strong co-ordinate bonds with zinc (such as carbonyl or mercapto group) were designed.

Captopril, a well known antihypertcnsive agent is an outcome of this approach.

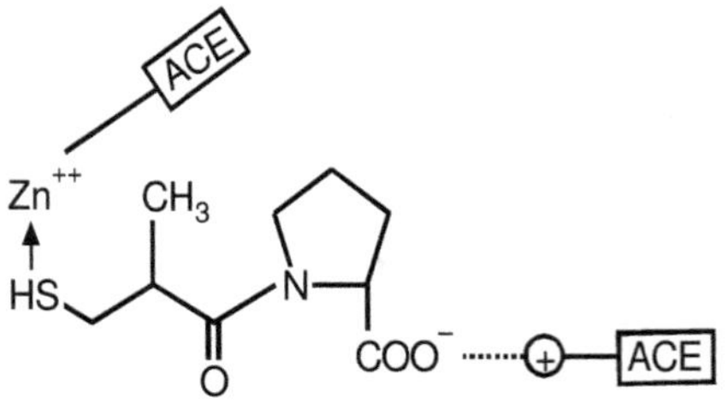

Fig. 2.2 : Interaction of Captopril with the Active Sites of ACE

Enalepril is a second generation, non-sulfhydryl ACE inhibitor. Chemically it belongs to the group of substituted N-carboxymethyl dipeptide which can inhibit metallodipeptidyl carboxypeptidases, despite lack of Zn^{++} sulfhydryl interaction.

Since highly lipophilic replacements enhanced the binding of the drug to the enzyme, more lipophilic ACE-inhibitors than the captopril were synthesized. Examples include,

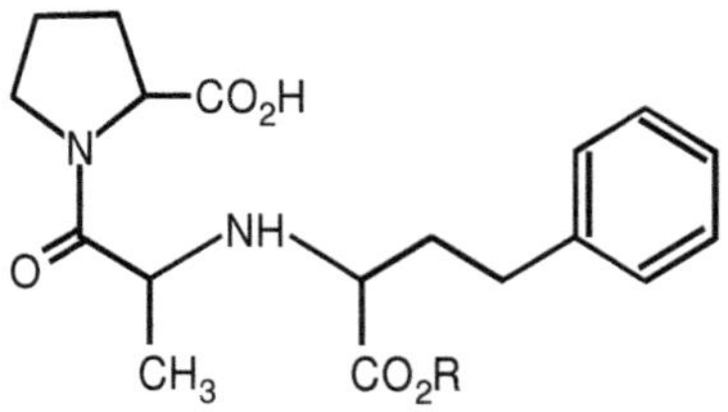

Enalepril
(R = C_2H_5)

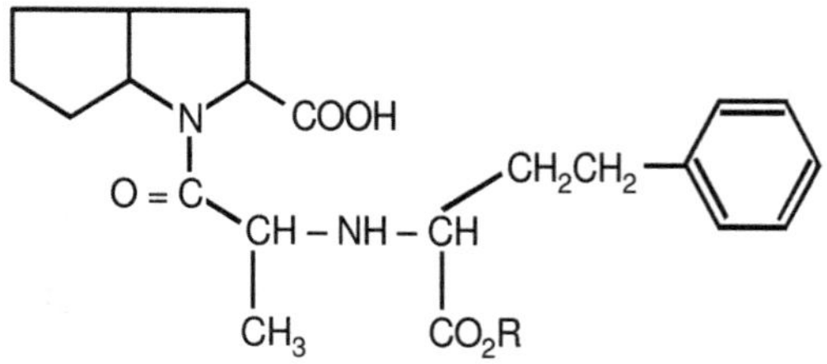

Ramipril (Hoechst); R = C_2H_5
Ramiprilal; R = H

2.18 INTEGRASE INHIBITORS

The enzyme, viral endonuclease (integrase) catalyzes the incorporation of viral DNA into the host cell genome. Drugs that interfere with the structure and function of retroviral mRNA transcribed from integrated DNA in infected cells could be of therapeutic value in AIDS. Ribaverin and doxorubicin are the examples of integrase inhibitors.

2.19 GLYCOSIDASE INHIBITORS

The enzyme, glycosidase participates in the final step in the HIV-life cycle to cleave off glucose units from the oligosaccharide chain. It catalyses the processing of the surface glycoproteins and thus helps in the maturation of infectious viral progency. The glycosidase inhibitors include polyhydroxylated compounds such as castenospermine and N-butyldeoxy nojirimycin.

❖❖❖

3

ANTI-AIDS AGENTS

3.1 INTRODUCTION

The Acquired Immuno Deficiency Syndrome (AIDS) was first reported in 1981 as a clinical syndrome consisting of opportunistic infection and/or neoplasia associated with unexplained immunodeficiency among a group of previously healthy homosexual males. AIDS originated in central Africa in a certain species of monkey. The virus then changed and spread to humans. Since the discovery of AIDS in 1981 in the United States, the disease has grown into pandemic proportions around the globe. By 1993, there were an estimated 14 million HIV-infected people throughout the world.

AIDS is the end stage disease representing the irreversible breakdown of immune defence mechanisms. The immune competence of the patient is completely lost. As a result, chemotaxis, antigen identification and the functioning of monocytes and macrophages are gradually diminished. The patient is vulnerable to attack by serious infectious organisms in the environment. AIDS is defined as the occurrence of either a life threatening opportunistic infection or development of Kaposi's sarcoma (i.e., parasitic infection of lungs with symptoms similar to those of other forms of severe pneumonia) in a person younger than 60 years and has no underlying immuno suppressive cause.

The patient is susceptible to the attack of infections with relatively avirulent micro-organisms as well as to lymphoid and other malignancies. The commonly seen infection in AIDS patients include oral candidiasis, herpes zoster, hairy cell leucoplakia, salmonellosis, P. carinii pneumonia, toxoplasmosis, cytomegalovirus infection or tuberculosis. Lymphoid and other malignancies may also be present. AIDS takes 6 months to 5 years or more to develop after contact with the infectious agent. The major symptoms seen in an AIDS patient include swollen glands (lymph nodes) in neck, armpits or groin; weight loss, fever or night sweats, chronic diarrhoea, purple spots on the skin, fatigue, cough and shortness of breath. Death is caused either by cancer or one of many infections in the body.

The first human retrovirus, called human T-cell leukaemia virus type I (HTLV-I) was isolated in 1979 by Gallo and associates. The first case of AIDS patient was detected in 1981 in New York. Thereafter, efforts were identified to isolate the infecting agent of AIDS. A retroviral cause for AIDS was first established by French researchers, led by Luc Montagnier who isolated a virus from a West African patient suffering from lymphadenopathy in 1983 at Pasteur Institute, Paris. It was found to be a retrovirus. It was named as Lyphadenopathy Associated Virus (LAV). This was followed by many reports describing the isolation of aetiological agents in AIDS. All these agents were described under the term, AIDS-related viruses (ARV). In 1986, the International Committee on Virus Nomenclature had coined the terms, 'Human Immunodeficiency Virus, (HIV) for these infective agents, in order to avoid confusion.

3.2 STRUCTURAL FEATURES OF HIV

Human immunodeficiency virus belongs to the lentiviridae family of pathogenic human retroviruses, which rely on RNA to encode their genetic message. It is an example of a thermolabile enveloped virus having a diameter of 90-120 nm. On electron microscopy, it has a characteristic dense, cylindrical nucleoid containing core proteins, two copies of single stranded viral RNA and reverse transcriptase surrounded by a lipid envelope. The reverse transcriptase of HIV-1 has been shown to be Mg^{++} requiring RNA-dependent DNA polymerase that is responsible for replicating the RNA viral genome. The surface of lipid envelope consists of two major glycosylated proteins, gp 41 and gp 120.

Minor antigenic differences in both core and envelope antigens are reported between isolates from different patients as well as from the same patient. Two major forms of HIV have been described, HIV-1 and HIV-2. Despite the marked heterogeneity in envelope structure and ability to propagate, HIV-2 has a more restricted geographic distribution and has been mostly isolated from several patients in Western Africa, as well as from several patients in Europe and South America. The clinical manifestations in patients infected with HIV-2 are identical to their HIV-1 counter parts.

The first step in the retroviral replication cycle is the specific interaction of the outer membrane component of virion envelope glycoprotein with a specific cell surface receptors. Three distinct retroviral receptors have been defined thus far, i.e. the glycoprotein receptor for HIV-1, for ecotropic Murine Leukaemia Virus (MLV) and for Gibbon Ape Leukaemia Virus (GALV).

The virus appeared to replicate selectively in $CD4^+$ lymphocytes. Binding of HIV-1 to $CD4^+$ cells involved the formation of a high-affinity complex between the CD4 molecule and gp 120 with a dissociation constant of approximately 4×10^{-9} M. Following binding to the CD4 molecule, HIV is internalised and uncoated. HIV infection of monocytes and macrophages may result in defective chemotaxis, altered monokine production, enhanced release of interleukin-1 (IL-1), tumour necrosis factor (cachectin), or other pyrogens, and by this means lead to certain aspects of HIV infection including impaired pulmonary resistance to opportunistic disease.

The HIV virus can remain silent over a long period of time. Under favourable conditions, viral replication occurs by increased rate of synthesis of viral RNA and other components. Since HIV virus affects the functioning of immune system, the symptoms associated are mainly due to the failure of immune responses rather than due to viral cytotoxicity. The T_4-lymphocytes serve as suitable host cell for HIV viruses. The major damage occurs to T_4-lymphocytes. T-cells decrease in the number. This results into a lack of secretion of activating factors from T_4-lymphocytes. This is a contributing factor for the failure of immune system.

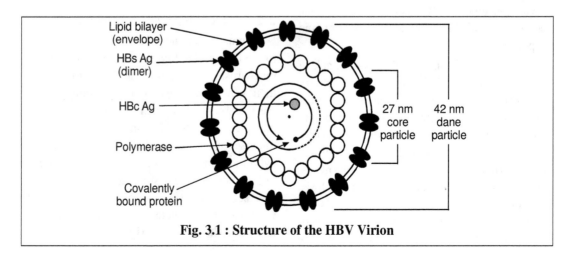

Fig. 3.1 : Structure of the HBV Virion

In an infected person. HIV viruses can be detected into saliva, tears, urine, cervical secretions, semen, breast milk, blood, lymphocytes and cell free plasma. Such factors as frequent exposure to sperm, rectal exposure to sperm, and / or amyl nitrate and butyl nitrate poppers, which were used to enhance sexual performance, were considered potential causes of AIDS.

3.3 EPIDEMIOLOGY OF HIV VIRUS

AIDS virus may be transmitted by following possible routes :

(a) Through sexual contacts in both, homosexuals and heterosexuals.

(b) Through transfusion of blood (haemophilia transfusion of whole blood, red blood cells, platelets and plasma), blood products or other body products.

(c) Through the donation of tissue or organ.

(d) Through certain infections and / or injuries.

(e) From infected mother to baby.

Exposure measures for HIV include sexual activities, contraceptive practices, drug use patterns, obstetric history, cultural factors, nosocomial injuries and serologic measures. AIDS is an increasing worldwide epidemic. The prevalence rate of HIV-infection may remain high in homosexual men, parenteral drug users, female prostitutes, haemophilia patients, military recruit applicants and volunteer blood donors. The use of condoms clearly reduces but does not eliminate, the risk of heterosexual transmission of HIV.

In the case of intravenous drug abusers, increased exposure to foreign tissue antigens might occur when recipients used dirty needles contaminated with small amounts of blood from previous users. The increase in T-suppresser cells is presumably due to frequent antigenic stimulation. The risk of being infected with HIV is closely linked to both the frequency of drug injection and the sharing of needles or injection with previously used needles.

Two procedures have reduced markedly the risk of haemophilics being infected. The report that HIV is heat-labile, heat-treated products greatly reduced but did not eliminate HIV among haemophilic. The added step of screening and eliminating HIV-antibodies from donated blood and plasma has reduced HIV-transmission through blood products to almost nil. As a general rule, blood products with a high risk of transmitting hepatitis B virus are also likely to transmit HIV.

Similarly, during the prolonged nursing care of HIV-infected person, the nurses and other health care workers may get infected either due to

(a) Careless handling and disposal of sharp instruments.

(b) Or repeated exposures to blood, urine, faeces and gastric contents of infected patients.

Hence, broader use of gloves, masks and protective garments by hospital personnel and / or mandatory HIV screening of patients may be appropriate.

Majority of cases of HIV infection in children, occur by transplacental passage of HIV in pregnant, infected women. In addition, virus transmission to baby by breast-feeding from infected mother is also reported. Estimates of the HIV infection rate in babies born to seropositive women range from 25% when the mothers are largely asymptomatic, to 65% when the mothers have had a previous baby with AIDS.

HIV can also be transmitted from HIV-infected donors by transplantation of kidneys. Thus all potential organ, tissue and semen donors must be tested for HIV-antibodies. Patients with AIDS and related diseases often require dialysis. The United States Centres for Disease Control (CDC) mentioned that "standard blood and body fluids precautions and disinfection and sterilization strategies routinely practised in dialysis centres are adequate to prevent transmission of HIV".

Hypothetically biting insects could transmit HIV simply as "Flying syringes" carrying minute amounts of HIV - infected undigested blood from person to person.

Since the virus shows great affinity for the helper T-cells, an important armament in the arsenal of cellular immune system, the total number of CD_4^+ cells (T_4 count) is strongly predictive of AIDS, particularly if the count is below 300 CD_4^+ cells/μl. An increased risk of AIDS is also noted with thrombocytopenia, anaemia, monocytopenia and high levels of cytomegalovirus antibodies. Detection of HIV core (p24) antigen in serum may be strongly predictive of AIDS. Detection of a interferon in serum in high levels, appears to be a useful marker for AIDS.

Currently there are four ways to detect HIV infection :

(a) Isolating the virus by culturing cellular or body fluid samples.

(b) Noting the high levels of reverse transcriptase and HIV-proteins in target cells.

(c) Identifying HIV-specific nucleic acid sequences in cellular materials, and

(d) Identifying HIV-specific antigens and antibodies in serum or other body fluids.

The HIV-infection can also be predicted by signs and symptoms. Thus as per WHO, AIDS can be defined as the presence of disseminated kiposi's sarcoma or cryptococcal meningitis and the presence of one or more of signs which include weight loss, diarrhoea, fever, cough, general lymphadenopathy, general pruritic dermatitis, oropharyngeal candidiasis, chronic herpes simplex or a history of herpes zoster within 5 years.

3.4 LIFE-CYCLE OF HIV

The primary target cells of all known human retroviruses including HTLV-I, HTLV-II, HIV-1 and HIV-2, possess receptors for interleukin -2 (IL-2) and require this factor for proliferation.

All retroviruses were known to contain gag, pol and env genes as basic components of a replicating genome. HIV has as its major structural components a core of genomic RNA; group specific antigen (gag) proteins which play a role both in the structure of the core and assembly of the virion; a lipid bilayer, and an outside envelope glycoprotein.

The reverse transcriptase gene is one component of the pol region, and in general this region is expressed as a polyprotein that includes a protease, reverse transcriptase and an endonuclease (integrase). Human immunodeficiency virus integrase has two important biochemical steps comprising overall enzyme function : nucleolytic cleavage and strand transfer (integration) reaction. Incorporation of viral DNA into the host cell genome could be translated as the basis of life-long infection.

The life cycle of the human immunodeficiency virus (HIV) encompasses a number of steps adsorption, penetration, uncoating, reverse transcription of the viral RNA genome to double-stranded DNA, circularisation and integration of the proviral DNA in the cellular genome, transcription of the viral DNA genome to m-RNA and translation of the latter to viral proteins, processing of these proteins (proteolytic cleavage), myristylation and glycosylation), assembly and release of the new virus particles.

The major structural core protein of HIV-1 is the p24 protein. This, and the myristylated protein p18, comprise the major gag structural proteins.

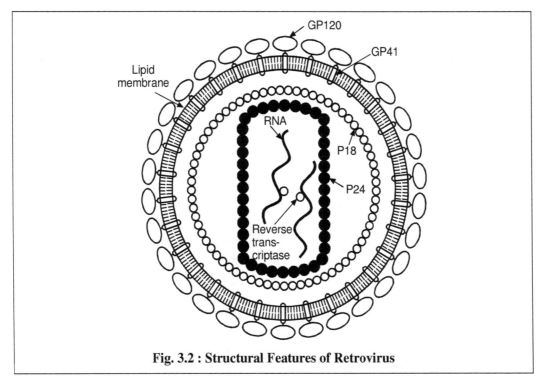

Fig. 3.2 : Structural Features of Retrovirus

Surrounding the viral core is a lipid membrane derived from the outer membrane of the host cell. Studding the outer membrane of the virus are the envelope glycoproteins, gp 120 and gp 4l.

The first step in the HIV infection is its binding to the helper/inducer T-cells at their cell surface proteins known as T4 or CD-4 antibodies. The cytopathic effect is thought to be mediated in part by an interaction between the T4 molecule and the HIV envelope protein that brings about lethal cell to cell fusion (syncytia) or a surface autofusion phenomenon that destroys the integrity of the cell membrane. The cytopathic effect of HIV in $CD4^+$ cells is a function of the density of the CD4 molecules on the surface of the cells. In fact, in HIV-seropositive patients, low T4 cell counts (less than 200/mm^3) is often an indication of the imminent development of AIDS with an opportunistic infection. In many patients, this rapid loss has coincided with marked increase in circulating HIV-antigens.

Thus the hallmark of AIDS infection clinically is a progressive deterioration of immune competence due to gradual loss of $CD4^+$ helper/ inducer lymphocytes. Beside T-cells, other cells expressing CD4 on their surface may also harbour HIV-1 and thereby act as a reservoir for the virus, thus extending the latency period associated with the infection. These include macrophages, monocytes and lymphoid cells. It was recently found that galactosyl ceramide and sulfatide receptors on colon and neural cells could also act as potential binding sites for HIV.

Following virus adsorption due to a high-affiniity, specific interaction between the viral gp 120 molecule and the target cell T4 (CD4) molecule, fusion of the viral and cellular membranes is believed to occur. This results in internalisation of viral core components.

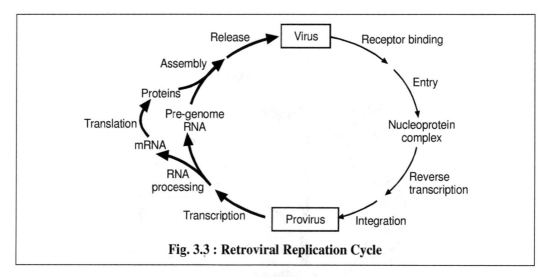

Fig. 3.3 : Retroviral Replication Cycle

Activation of the fusogenic potential of the retroviral envelop requires, complex conformational changes in the viral envelop proteins. This fusion is a pH-independent process.

After fusion, the viral uncoating leads to the partial or complete loss of envelope proteins and the virion membrane. This leads to the formation of a viral 'nucleoprotein complex' that is responsible to initiate the process of reverse transcription. The HIV-1 reverse transcriptase is a heterodimer consisting of three functional domains, namely

    (a) RNA-dependent DNA polymerase,

    (b) RNase H, and

    (c) Double stranded RNA-dependent RNase

Reverse transcription catalyzed by the viral RNA-dependent DNA polymerase generates a double stranded DNA copy of the viral RNA genome. This newly synthesized viral DNA through a series of events, is then integrated into the host cell genome by the help of the enzyme integrase. The viral DNA is transcribed to m-RNA and the viral genomic RNA using host cell RNA polymerases. Then, using the replication machinery of the host cell, other important enzymes and proteins, which are necessary for the formation, maturation and packaging of new virions are synthesized. The new virions are assembled at the cell surface where viral RNA, reverse transcriptase, structural and regulatory proteins and envelope proteins are assembled in a highly organised fashion. The budding virions are then cleaved off from a large peptide precursor by HIV-protease and infect other healthy cells completing the life cycle.

3.5 THERAPY OF HIV-INFECTION

Ideally, an anti-AIDS agent is expected to arrest the virulence and further infection of healthy cells without displaying toxicity towards normal cellular physiology. For example, the enzyme, reverse transcriptase does not exist in non-infected cells. Hence, reverse transcriptase inhibitors are the potential anti-AIDS agents. Drug related toxicities, emergence of drug-resistant viral strains and lack of total eradication of virus has necessitated the search for newer, potent and more effective anti-AIDS agents.

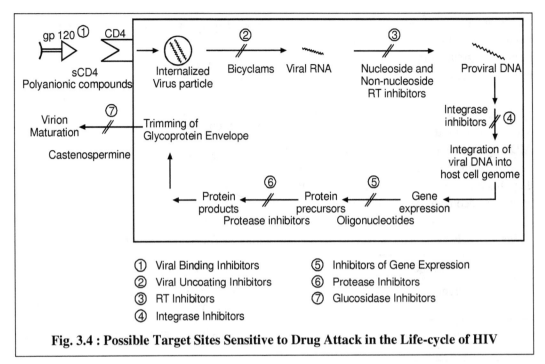

Fig. 3.4 : Possible Target Sites Sensitive to Drug Attack in the Life-cycle of HIV

A number of steps involved in HIV-replication cycle are potential targets for designing of anti-AIDS agent. Thus, an anti-HIV compound may exert its activity by inhibiting a variety of important steps in the viral life-cycle. It should be orally active, have a favourable pharmacokinetic profile and a wide safety margin. With AIDS added to the array of virus infections, the urgent need of an effective

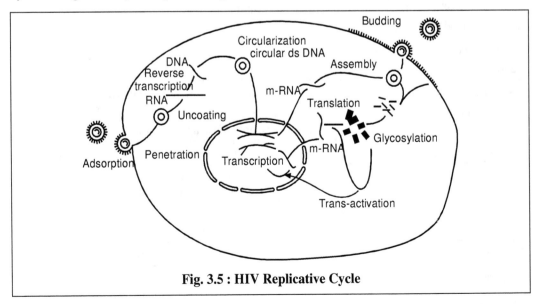

Fig. 3.5 : HIV Replicative Cycle

chemotherapy imparts an enormous momentum to the development of anti-AIDS agents. A great number of compounds have been developed.

Based on a more detailed knowledge of SAR studies of the different classes of anti-AIDS agents, combined with a better insight in their mechanism of action and the viral targets they interact with, the design of anti-AIDS drugs has become more rationally defined.

3.6 VIRAL BINDING (ADSORPTION) INHIBITORS

The HIV-1 binds to the target cell through a high affinity, specific interaction between the viral gp 120 molecule and the target cell T4 (CD4) molecule. Attempts were made to design compounds which can interfere with the CD4/gp 120 interaction to inhibit the transmission of HIV-1 from the infected cell to the healthy cell. Therapeutic agents could be designed to alter the lipid composition of the viral surface or target cell surface to reduce viral infectivity or cytopathic effects.

Table 3.1 : Selected Stages of HIV Replication that may be Targeted for Therapeutic Intervention

Stage	Possible intervention
Binding to target cell.	Antibodies to virus or cellular receptors genetically-engineered soluble CD4 proteins.
Fusion of virus with target cell	Antibodies or drugs that block the fusogenic domain of the virus.
Entry into target cell and uncoating of RNA	Drugs (by analogy with calmodulin antagonists)
Transcription of RNA to DNA by reverse transcriptase	Reverse transcriptase inhibitors (e.g. AZT and other dideoxy or didehydro-dideoxynucleoside congeners)
Degradation of RNA by RNase activity (encoded by viral pol gene)	RNase H inhibitors
Integration of DNA into host genome	Agents that inhibit pol-encoded integrase function.
Transcriptional efficiency / translation of viral RNA	Inhibitors of tat protein; mutant tat protein molecules; TAR inhibitors : "Pseudo" TAR molecules; rev inhibitors; anti-sense against tat or rev;
Ribosomal frameshifting	Ribosomal frameshift inhibitors castenospermine.
Viral component production	Myristylation, glycosylation inhibitors (e.g.castenospermine and inhibitors of trimming glucosidase) : Protease inhibitors (e.g. synthetic peptide analogues : aspartyl protease-specific inhibitors)
Packaging	Antisense construct against the gene.
Viral budding	Interferons or interferon inducers; antibodies to viral antigens which may be associated with viral release.

(a) Soluble CD4 (S CD4) derivatives :

It was reported that truncated soluble CD4 (SCD4) molecule is capable of inhibiting viral binding because of the presence of same binding sites as are present on the intact CD4 molecule. However, SCD4 failed to show clinical utility due to short half-life. Hence, hybrid molecules of SCD4 and IgG were prepared to increase the plasma half-life of SCD4 more than 100 fold.

(b) Polyanionic compounds :

The antiviral properties of polyanionic substances such as polyacrylic acid, polymethacrylic acid, polyvinyl sulphate, dextran sulphate, heparin are because of their ability to interfere with the virus adsorption process.

Dextran sulphate (DS) failed to reveal any anti-AIDS potential in clinical trials because of its metabolic pattern. Glycosidic bonds present in the DS skeleton undergo in-vivo hydrolysis. This problem of hydrolytic cleavage can be overcome by using a polymethylene hydrocarbon skeleton, while keeping the sulphate groups intact to provide the essential anionic moiety. This is the basis of development of a sulphated copolymer of acrylic acid and vinyl alcohol (PAVAS) and sulphated polymer of vinyl alcohol (PVAS). Similarly the sulphate groups present on carbohydrate skeleton in DS may undergo in vivo desulphation. This can be prevented by replacing the sulphate group by a metabolically stable anionic moiety like, sulphonic acid. This resulted in potent anti-HIV-1 aliphatic (PVS) and an aromatic (PSS) sulphonic acid polymer.

Out of various naphthalenesulphonic acid derivatives prepared, a bis derivative (1) and a tris derivative (2) showed pronounced antiviral activity in-vitro. Also the anionic compounds, Evans Blue and aurintricarboxylic acid (an anionic triphenylmethane dye) represent two interesting leads in the development of future anti-AIDS agents.

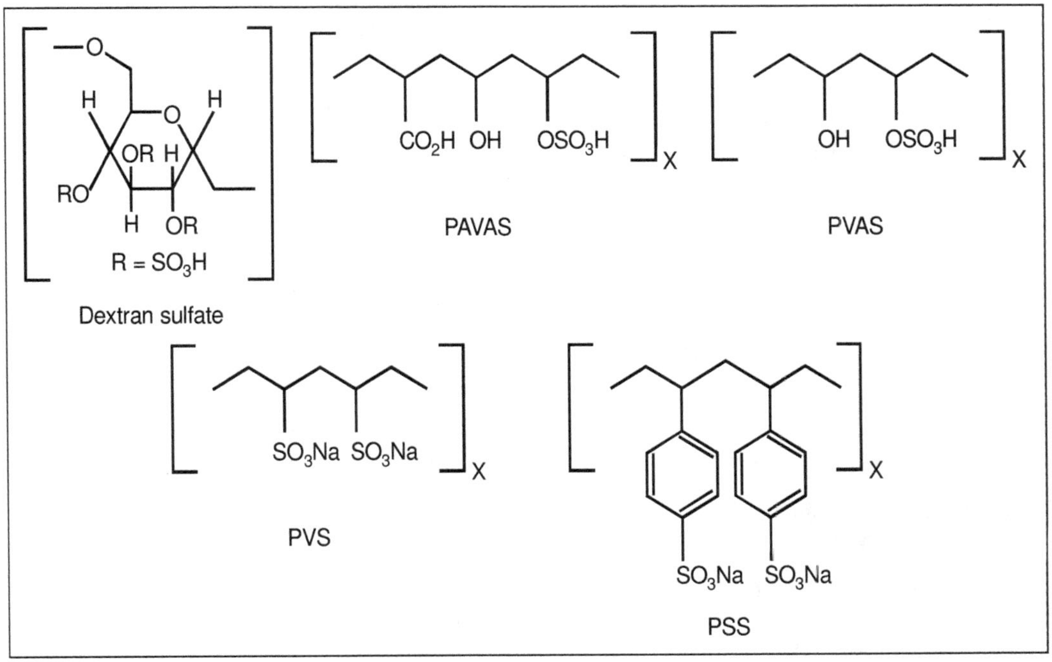

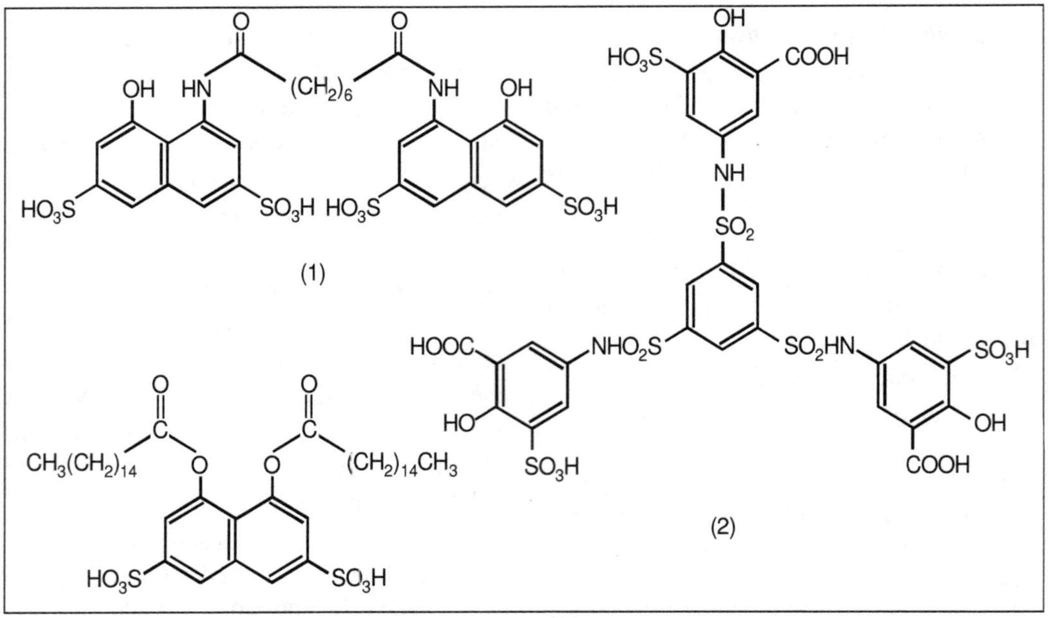

(1)

(2)

3.7 VIRAL UNCOATING INHIBITORS

After binding to a cell. HIV enters the target cell by a fusion process.

To date, bicyclams remain the only class of compounds having retroviral uncoating inhibitory activity. They showed a potent and selective inhibitory response and prevent the spread of infection to healthy cells. Other drugs could be developed to block this step just as calmodulin antagonists block the entry of Epstein-Barr virus into B cells.

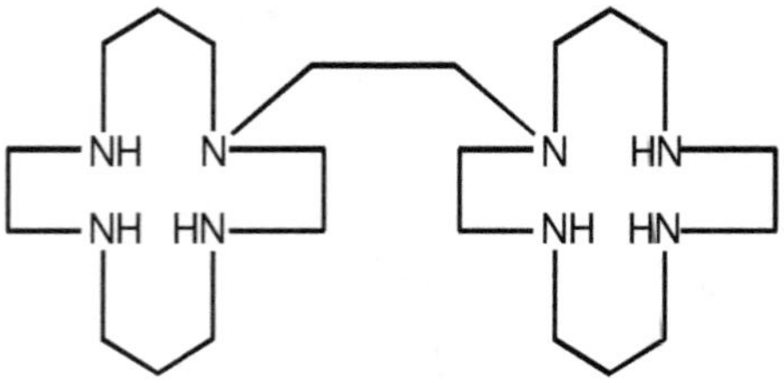

Bicyclam

3.8 REVERSE TRANSCRIPTASE INHIBITORS

Uncoated viral RNA is used as a template for the production of DNA by reverse transcriptase. Since HIV replication is the main factor in both the initiation and progression of AIDS, inhibition of reverse transcriptase is an attractive target for drug development. Suramin (a hexasulphonate naphthylurea derivative) a drug that has been used for many decades to treat African trypanosomiasis (sleeping sickness), was the first compound found effective in blocking reverse transcriptase activity of various animal retroviruses.

As its antiviral action is reversible, long-term administration of suramin may be necessary to achieve any clinical benefit. Upon prolonged treatment, suramin proved rather toxic, some of its less toxic derivatives may be more useful. Retroviral reverse transcriptase possesses an inherent RNase H activity that specifically degrades the RNA of the RNA-DNA hybrid. The C-terminal region of reverse transcription protein is a domain with RNase H activity. Theoretically, inhibition of this process would suppress viral replication. The reverse transcriptase of HIV has been purified and seems to exist as a p51 and p66 molecule.

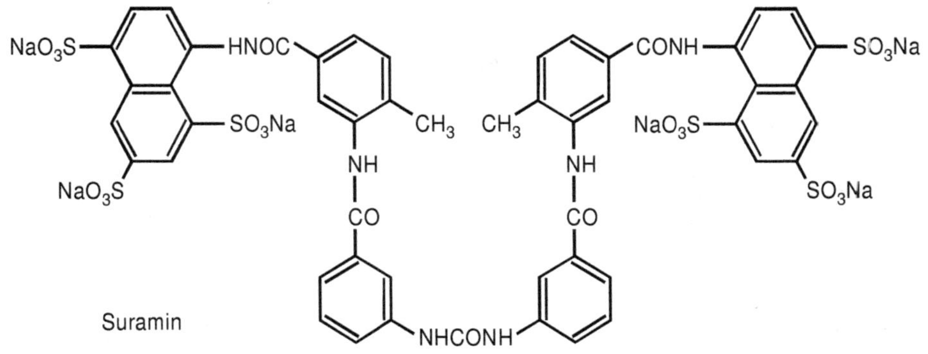

Suramin

(a) Nucleoside reverse transcriptase inhibitors :

The reverse transcription and other steps of the replicative cycle involve nucleic acids. Thus it is not unexpected that nucleoside derivatives may interfere with them producing a selective antiviral activity. The 2',3'-dideoxynucleosides and 3'-azido-3'-deoxythymidine are the most potent and selective anti-HIV examples from this series. 3'-dideoxynucleosides are successively phosphorylated in the cytoplasm of a target cell to yield 2',3'-dideoxynucleosides -5'-triphosphates, which become analogues of the 2'-deoxynucleoside-5'-triphosphates that are the natural substrates for cellular DNA polymerases and reverse transcriptase. Such analogues could compete with the binding of normal nucleotides to DNA polymerases (with high relative affinity for reverse transcriptase) or could be incorporated into DNA and bring about DNA chain termination because normal 5' → 3' phosphodiester linkages cannot be completed. Dideoxynucleotide analogues can serve as substrates for the HIV reverse transcriptase to elongate a DNA chain by one residue, after which the chain is terminated.

The AZT undergoes anabolic phosphorylation in human T-cells to a nucloside-5'-triphosphate which can compete with thymidine-5'-triphosphate (TTP) and serve as a chain-terminating inhibitor of HIV-reverse transcriptase. A form of partial pyrimidine depletion is likely to contribute to bone marrow suppression, a main side effect of AZT.

The discovery of 3-azido-3-deoxythymidine (AZT) as a reverse transcriptase inhibitor, vigorous efforts have been directed toward the development of nucleoside analogues. They act as RT inhibitors after undergoing in-vivo phosphorylation to generate the triphosphate derivative. This intracellular phosphorylation is important for drug activation and is achieved by cellular kinases. These triphosphate may inhibit the reverse transcriptase in competition with the triphosphates of natural nucleosides (i.e., dTTP, dCTP, dATP, dGTP). Since the 3-hydroxyl group is absent in the 2',3'-dideoxynucleosides which is responsive for the elongation of the DNA, this leads to the shut-off of viral DNA synthesis. Similar drugs belonging to 2',3'-deoxythymidine (ddT), deoxyinosin (ddI) and deoxycytidine (ddC) are undergoing clinical trials in patients with AIDS and AIDS related complexes (ARC). The key toxicity in case of ddC is peripheral neuropathy.

2', 3'-Dideoxynucleosides

Thymidine kinase catalyses the phosphorylation of AZT to its 5'-monophosphate derivative very efficiently. This conversion is not a rate-limiting step for AZT as it is for many 2', 3'-dideoxy nucleosides. The 5'-monophosphate then gets converted to diphosphate and triphosphate form.

A short-term (6 week) treatment with AZT led to clinical, virological and immunological improvement but the long-term use of AZT is associated with severe toxicity (anaemia, leukopenia due to bone marrow suppression) and decline in immune response. Immunologic deterioration may be due to (a) AZT-toxicity to homopoietic system, and (b) emergence of drug-resistant HIV-variants.

Structure activity relationship :

(1) It is now established that at the 3' position in the 2',3'-dideoxy skeleton, a substitution of azido, fluoro or hydrogen is allowed, only when coupled with an appropriate purine or pyrimidine base. The incorporation of 2', 3'-double bond is also permissible as it occurs in D4T.

(2) 2', 3'-dideoxynucleosides face stability problems when they are exposed to gastric acid through oral route. The substitution of electronegative atom at 2' or 3' position stabilizes the drug towards acidic pH.

(3) The anti-AIDS activity of AZT is also increased by incorporating the cyanide group at 3rd position.

(a) 2', 3' - dideoxy - β - D - glyceropent - 2 – enofuranozyl nucleosides

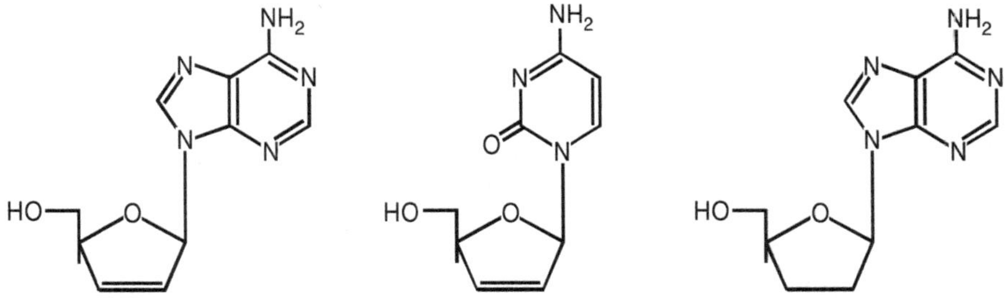

(b) Carbolic nucleosides :

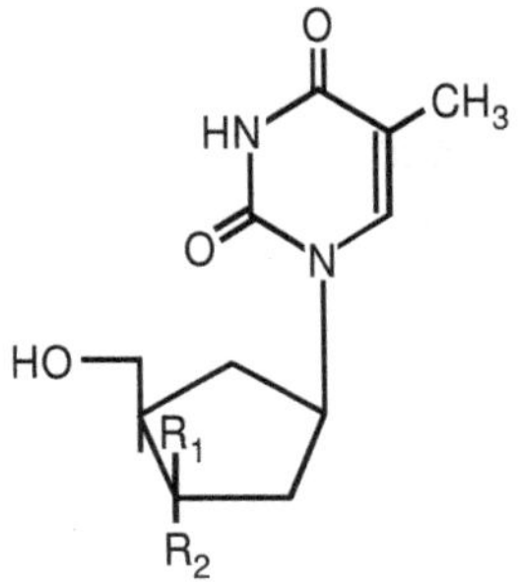

(1) $R_1 = -H; R_2 = N_3$
Carbocyclic - 3 - azido
2', 3'-dideoxythymidine

(2) R_1 epimer = N_3; $R_2 = -H$

(c) Acyclic nucleosides :

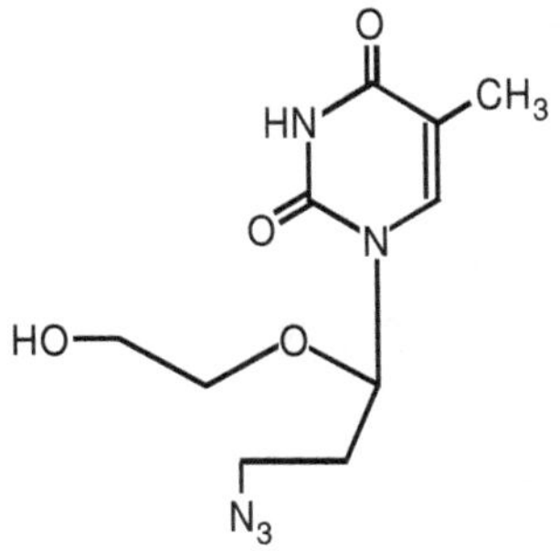

3-azido-2', 3'-dideoxycytozide (AZT analogue)

(d) Miscellaneous nucleosides :

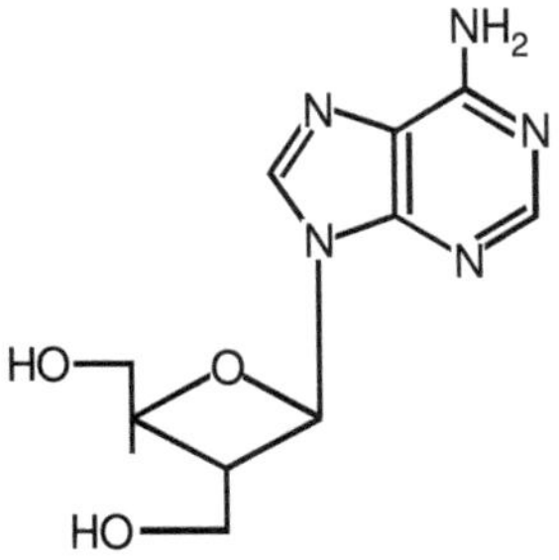

Oxetanosin from the
cultures of Bacillus
megatezium

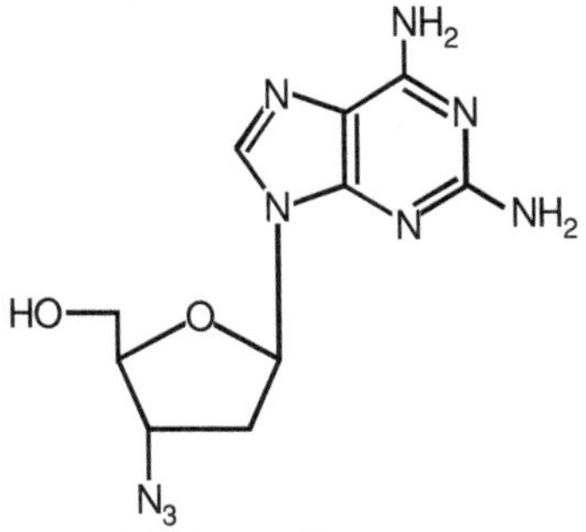

3'-azido-2', 3'-dideoxy
2, 6-diaminopurineriboside
(Az dd DAPR)

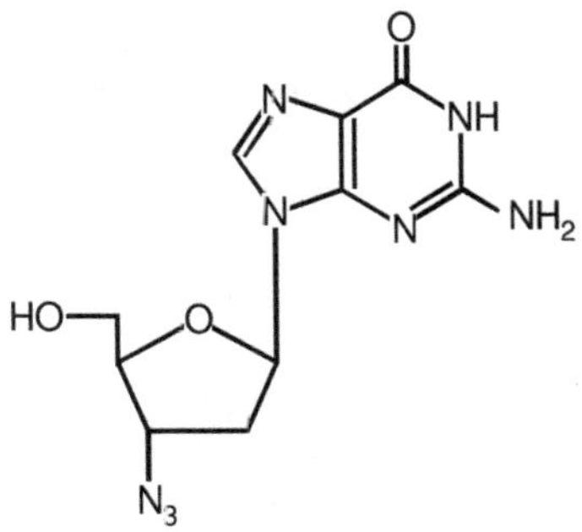

3'-azido-2', 3'-dideoxy
guanosine
(Az dd Guo)

(4) Other important categories from this class include,

    (a) 2', 3', -dideoxy-β-D-glyceropent-2-eno furanozyl nucleosides.

    (b) Carbonic nucleosides in which the furanose ring is replaced by a cyclopentane ring. They act as inhibitors of the kinases. Thus the formation of nucleotides from nucleosides and the incorporation of nucleotides into DNA can be prevented.

    (c) Acyclic nucleosides which are more stable toward gastric acid. Hence, they are orally effective.

    (d) Miscellaneous nucleosides from microbial sources.

The drug related toxicities have restricted the long-term use of nucleoside anti-AIDS agents. The side-effects observed with AZT treatment include, oedema, ulceration, nail pigmentation, macrocytic anaemia, leukopenia, myopathy and meningoencephalitis. Similarly, prolonged use of DDI leads to painful peripheral neuropathy, pancreatitis and hepatic failure. In the treatment with DDC, cardiomyopathy, pancreatitis and ulceration are reported to occur.

The emergence of drug resistant strains of HIV has also limited the clinical utility of nucleoside agents. Viral resistance develops due to multiple mutations in the viral genome and it results into reduced sensitivity towards the drugs. For example, mutations at amino acid residues 67, 70, 215 and 219 in the enzyme reverse transcriptase are implicated for AZT resistance. A single Leu to Val mutation at position 74 causes DDI resistance while a single Thr → Asp mutation at position 69 confers DDC resistance. Similarly, the phosphorylation reactions crucial to the activation of the nucleoside analogues are catalysed by host-cell kinases. If the relevant kinases are lacking in the host cell the retrovirus will appear resistant to the nucleoside analogues.

(b) Non-nucleoside reverse transcriptase inhibitors :

These agents have binding sites on reverse transcriptase which are distinct to that of nucleoside inhibitors. Sulphonic acid polymers display excellent inhibitory activity against both of the viral reverse transcriptase. These observations suggest the need of prodrug modification to mask the polarity of sulphonic acid groups to facilitate cellular penetration.

Non-nuceloside reverse transcriptase inhibitors

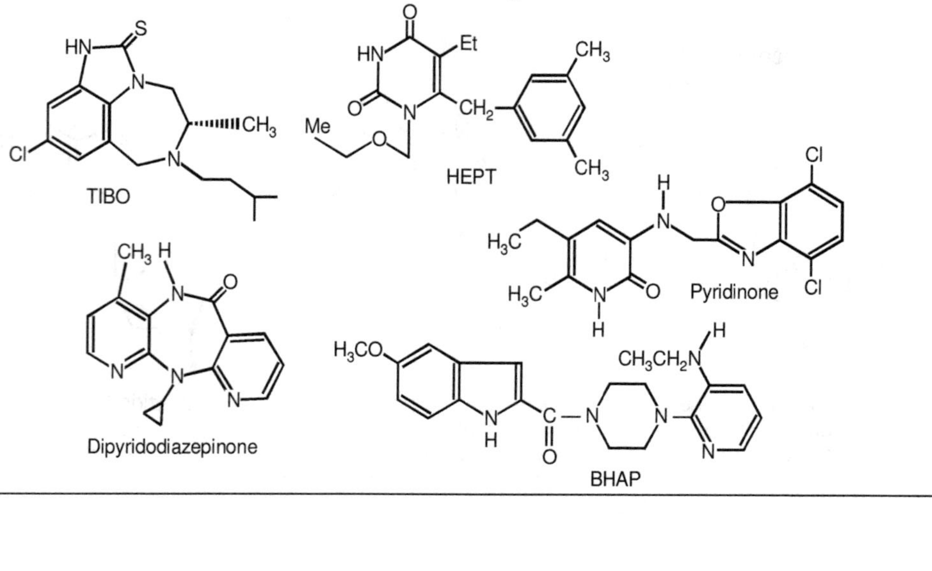

3.9 INTEGRASE INHIBITORS

The enzyme viral endonuclease (integrase) catalyses the incorporation of viral DNA into the host cell genome. Drugs that interfere with the structure and function of retroviral mRNA transcribed from integrated DNA in infected cells could be of therapeutic value in AIDS. One drug, ribaverin, acts as a guanosine analogue, that interferes with the 5'-capping of viral mRNA in other viral systems. A variety of compounds including DNA topoisomerase inhibitors, mono and bifunctional intercalators and antimalarials were evaluated for their integrase inhibitory activity. Out of them, doxorubicin, a potent topoisomerase inhibitor and anti-tumour agent was found to be a potent integrase inhibitor.

3.10 GENE EXPRESSION INHIBITORS

Once the viral DNA is incorporated into the host cell genome, the host genetic machinery will continue to produce viral gene products. The antisense oligonucleotides can effectively inhibit the gene expression. Since they contain a region complimentary to a segment of genome or mRNA, they interfere with gene expression.

Basically, this approach encompasses short sequences of DNA (sometimes chemically modified, to improve cell penetration and resistance to enzymatic degradation) whose base-pairs are complementary to a vital segment of the viral genome. In theory, such antisense oligodeoxy nucleotides could block expression of the viral genome through a kind of hybridization, arrest of translation or possibly interfere with the binding of a regular protein such as tat- III.

Antisense oligonucleotides have shown inhibitory activities against HIV-1 replication in chronically infected cells, syncytia (infected cells form a cluster with non-infected cells) and reverse transcriptase.

Bioisosteric replacement of phosphodiester linkages with sulphur and amino groups to produce phosphorothioates and phosphoramidates have been made to overcome the problem of exonuclease mediated hydrolytic cleavage of oligonucleotides.

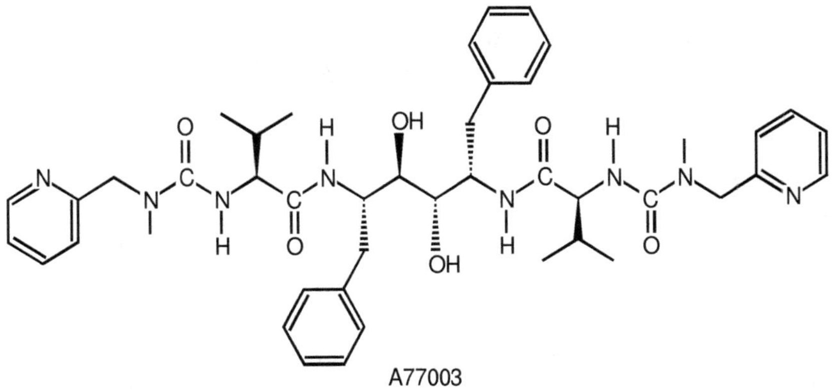

A77003

3.11 PROTEASE INHIBITORS

The final stages in the replicative cycle of HIV involve crucial secondary processing of certain viral proteins by a protease (a function of one of the pol gene products) and myristylating and glycosylating enzymes (provided by host) as a prelude to assembly of infectious virions.

Chemically, HIV protease is a homodimeric aspartyl protease which degrades large polypeptide precursors into smaller functional protein fragments required for the packaging and infectivity of budding virions. The active site of HIV-protease consists of a catalytic triad of Asp-Thr-Gly. Therefore, additional strategies for the treatment of AIDS might involve certain kinds of protease inhibitors or drugs that alter myristylation and glycosylation steps in the synthesis of viral components.

Beside the peptide based protease inhibitors (e.g. A 77003) attempts were made to synthesize non-peptide protease inhibitors (e.g. sulphonic acid azodyes).

The computer aided molecular modelling helped to develop the three dimensional structure of protease. It leads to identify haloperidol as a potent protease inhibitor but at toxic dose.

3.12 GLUCOSIDASE INHIBITORS

The enzyme. glucosidase participates in the final step in the HIV-life cycle to cleave off glucose units from the oligosaccharide chain. It catalyses the processing of the surface glycoproteins and thus helps to the maturation of infections viral progency. The glycosidase inhibitors include polyhydroxylated compounds such as castenospermine and N-butyldeoxy nojirimycin.

Finally, retroviruses are released by a process of vital budding, which may be inhibited by interferons.

Table 3.2 : Antiviral Drugs Found Active Against HIV

Suramin derivatives	Evans Blue
Aurintricarboxylic acid (ATA)	Ribavirin
Foscarnet (Phosphonoformate, PFA)	Inteferon
D-Penicillamine	HPA-23 (ammonium 21-tungsto-9-antimoniate)
Rifabutin (Ansamycin)	Amphotericin β methyl ester
Dithiocarb (Diethyldithiocarbamate sodium salt)	Glycyrrhizin
Heparin and dextran sulphate	Avarol (a sesquiterpenoid hydroquinone)
AL-721 (lipid mixture composed of glycerides, phosphatidylcholine and phosphatidylethanolamine in a 7:2:1 ratio)	Peptide T (octapeptide : (Ala-Ser-Thr-Thr-Thr Asn-Tyr-Thr)
2-Deoxy-D-glucose and other glycosylation inhibitors (i.e. castenospermine)	Oligodeoxynucleotide phosphorothioates
Azidothymidine	2', 3'-Dideoxycytidine
2', 3'- Dideoxycytidine	2', 3' -Dideoxy-5- fluorocytidine
3'-Fluoro-2', 3'-dideoxycytidine	2', 3'-Dideoxythymidine
2', 3'-Dideoxythymidinene	3'-Fluoro-2', 3'-dideoxythymidine
3'-Fluoro-2', 3'-dideoxyuridine	2', 3' -Dideoxyadenosine
2', 3' -Dideoxyinosine	3'-Azido-2', 3'-dideoxyadenosine
2'- 3'-Dideoxy-2, 6-diaminopurineriboside	2', 3'-Dideoxyguanosine
3'-Azido-2', 3'-dideoxyguanosine	3'-Azido-2' 3'-dideoxy-2, 6-diaminopurineriboside

3.13 ANTI-AIDS VACCINE

In order to booster immunity in immuno-deficient AIDS patients, efforts are being made to develop a safe and efficacious vaccine against AIDS.

The development of an effective vaccine against HIV-1 may require immunisation protocols that elicit cytolytic-T-lymphocytes (CTL) in addition to neutralising antibodies. The vaccination has shown to elicit the functionally heterogeneous $CD4^+$-T-cell response that include clone with antigen specific major histocompatibility complex (MHC) restricted cytolytic activity. These clones are capable of lysing target cell expressing the target HIV-1 envelope gene and thus be active against HIV-1 infected cells in-vivo.

Recent studies shows that HIV vaccine consisting of HIV-proteins may reduce the loss of $CD4^+$ cell and stabilizes the clinical state and improves the immune response against HIV following the exposure to viral antigens. Because of the highly divergent nature of human HIV, the biggest concern at the present time is whether or not a single vaccine will be effective in neutralising different HIV-isolates.

Combination Therapy of Aids :

The therapy of AIDS is a continuous long-term process. This invites the problem of drug related toxicities and emergence of viral resistance which have limited the clinical utility of most of anti-AIDS agents. Convergent combination therapy using a three-drug regimen comprising of AZT, DDI and pyridinone has shown success in cell cultures by completely attenuating HIV-1 replication.

Combination therapy may also result in :

(a) Enhanced activity, especially in compounds that interact at different steps of HIV-1life cycle. Similarly, synergistic action may also be seen in those compounds that interact with the same target enzyme (i.e. reverse transcriptase) but differ in pharmaco-kinetic behaviour.

(b) Diminished toxicity because the combination therapy allows reduction in drug dose, provided that agents having different toxicological behaviour are combined.

(c) Decreased risk of emergence of drug-resistant variants.

Various combinations of anti-HIV agents were developed which include

retrovir + acyclovir (Mitsuya and Broder, 1987)

retrovir + dextran sulphate (Ueno and Kuno, 1987)

retrovir + poly (I) Poly (C_{12}, u) (Mitcell, 1987)

retrovir + human interferon α 2A (Hartshorn, 1987)

foscarnet + human interferon α 2A (Hartshorn, 1986)

A combination of antiretroviral therapy coupled with bone marrow transplantation, lymphocyte replacement or stimulation of bone marrow precursor cells by colony-stimulating factors might be successful in certain AIDS patients.

3.14 FUTURE DEVELOPMENTS IN ANTI-AIDS THERAPY

(a) New leads in anti-AIDS drug design include inhibitors of Tat, a regulatory protein needed for HIV-1 replication and tumour necrosis factor (TNF) which might show an up-regulating effect on HIV-replication.

(b) The presence of cellular glutathione and other thiols like cystine is essential for normal T-cell physiology. The depletion of cellular thiols is observed in AIDS patient. N-acetylcysteine (NAC) elevates the cellular concentration of cystine and prevents HIV-1 activation in latently infected cells. It thus helps to restore the normal T-cell functions in AIDS patients.

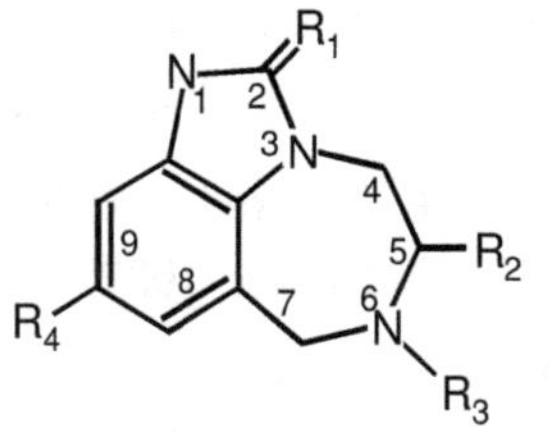

Tetrahydro-imidazo [4, 5, 1-jk] [1,4] – benzodiazepin – 2 (1H) – one and – thione (TIBO) derivatives.

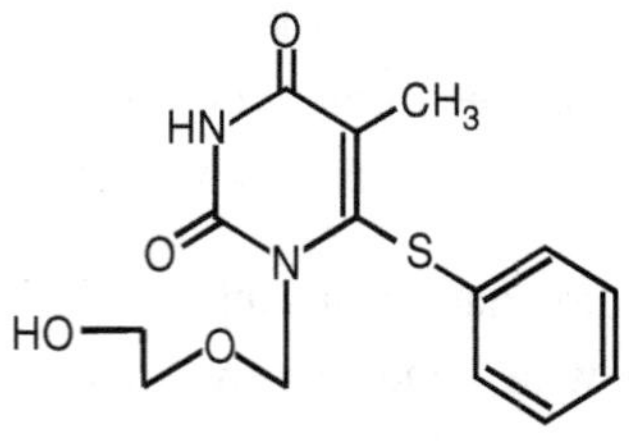

1-[(2-hydroxyethoxy) methyl]-6-phenylthiothymine

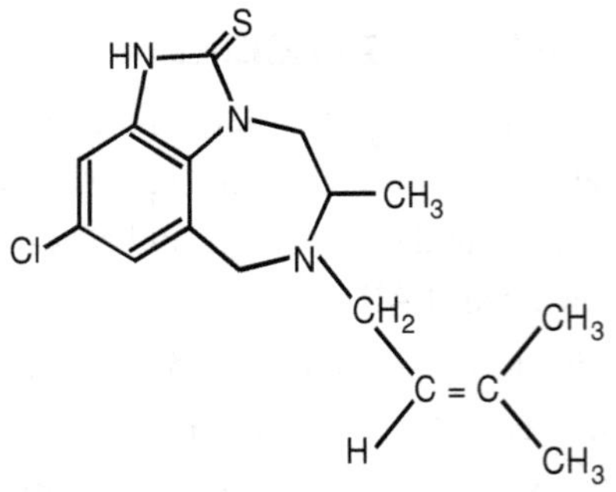

Tetrahydroimidazo-benzodiazepinone and thione (TIBO) derivatives

3.15 IMMUNOPATHOGENESIS OF AIDS VIRUS

Although all compartments of the immune system are at least indirectly affected in patients with AIDS, impaired T-cell mediated responses appear to have the greatest clinical consequences. High-level HIV envelope expression on infected cells results in cell fusion with neighbouring uninfected T4 cells by direct binding of a gp 120-CD4 complex, Such syncytia (cell to cell fusion) can be comprised of literally hundreds of infected and uninfected cells. The progressive recruitment of T4 cells to form syncytia with HIV-1 expressing cells in blood, lymph node and other tissues, could lead to substantial T4 cell loss. In addition, it was shown that cell free gp 120 can adsorb to $T4^+$ cells and there serve as an effective antigen for mediating antibody-dependent cell mediated cytotoxicity. Sub-populations of $CD8^+$ cells, particularly the $CD8^+$ Leu 7^+ and the $CD8^+$ Leu 8^- subsets have been reported to be substantially increased in HIV seropositive patients. The expansion of $CD8^+$ population may represent the generation of cytotoxic reactions. Thus, autoimmune recognition and destruction of host cells represent the irreversible breakdown of immune defence mechanisms.

Table 3.3 : Immunologic Abnormalities in AIDS

(a) T-cells

CD4$^+$ cell depletion.

Decreased proliferation to soluble antigen.

Decreased helper response for PWM induced immunoglobuline synthesis.

Impaired delayed type hypersensitivity.

Decreased γ-interferon production in response to antigens.

Decreased proliferation to T-cell mutagens, alloantigens and anti-CD 3.

Decreased AMLR response.

Decreased cell mediated cytotoxicity to virally infected cells.

Decreased IL-2 production.

Lymphopenia.

(b) B-cells

Polyclonal activation with hypergammaglobulinemia (IgG, IgA, and IgD), increased spontaneous plaque forming cells, and proliferation.

Decreased humoral response to immunization.

Circulating autoantibodies

(c) Macrophage/monocytes

Decreased chemotaxis

(d) Natural killer cells

Decreased cytotoxicity

(e) Other humoral responses

Increased acid labile γ-interferon production.

Increased soluble immune complexes

Decreased α_1-thymosin.

A small percentage of cells appears to be actively producing virions. Significant cell losses could occur over the time due to viral persistence, reactivation of latent virus and progressive dissemination to uninfected cells. A likely prerequisite for lymphodepletion, however would be concomitant failure of hematopoietic organs to regenerate the depleted lymphocytes.

The HIV can remain silent over a long period of time. Under favourable conditions, viral replication occurs by increased rate of synthesis of viral RNA and other components. Since AIDS-virus affects the functioning of immune system, the symptoms associated are mainly due to the failure of immune responses rather than due to viral cytotoxicity. Later in the course of their disease, AIDS patients get depleted of all lymphoid cells, including the CD8$^+$ population. This may be caused by severe bone marrow depression. As a result, AIDS patients are particularly prone to develop opportunistic infections and neoplasms.

Pneumocystis carinii pneumonia is the predominant opportunistic infection and the immediate cause of death in the majority of AIDS patients. The aggressive form of Kaposi's sarcoma may be due in part to a T-cell defect.

The hallmark of HIV-1 infection in infected persons is a progressive depletion of T4 (CD4) bearing lymphocytes, eventually leading to immunodeficiency and secondary infections and neoplasms.

An increased susceptibility to certain bacterial pathogen is seen in AIDS patients, particularly within the pediatric population. Many of these bacterial infections affect the respiratory and gastrointestinal systems. In addition to the immunologic abnormalities induced by HIV itself, other organisms concomitantly infecting these patients may depress immune function. This may contribute to the morbidity and mortality of patients, especially at the later stages of their illness. As a result, in patients coinfected with these organisms, HIV viremia may be amplified and depletion of CD4$^+$ cells may be accelerated.

The general course of HIV-1 disease is characterized by a protracted, progressive T4 cell loss with an estimated mean period from time of infection to the development of clinical AIDS to be more than 5 years. Depending upon the type of infection and the organ most affected, different patients may complain about different symptoms. The prominent organs affected involve.

(i) Gastrointestinal tract :

It is most susceptible for the attack of organisms like mycobacteria, salmonellae, cryptosporidium, adenoviruses and isospora. Prominent symptoms include mouth thrush, dysphagia, abdominal pain, diarrohoea, gingivitis, herpetic stomatitis, and hairy leukoplakia. Chronic colitis is seen mainly in male homosexuals.

(ii) Cutaneous signs :

These include candidiasis, impetigo, herpes lesions, prurigo, xeroderma, folliculitis, seborrhoeic dermatitis and mulluscum contagiosum.

(iii) Respiratory system :

This system becomes vulnerable for the attact of P carinii, M. tuberculosis and M. avium. Major symptoms include fever, dyspnoea. dry cough and pneumonis.

(iv) Central nervous system :

Dementia and impairment of CNS functions are reported to occur because of the ability of HIV virus to enter into CNS. Besides this toxoplasmosis, cryptococcosis and lymphomas of CNS are also reported to occur.

Infection with the Human Immunodeficiency Virus (HIV) and AIDS are urgent problems worldwide with broad social, cultural, economic, political, ethical and legal implications. Sexual intercourse is the predominant mode of transmission of HIV-infection. Atleast one-fifth of all people with AIDS are in their twenties who are most likely to have become infected with HIV as adolescents. Because at present, there is no cure for HIV-infection, primary prevention through education must be a major aim of any public health programme.

Rapid changes in society - urbanization, industrialization, increased travel, the spread of non-traditional values through the mass media, the decline of the influence and support of the joint family are some of the major contributory factors in the spread of HIV or sexually transmitted infection. Knowledge about transmission and means of prevention will help to develop the skills and resources to avoid it. Such education needs to be given to young people before they have their first sexual experience, so that they can protect themselves from infection.

Treatment of HIV infection consists of four important phases. The first phase deals with control of infections and malignancies associated with the patient. The treatment is infection specific. For example, in AIDS patients with Pneumocystis carinii infection, cotrimoxazole is given orally. Pentamidine may also be used either i.m. or i.v. in the does of 4 mg/kg body weight per day. Toxoplasma gondii is a protozoal organism that affects mainly heart, lung, liver, spleen and CNS. Drugs of choice include pyrimethamine (25 mg/day) and sulfadiazine (2 g perday) orally. Folinic acid may be used in the dose of 10 mg per day to prevent hematologic abnormalities. Besides this, Mycobacterium avium intracellulare is found in 50% patients with AIDS. It affects mainly GIT, lung and other tissues. To correct most of these infections, interleukin-2 is commonly used agent. It is a potent lymphokine responsible for the activation of various components of immune system.

The second phase of the treatment consists of employing general measures to cool down imaginary anxiety and fear experienced by the patients. The infected person must be reassured that he can resume a normal life if proper precautions and treatment are taken. The high risk factors must be identified and eliminated. This is to be supported by health education.

The third phase of the treatment deals with measures to improve the functioning of immune system. A large number of antiviral agents (e.g., α-interferon, ribavirin, suramin, etc.). This can be supplemented by administration of immunoenhancers like interleukin-2, thymic factor, leucocyte transfusion or by the transplantation of bone-marrow.

The last phase of the treatment consists of administration of anti-HIV agent. Zidovudine (azidothymidine) is the only drug available. It is an orally effective antiviral agent beneficial in the treatment of AIDS and AIDS related syndromes. Adverse effects include headache, leukopenia and macrocytic anaemia.

Efforts are being continued to develop a vaccine, effective in the treatment of AIDS. However, prospects for such a vaccine in the near future are unfortunately dim.

As the problem of AIDS affects more and more countries and greater number of people, provision for information and education has become a major weapon against the disease.

Table 3.4 : Infections in Patients with AIDS

Micro-organism	Location	Clinical manifestations
Protozoa		
Pneumocystis carinii	Lung, spleen, lymph node, eye, disseminated	Pneumonia, splenomegaly, lymphadenopathy, choroiditis
Toxoplasma gondii	Brain, eye, heart, adrenal, disseminated	Meningoencephalitis, chorioretinitis, myocarditis
Cryptosporidium	Intestine, gallbladder, bile ducts, respiratory epithelium	Diarrhoea, cholecystitis, sclerosing cholangitis
Entamoeba histolytica	Intestine	Diarrhoea
Giardia lamblia	Intestine	Diarrhoea
Acanthamoeba	Brain	Meningoencephalitis
Fungi		
Candida	Oropharynx, oesophagus, trachea, bronchi, lung	Thrush, oesophagitis, tracheobronchitis, pneumonia
Cryptococcus neoformans	Brain, lung, lymph node, bone marrow, skin, blood, urine, disseminated	Meningoencephalitis, pnenumonia, lymphadenopathy, fungemia
Histoplasma capsulatum	Lung, liver, spleen, lymph node, adrenal, bone-marrow, eye, skin, blood, urine, disseminated	Pneumonia, hepatosplenomegaly, lymphadenopathy, chorioretinitis, pancytopenia, fungemia

Coccidioides immitis	Lung, brain, lymph node, liver, spleen, skin, blood, urine, disseminated	Pneumonia, meningoencephalitis, hepatosplenomegaly, lymphadenopathy, fungemia
Bacteria		
Mycobacterium avivum	Lymph node, liver, spleen, bone marrow, intestine, lung, skin, adrenal, blood, urine, disseminated	Lymphadenopathy, hepatosplenomegaly, pancytopenia, pneumonia, diarrhoea, mycobacteremia
Nocardia spp.	Lung, pleura, pericardium, soft tissues, bone, brain, lymph node, spleen, kidney, disseminated	Pneumonia, empyema, pericarditis, retropharyngeal or subcutaneous abscess, draining sinus tract, encephalitis
Salmonella spp.	Intestine, blood	Diarrhoea, bacteremia
Shigella spp.	Intestine, blood	Diarrhoea, bacteremia
Listeria monocytogenes	Meninges, blood	Meningitis, bacteremia
Treponema pallidum	Lymph node, testis, brain	Lymphadenopathy, orchitis, neurosyphilis
Viruses		
Cytomegalovirus	Lung, adrenal, eye, brain, peripheral nerve, intestine, liver, seminal vesicle, blood, disseminated	Pneumonia, chorioretinitis, meningoencephalitis, rediculitis with polyneuropathy, diarrhoea, viremia
Herpes simplex	Mucocutaneous, oesophagus, bronchus, lung, disseminated	Ulcerative mucocutaneous lesions, oesophagitis, bronchitis, pneumonia, encephalitis
Herpers zoster	Mucocutaneous, disseminated	Multiple dermatomal zoster, Herpes zoster ophthalmicus
Hepatitis-B	Liver	Antigenemia
Polyomavirus	Brain	Progressive multifocal leukoencephalopathy
Poxvirus	Mucocutaneous	Molluscum contagiosum
Papillomavirus	Mucocutaneous	Condyloma accuminatum, oral hairy leukoplakia
Helminths		
Strongyloides stercoralis	Intestine, lung, brain, disseminated	Diarrhoea, pneumonia, meningoencephalitis, recurrent poly microbial bacteremias

3.16 PREVENTIVE MEASURES OF AIDS

Priority must be given to preventive measures and that sufficient research facilities must be made available. HIV has been isolated from cervical secretion, vaginal secretion and semen. The prevalence of HIV among homosexual men is high. Men and women who are at risk for HIV and who remain sexually active should avoid all contact with semen, genital secretions, and blood. Semen does harbour HIV and oral-genital contact may therefore carry a risk for infection with HIV. Since, saliva has been reported to harbour HIV, deep kissing must be discouraged.

The number of sexual partners, sexual contact with female prostitutes and the presence of other sexually transmitted diseases (STD) have been associated with increased risk of HIV infection.

(a) Barrier contraceptive :

Condom use has been shown to decrease the risk of transmission of organisms that may be present in semen, including chlamydia trachomatis, hepatitis-B virus, mycoplasma bominis, Neisseria gonorrhoea, Trichomonas vaginalis, and Ureaplasma urealyticum. A condom may be helpful in prevention of these STDs if lesions are on the penis or female genitalia or if an infectious discharge is present. HIV may be derived from blood lymphocytes during menstruation or sequestered in inflammatory lesions. Latex condoms do not allow the leakage of HIV. They must be used to avoid all contacts with semen, pre-ejaculated fluid, vaginal and cervical secretions, any genital or oral lesions and genital tract in general.

To be effective, condoms must be used routinely and correctly and must remain intact.

(b) Spermicides :

Spermicides provide a chemical barrier for prevention of STDs. Although spermicides are generally not irritating to the urethral mucosa or vagina, allergic reactions and irritation have been described.

Nonoxynol-9 can inhibit HIV replication and kill lymphocytes. Spermicides may cause deterioration of latex and therefore potentially increases the risk of breakage of latex condoms.

The ever increasing spread of HIV-infection and the corresponding exponential increase in AIDS probably represents the greatest future threat to the health of the society. Since, the risk of HIV infection is greater in sexual activities, the informative and educational campaigns are important to induce a wide population to change their sexual behaviour. For the purpose of planning the health services more efficiently, blood samples of suspected persons, should be checked at regular intervals (e.g. every 6 months) for HIV-antibodies.

In most of the cases, the parents often refuse to take back AIDS infected child to home. Such babies are born and die in hospitals after intensive treatment and care. Similarly, the HIV-infected person is also not accepted by the society. He suffers from 'rejection syndrome' during his remaining life span. Though a number of anti-AIDS drugs are now available, HIV-infected person needs sympathy and love. Trained personnel are also required even for outside of hospital, due to the possibly severe changes in the neurological and mental condition of the patient.

4

MICROBIAL BIOCONVERSIONS IN STEROIDS

4.1 INTRODUCTION

Micro-organisms employ both constitutive and inducible enzymes to degrade and synthesize a variety of chemical compounds, not only for their viability and reproduction, but also for their metabolism. A metabolic intermediate or product, found in most of the living systems, essential for growth and life and biosynthesised by a limited number of biochemical pathways is known as general metabolite. While a metabolic intermediate or product found as a differentiation product in restricted taxonomic groups, not essential for growth and life of producing organism and biosynthesised from one or more general metabolites by a variety of pathways is known as a secondary metabolite. Most of the secondary metabolites are produced by bacteria, fungi and plants. Strange natural products were derived from primary intermediates of normal metabolism.

Metabolic products which can not be further degraded may usually be isolated from fermentation medium. Such chemical reactions mediated by micro-organisms or their enzyme preparations are called as biotransformations. They are carried out either with pure cultures of micro-organisms, with plant cultures or with purified enzymes. Microbial enzymes cover nearly all types of chemical reactions.

4.2 CHARACTERISTICS OF BIOTRANSFORMATIONS

Biotransformations have following characteristics common to all enzyme catalysed reactions :

(a) Regiospecificity :

The substrate molecule is usually attacked at the same site, even if several groups of equivalent or similar reactivity are present. For example in the second step of commercially synthesized ascorbic acid, D-sorbitol is converted to L-sorbose by highly selective dehydrogenation with Acetobacter soboxydans. Among the six hydroxyl groups of D-sorbitol, microbial oxidation takes place exclusively at position 2, producing L-sorbose as only product in higher yields.

(b) Reaction specificity :

The catalytic activity is usually restricted to a single reaction type. It means that side reactions are not expected as long as one enzyme is involved in particular biotransformation.

(c) Stereospecificity :

Since the reactive centre of an enzyme provides an asymmetrical environment, it can easily make differentiation between enantiomers of a racemic mixture. Therefore only one or at the most preferentially one of the enantiomers is attacked. Similarly, if an enzyme reaction produces a new asymmetric centre, usually only one of the possible enantiomers is formed resulting into optically pure compound. In the case of a drug containing one chiral centre, administration of a racemic form allows delivery of 50% less active compound.

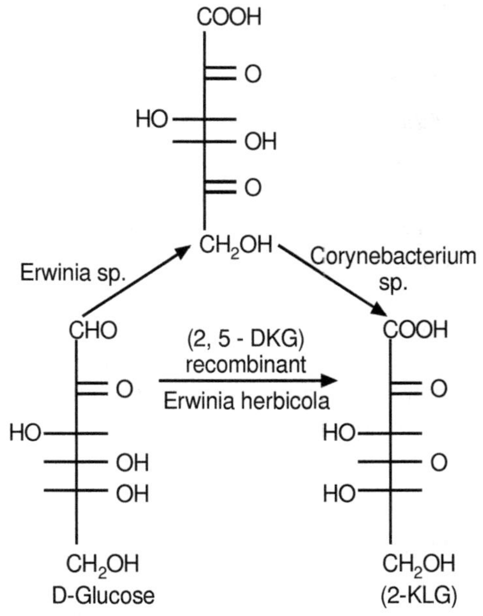

Most pharmaceutical companies started to develop a drug into a single enantiomeric form. Since, pure chemical reactions fail to achieve this goal, biotechnology has been routinely utilised in many of the chiral synthesis. For example, naproxen and ibuprofen have been resolved by enzymatic approach. Similarly, in the synthesis of vitamin C, a number of bacterial species from Coryneform group have been used to carry out microbial conversion of 2,5 - diketo -D-gluconic acid (2,5-DKG) into 2-keto- L-gluconic acid (2-KLG), a key intermediate in vitamin C synthesis.

Relatively mild operational conditions needed for microbial bioconversions hindered the practical applicability of microbial enzymes in chirotechnology. Similarly, the biocatalysts selected, are prone to have low stability. In such cases the presence of substantial amount of organic solvent in the reaction medium may help to optimise enzyme properties to get enhanced stability, altered substrate and enantiomeric specificities and their ability to catalyse unusual reactions. In the selection of a suitable solvent, certain properties like solvent density, viscosity, surface tension, flammability, cost and toxicity need to be taken into consideration.

(d) Mild reaction conditions :

Activation energy of chemical reaction is distinctly lowered by interaction of substrate and enzyme, thus biotransformation takes place under mild conditions such as pH near neutrality, room temperature and at normal pressure. Therefore, even a labile compound may be converted using low energy consumption without undesired decomposition or isomerisation.

(e) Functionalization at non-activated carbon :

Microbial biotransformations can selectively introduce functional groups at certain non-activated positions in a molecule, which can not be attracted by chemical reagents. For example, cortisone acetate was initially prepared in very low yields from deoxy cholic acid by a chemical synthesis requiring 31 steps. About nine steps were necessary to convert hydroxy group at C_{12} to keto group at C_{11}. Several years later, much shorter pathways were made available by direct microbial C_{11}-hydroxylation of precursors readily available by chemical degradation of inexpensive diosgenin or stigmasterol.

4.3 ELIMINATION OF SIDE REACTIONS

In biotransformations, side-reactions are likely to occur if the substrate or its product is attacked by undesired enzymes present in the cell. To simplify the isolation of main product from the fermentor, suppression of such side-reactions is necessary. In order to eliminate side-reactions selectively, one has to provide conditions suppressing the activities of undesired enzymes, while maintaining the desired activity in the biotransformation. The selective inactivation of enzymes which are responsible for side reactions may thus be achieved by physical (heat) and/or chemical treatments of biomass (pH shift with acid or alkaline solution) with detergents or organic solvents.

4.4 PRODUCT ISOLATION

The biotransformation products are low or medium molecular weight compounds. They are dissolved or suspended in fermentation medium and can be isolated from whole broth or, if preferable, from supernatant after removal of biomass by filtration or centrifugation. Lipophilic products are usually separated by extraction with organic solvents and concentrated by solvent removal in vacuum evaporator.

4.5 MICROBIAL BIOCONVERSIONS

Micro-organisms can be used to catalyse chemical reactions which otherwise are very difficult to occur. For example, 11-hydroxylation in steroids. Microbial enzymes are highly versatile in nature. Micro-organisms are more adoptogenic than higher cells. They immediately decompose or metabolise the substrate. In addition, they can develop new enzymes for metabolism or decomposition of any chemical which is first time coming into contact with micro-organisms. Enzymes are available for catalyzing any type of chemical modifications in the structure. The success depends on how skillfully one select proper micro-organism for particular conversion.

4.6 POTENTIAL USES OF MICROBIAL BIOCONVERSIONS

Current fields of use of micro-organisms are limited to those in agriculture, chemical industries and pharmaceuticals. The biotransformations may be used for the degradation of toxic pollutants. Mixed cultures of micro-organisms with unexpected metabolic activities may be further endowed with additional capabilities through genetic engineering, to clean up the toxic wastes such as polychlorinated biphenyls, chlorinated phenols and chlorinated benzenes. For this, mixed cultures are often efficient. Recent application of extracellular microbial lipases in hydrolysis of racemic ester to yield optically pure enantiomers, provided several industrial processes for manufacture of chiral synthones. Since, the desired therapeutic activity resides mainly in one of the enantiomer, the presence of another enantiomer in the drug invites the occurrence of unwanted side-effects. For example, in captopril, the S-form is 100 times active than R-enantiomer.

4.7 COMMERCIAL APPLICATIONS FOR MICROBIAL BIOCONVERSION

Microbial bioconversions are routinely used in commercial production of a variety of drugs. Important examples include,

(a) Vitamins :

Vitamin B_{12} can be obtained by combination of cobalamin with cobalt salt. The reaction is catalysed by Streptomyces olivaceous, Streptomyces gresious, Bacillus megaterium, Pseudomonas denitrificans or Propionibacterium shermanii. Merck, USA produced higest yields of vitamin B_{12} using cheapest source of energy viz. Beet molasses using Pseudomonas denitrificans.

Similarly, Eremothecium ashbyii, Ashbya gossypii, Clostridium species or Candida species may be used in the production of riboflavin.

In the production of vitamin C, the conversion of D-sorbitol to L-sorbose is catalysed by Acetobacter suboxydense.

(b) Steroids :

The C-17 side-chain cleavage can be done properly but in poor yields by any chemical reaction. however micro-organisms cleave this side-chain with high efficiency.

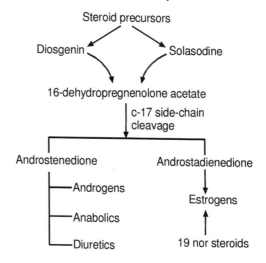

(c)

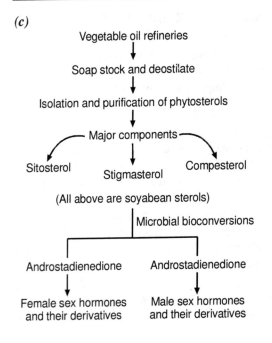

(d) Citric acid can be produced by microbial bioconversions using Aspergillus niger.

(e) Other specialised synthesis involving microbial introduction of 16 α-hydroxyl group into 18-hydroxy cortisone and 18-hydroxyl group for preparation of aldosterone remain useful biotechnological application though on a limited scale. Similarly, special synthetic use of micro-organisms lies in preparation of isotopically labelled steroids for other metabolic studies.

The world steroid drug industry, till was based mainly on Mexican diosgenin extracted from tubers of wild Dioscorea species. Other precursors include stigmasterol, cholesterol, sitosterol and hecogenin.

Steroid history dates back to 1773 with the isolation of cholesterol from gall stones. There was a long dormant period before the interest in cholesterol was revived in 1903 by the study of testicular, ovarian, bile and adrenal extracts, and the urine of a pregnant mare. At the same time, chemists were determining structures of cholesterol, bile acids and hormones. During 1929 to 1935 most of the initial difficulties were overcome and it was in this period that the isolation, characterisation and structure determination of estrone, progesterone and testosterone were accomplished, structures of cholesterol and bile acids were also determined.

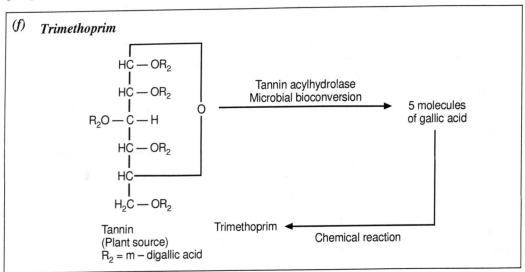

Inspite of large scale production, cost of synthetic hormones due to multiple chemical steps involved was more that $ 100,000 per kg. The cost of progesterone obtained even from plant sterol (stigmasterol) was around $ 80,000. Further search proved fruitful in 1939, when Russel Marker discovered that the tubers of a wild Mexican plant Dioscorea mexicana was a good source of diosgenin. Progesterone from diosgenin brings the price down to less $ 2,000 per kg. Diosgenin does not contain any keto or hydroxyl group at position 11 or 12 and could not, therefore, enter the synthesis of cortisone. Thus its use was limited to conversion of sex hormones alone. This led to hecogenin which has oxygen at 12th position. An outstanding advance in the steroid field came in 1949, when it was discovered by Peterson of Upjohn company that 'enzymes could selectively hydroxylate C-11 carbon atom of steroid molecule with ease'. Upjohn later developed an efficient route to progesterone from stigmasterol which brought down the price of progesterone to less than $ 200 per kg-within the reach of common man. The Merck deoxycholic acid process to cortisone in 37 steps was greatly simplified to 11 steps including microbial 11α-hydroxylation step by Upjohn. Another significant move was made in 1952 with the introduction of 19 nor super hormones and the introduction of highly active female sex hormones as oral contraceptives in 1955. Cholesterol from wool industry and stigmasterol and sitosterols from soap industry not only due to as cheap byproducts but also due to efficient microbial conversions, eliminate a number of chemical steps with cheaper and better yields of intermediates and steroidal drug.

Other steroidal precursors :

The steroid drug precursors other than diosgenin fall into :

- (i) ***Vegetable sources :*** Solasodine, hecogenin, stigmasterol, sitosterols and ergosterol.
- (ii) ***Animal sources :*** Cholesterol and bile acids (e.g., deoxycholic and cholic acids).
- (iii) ***Non-steroidal precursor :*** Squalene.

(a) Solasodine (N-analogue of diosgenin) :

It is present in the form of its glycosides in several genera belonging to the *Solanaceae* and *Liliaceae* families (leaves of Solanum aviculare and ripe fruits of S. khasianum)

(b) Hecogenin :

It is a steroidal sapogenin present in the form of its glycoside, heconin. Commercially, obtained from sisal juice, a by-product of sisal fibre of Agave sisalana, A. rigida and A. fourcroydes. Because of its additional C-12 oxygen function, it can be used only in one group of steroids namely corticosteroids.

(c) Stigmasterol :

The principle sources are the calabar or ordeal bean (Physostigma venenosum) and soyabean oil.

(d) Sitosterols :

It consists of very complex mixtures of α, β and γ sitosterols. The major sources of β-sitosterol are cotton seed oil, sugarcane wax and tall oil. γ-sitosterol is obtained from soysterols.

(e) Cholesterol :

Commercial sources are sheep wool grease, cattle spinal cord and cattle brain.

Microbial degradation of sitosterol and of cholesterol yield C19 steroids, used for production of other C19 steroid sex hormones, anabolic agents and for conversion to C18 estrogens or for resynthesis of C21 steroids as well.

(d) Deoxycholic and cholic acids :

Ox bile is the usual commercial source.

(g) Ergosterol :

It is the most common of fungal steroids called mycosterols. It occurs in most fungi including yeast, in lichens, algae and some vegetable oils. The main source of ergosterol is a yeast Saccharomyces cerevisiae.

(h) Miscellaneous precursors :

Smilagenin and its 25–S epimer sarsapogenin, tigogenin and tomatidine, cordylagenin, cannigenin and brisbegenin, conessine and holarrhimine, constitute the miscellaneous precursors.

Stigmasterol is converted to pregnenolone acetate which is subjected to a fermentation process that does the hydrolysis, oxidation and rearrangement to produce progesterone in excellent yields.

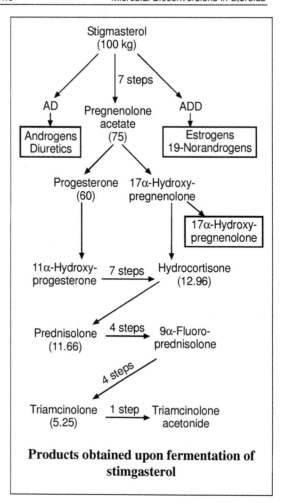

Products obtained upon fermentation of stimgasterol

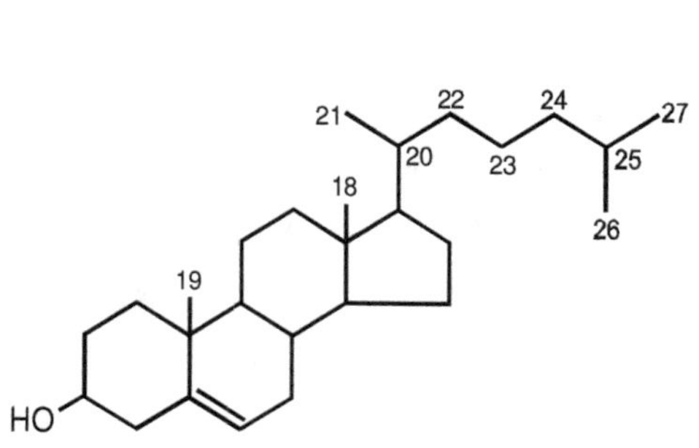

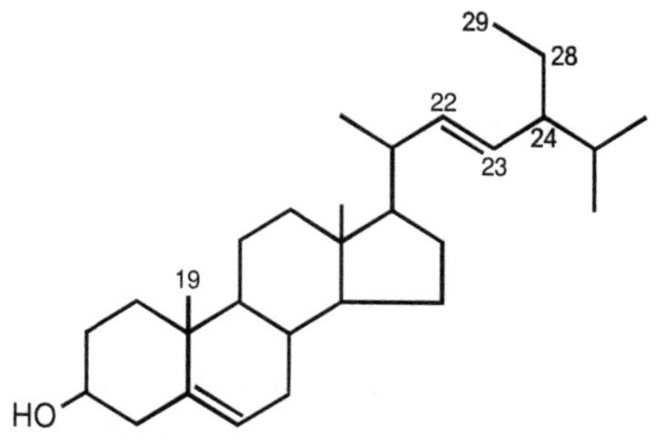

β-Sitosterol

Diosgenin

Solasodine

Hecogenin

Deoxycholic acid

Cholic acid

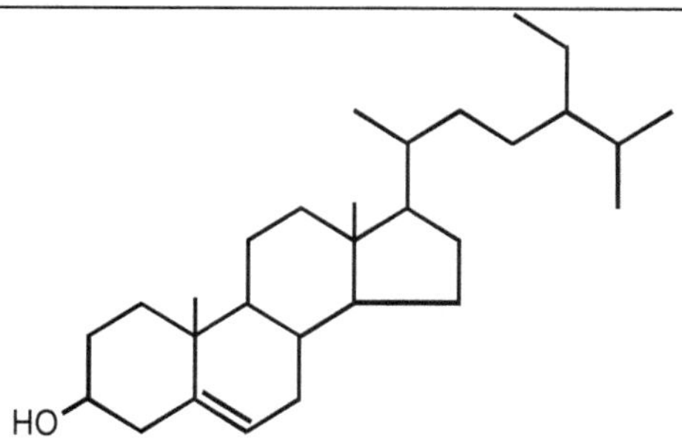

Some important steroid drug precursors

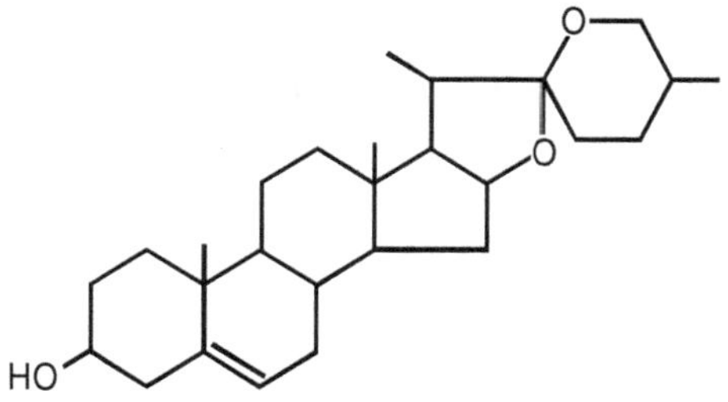

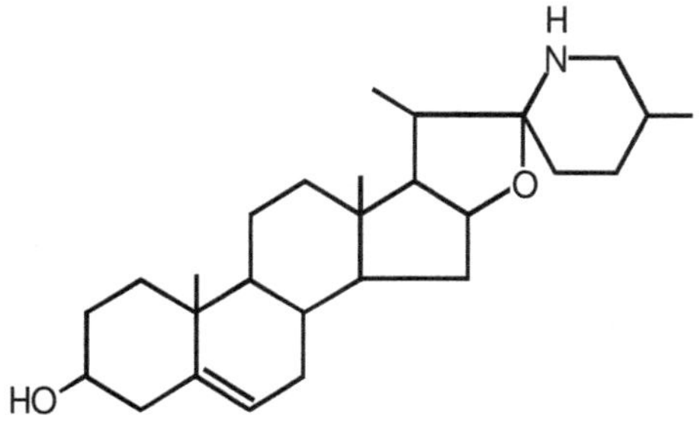

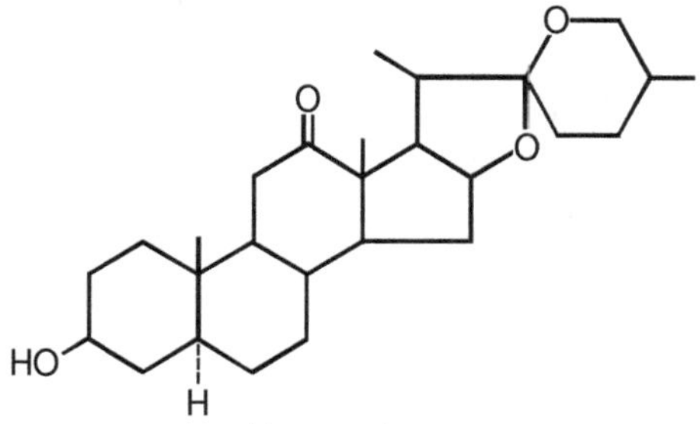

There are currently two major biotechnology applications dealing with steroids. They include :

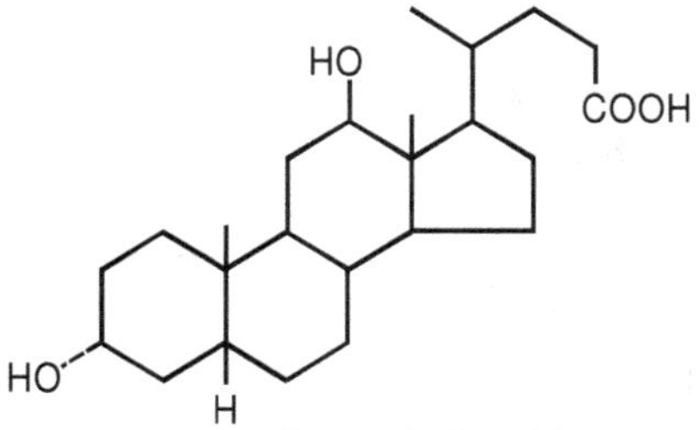

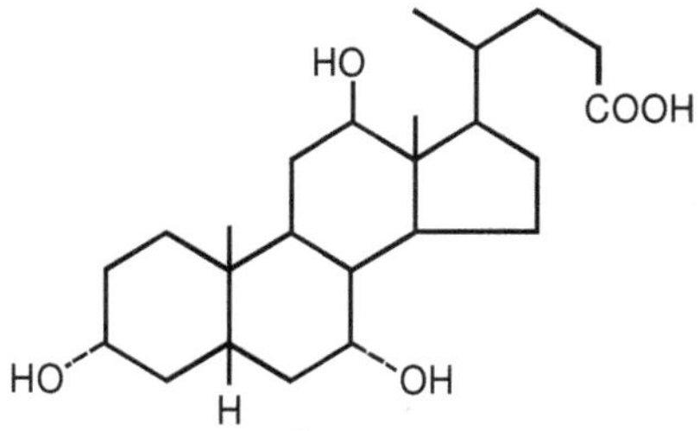

(a) Use of microbial agents for processing of raw materials or precursors into useful intermediates for general steroid production.

(b) Specific transformations of steroid intermediates to finished products. For example, the conversion of plant saponins to sapogenins (i.e. dioscin to diosgenin) using microbial hydrolysis illustrates first category. All these microbial biconversion may be utilized in commercial production of steroidal agents.

Micro-organisms used in much of the worlds investigation are from the important depositories such as,

1) **ATCC :** American type culture collection.

2) **CBS :** Central bureau voor schimmel culture bureau (Netherlands).

3) **IFO :** Institute for fermentation – Osaka.

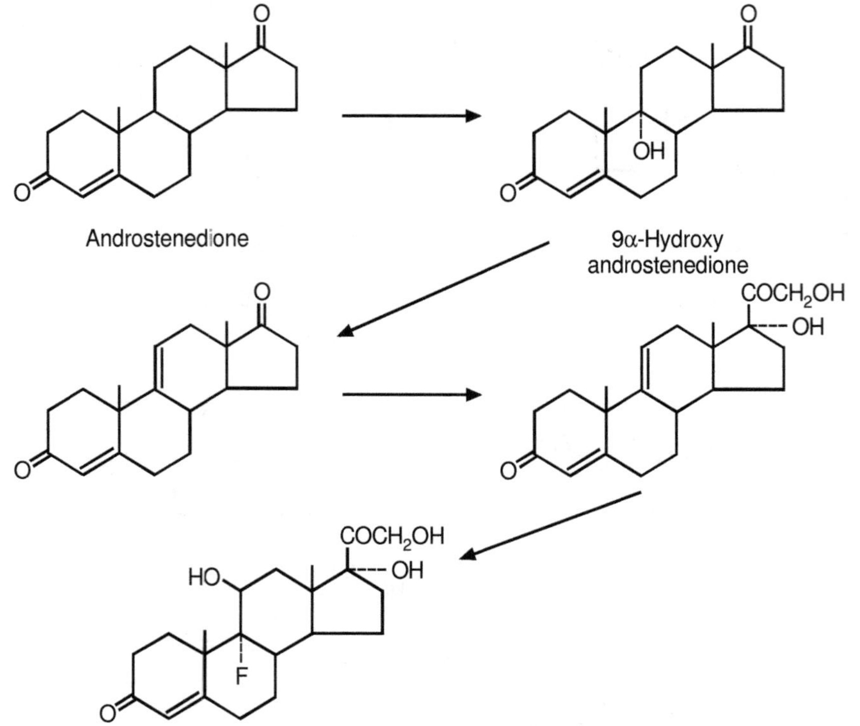

Androstenedione

9α-Hydroxy androstenedione

9α - Fluorohydrocortisone

4) **NRRL :** Northern Regional Research Laboratories U.S. Army (QN).

5) **WC :** Waksman collection. Rutgem University - New Bronswick N. J.

6) **GTCC :** German Type Culture Collection.

Even though a culture is available from one of these depositories, production cultures are strains developed by manufacturing companies after very extensive strain selection and improvement. Both natural mutant organism and those derived by treatment with mutagens, irradiation etc. have been evaluated.

4.8 STEROIDAL BIOCONVERSIONS

Drug undergoes metabolism in body. Metabolic transformations or biotransformations are enzyme reactions in which, drug may undergo a wide variety of oxidation, reduction and hydrolysis reactions.

The enzyme systems responsible for this metabolism are identified as :

(1) Microsomal enzymes from endoplasmic reticulum of liver and other tissues.

(2) Non-microsomal enzymes (present in the mitochondria, lysosomes or cytoplasm of the tissues or in the blood plasma).

(3) Reactions catalysed by intestinal microflora.

A battery of enzyme system of similar pattern is also found to be present in microorganisms. In fact, microorganism functions as a convenient source of required enzymes. Considerably later, when it was observed that microorganisms also metabolise the steroid compound in the similar fashion as does a human; they were used as aid to solve practical problems encountered in steroidal chemical synthesis.

The total chemical synthesis of one steroid from another, required many steps and the process may be costly and may provide poor yields because of certain rather difficult steps in the process. This was the problem with the synthesis of steroidal anti-inflammatory agents. An introduction of oxygen function at C-11, consumed 7-10 steps. So, the search for the improved methodology of steroid chemistry and opening of a new avenue to the synthesis was urgently needed. A pioneering experiment in this field was reported in 1937 when Mamoli and Vercellone showed that a fermenting yeast may be used to reduce 17-Keto steroid to 17β-hydroxy steroid.

This approach served as an important guideline in the synthesis of male hormone, testosterone and female sex hormone, 17β-estradiol as well.

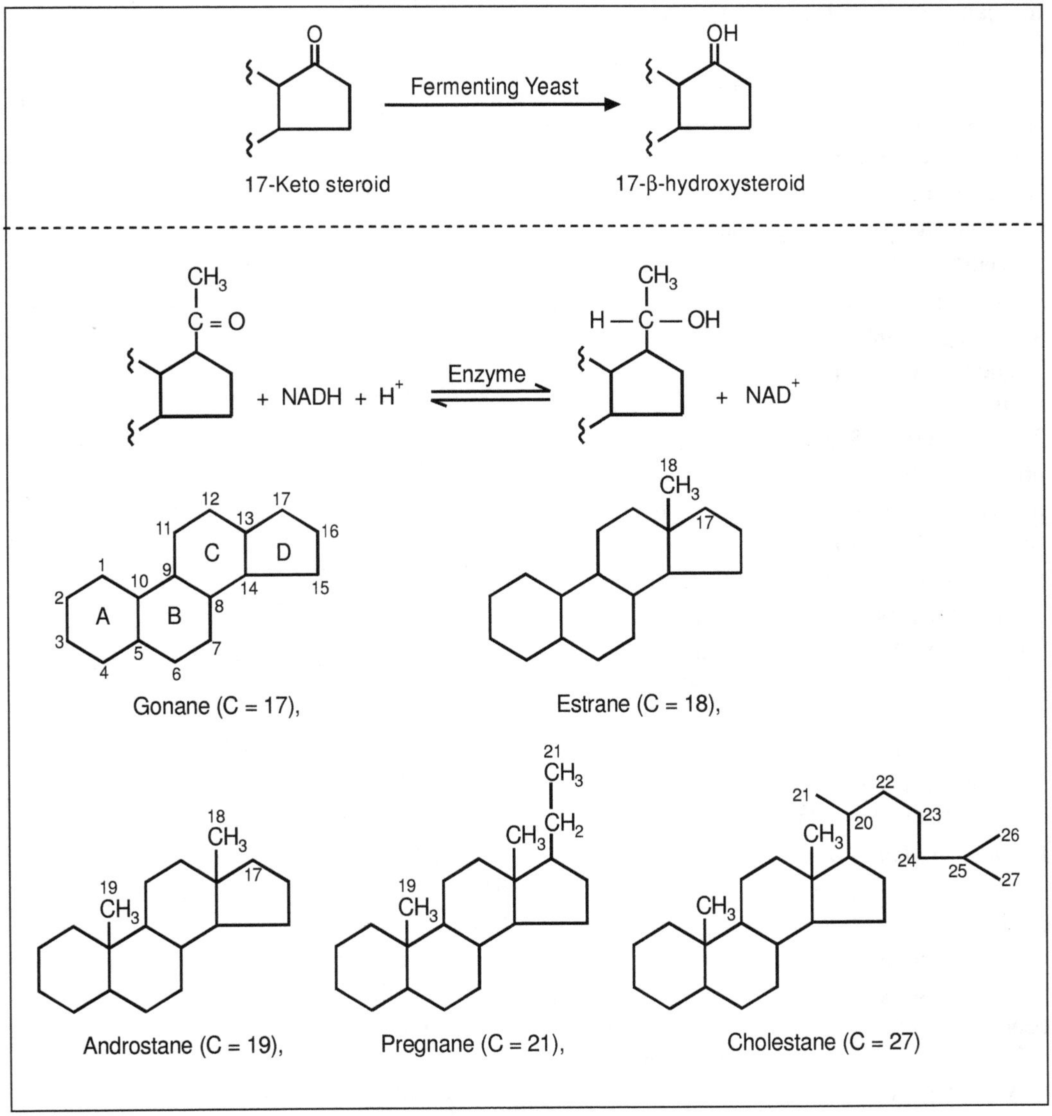

Thus, the above reaction and other similar transformations, which are difficult to carry out by chemical synthesis however proceed with an apparent ease when mediated by micro-organisms.

Advantages of microbial biotransformations over chemical synthesis :

(1) Steroid transformations are effected by fungi, bacteria, yeasts, protozoa and algae. These reactions are essentially detoxifying mechanisms employed by the micro-organisms.

(2) These transformations are sterio-specific i.e. specific organism must be used to carry out specific type of transformation e.g. Bacteria and yeasts are particularly active in oxidoreduction reactions, fungi are versatile specialist of hydroxylation.

(3) These transformations are site specific also e.g. streptomycetes are employed frequently as 16α-hydroxylators. In chemical synthesis one may usually get a mixture of 2 or 3 products. Separation of such a mixture presents a tedious job and may result into reduction in yield of the product. Thus, due to site specificity offered by microbes, the process proceeds with ease and efficacy.

(4) Microbial transformations of steroids now-a-days thus offer valuable tool in production of series of otherwise difficult accessible compounds.

(5) Microbial bioconversions often afford selective means of functionalizing remote and chemically inactivated positions.

Enzymes and microbial biotransformations :

(1) The micro-organisms display themselves as a convenient source of versatile enzyme systems.

(2) In some cases, coenzymes have also been recognised which may act on the substrate in the presence of main enzyme or may be engaged in the regeneration of active sites of the enzyme.

(3) NADH or another hydrogen source was expected to be present in oxido reduction reactions.

(4) Certain factors (oxido reductive system present in micro-organism) must be operating to regenerate back the oxidised form of NADH (i.e. NAD^+). This regeneration may be dependent upon the air oxygen.

(5) Alongwith NADP or NADH, other systems of flavin (or vitamin K type) were also reported to be operated in biotransformations.

(6) For efficient transformations to take place, oxygen must be placed in intimate contact with the cellular structure, so that the proper diffusion into the cell can occur efficiently.

(7) It is believed that these transformations take place within the culture cells and not in the medium surrounding the cells. Hence, to reach the culture cells, the solubility of a substrate in the medium and its rate of diffusion are the rate limiting steps.

(8) Multiple transformations in the same substrate may occur due to over abundance of different reactions specialised enzyme systems within the micro-organism e.g. Rhizopus arrhizus. So as per the need, inhibitory chemicals may be added to the culture media to supress the overactivity and to get selectivity of attack. On the similar lines, inducers of activity may also be used.

4.9 NUMBERING, NOMENCLATURE AND STERIO-CHEMISTRY OF STEROIDS

(1) Nearly all steroids are named as derivatives of any of the five basic steroidal rings.

(2) Solid lines denote groups above the plane of the nucleus (β-configuration) and dotted or broken lines denote groups behind the plane (α-configuration). If the configuration of the substituent is unknown its bond to the nucleus is drawn as a wavy line.

(3) The configuration of the H-atom at C-5 should always be indicated in the name.

(4) Circles were sometimes used to indicate α-hydrogens and dark dots to indicate β-hydrogens.

(5) Compounds with 5α-configuration, i.e. derived from 5α-cholestane belong to allo-series while compounds derived from 5β-cholestane belong to the normal series.

(6) If the double bond is not between sequentially numbered carbons, in such cases, both numbered carbons are to be indicated in the name.

(7) When a methyl group is missing from the side chain, this is indicated by the prefix not with the number of the C-atom which has disappeared.

(8) The symbol Δ is often used to designate a C=C bond in a steroid. If C=C is in between the 5 and 4, the compound is referred to as a Δ^4-steroid while if the C=C bond is in between the positions 5 and 10, the compound is designated as $\Delta^{5(10)}$ steroid e.g.

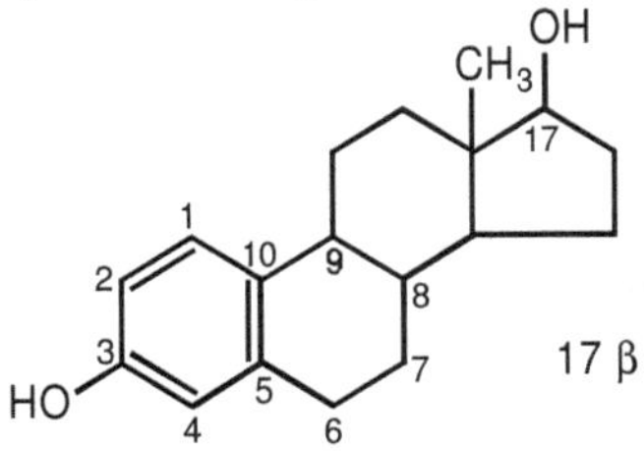

17 β - estradiol

(Estra – 1, 3, 5 (10) – triene – 3, 17 - β - diol)

Note : Since, 17β-estradiol contains 18 carbon atoms, it is considered as a derivative of Estrane, a basic nucleus.

The application of above rules can be illustrated in the following examples :

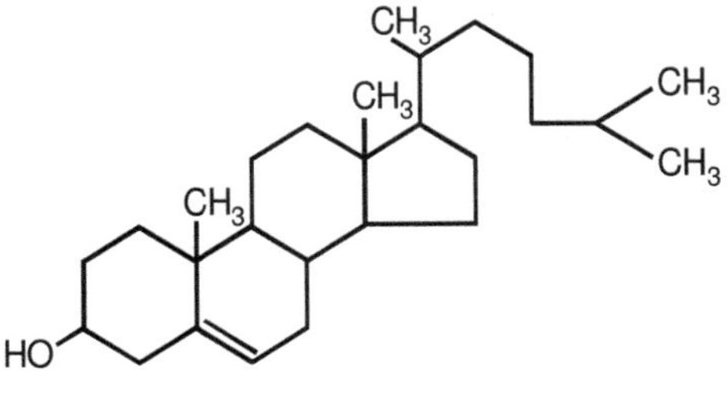

Cholesterol (Cholest-5-en-3-β-ol)

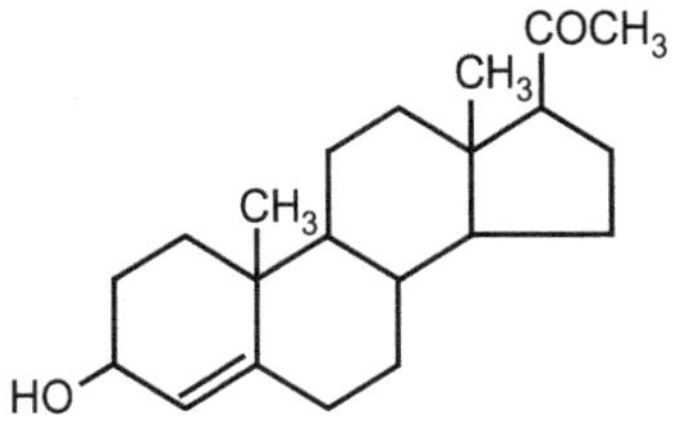

Progesterone (Pregn-4-ene-3, 20-dione)

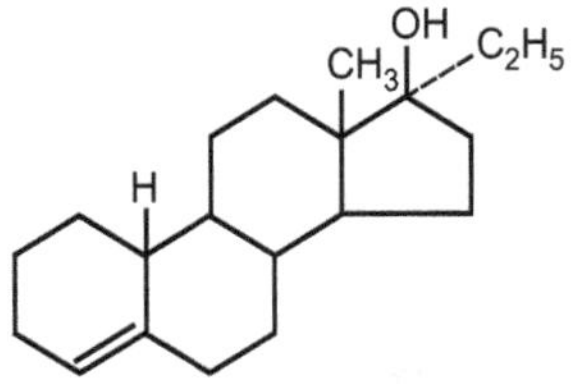

(17ethyl, 19 nor androst - 4 - en - 17ol) β

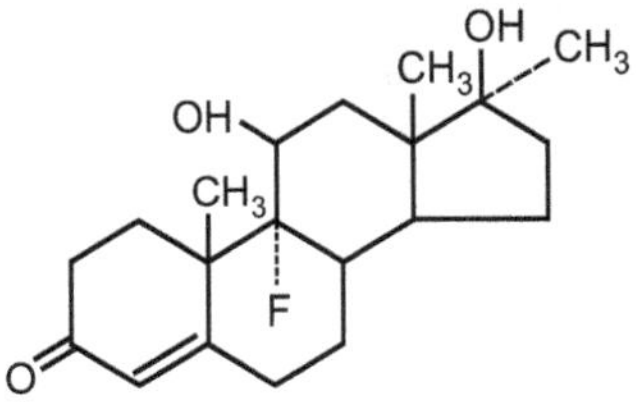

17methyl, 11, 17β dihydroxy - 9- fluoroandrost - 4 en - 3 - one   α

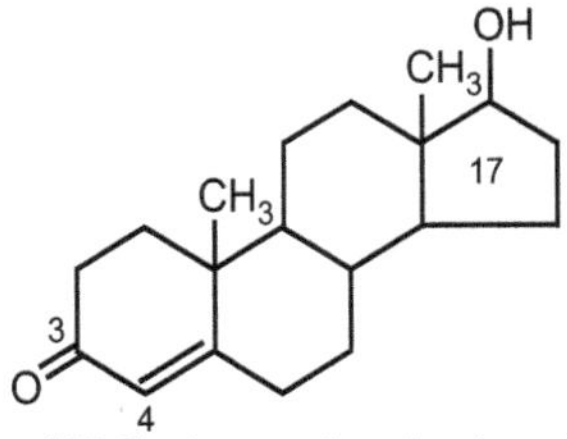

(17-βhydroxy - 4 androsten - 3 - one)

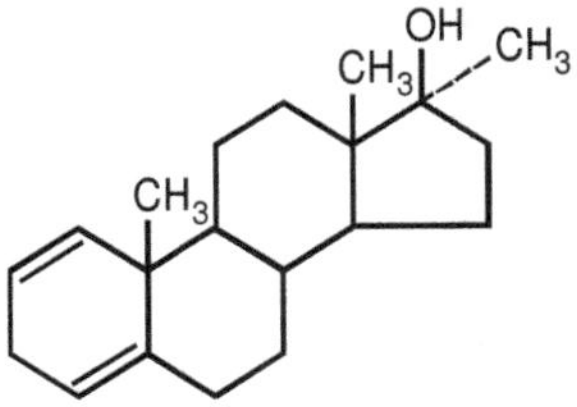

17 α-methyl, 17 β-hydroxy - androsta - 1, 4 - diene - 3- one

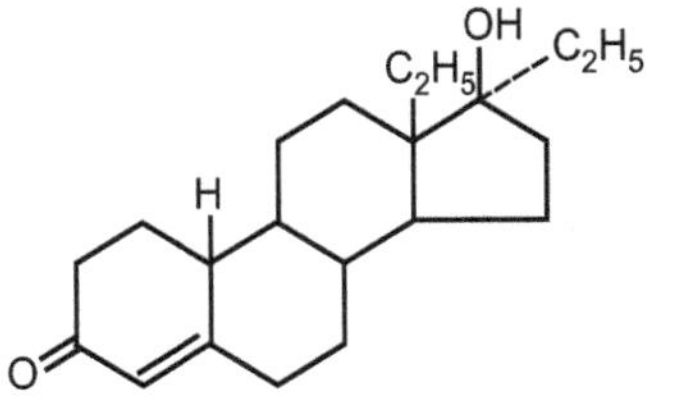

13-β17- diethyl - 17- hydroxy gon - 4 - ene - 3 - one

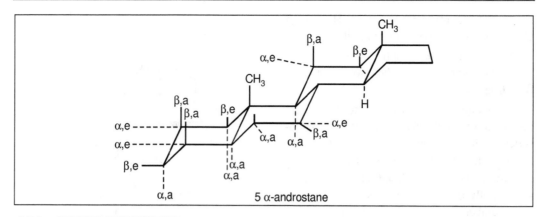

4.10 STERIOCHEMISTRY

(1) The absolute steriochemistry of the molecule and any substitutent is shown with solid (β) and dashed (α) bonds. An axial bond is perpendicular to the plane of molecule. An equatorial bond is horizontal to the plane of the molecule.

(2) The aliphatic side chains at positions 17, are always assumed to be of β-configuration.

(3) The terms cis and trans are occassionally used to indicate the backbone sterio-chemistry between rings. For example, 5α-steroids are A/B trans and 5β-steroids are A/B cis. The terms syn and anti are used analogously to trans and cis.

Conformation :

Cholestane, androstane and pregnane can exist into two conformations i.e.

(1) Chair form and
(2) Boat form

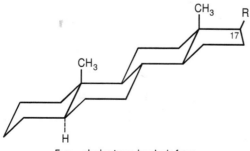

5 α – cholestane in chair form
R = side chain at C – 17

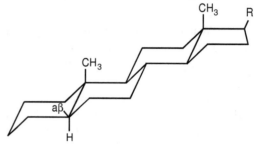

5 β – cholestane in chair form

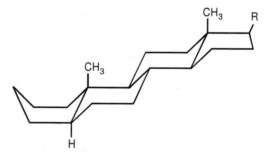

5 β – cholestane in boat form

Chair conformation is more stable than boat conformation due to less angle strains and hence all cyclohexane rings in the steroid nucleus exist in the chair conformation.

4.11 EARLIER WORK IN FIELD

(1) *Hydroxylation :*

Peterson and Murry (1950) made the original discovery of 11-hydroxylation on progesterone by using a fungus, particularly of the genera Rhizopus.

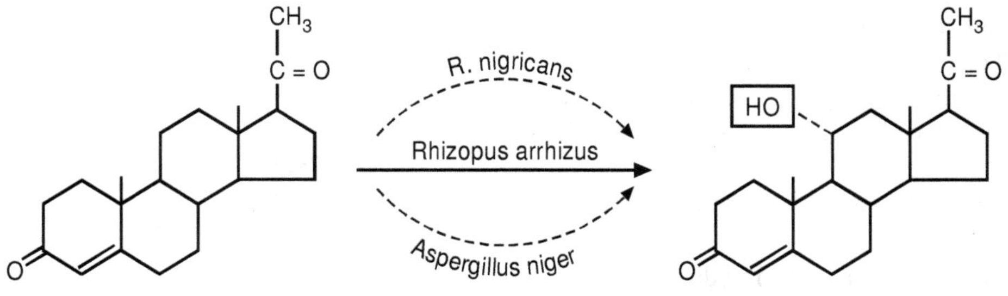

CH_3
$C = O$

R. nigricans

Rhizopus arrhizus

Aspergillus niger

HO

CH_3
$C = O$

Progesterone

11 α - hydroxy progesterone

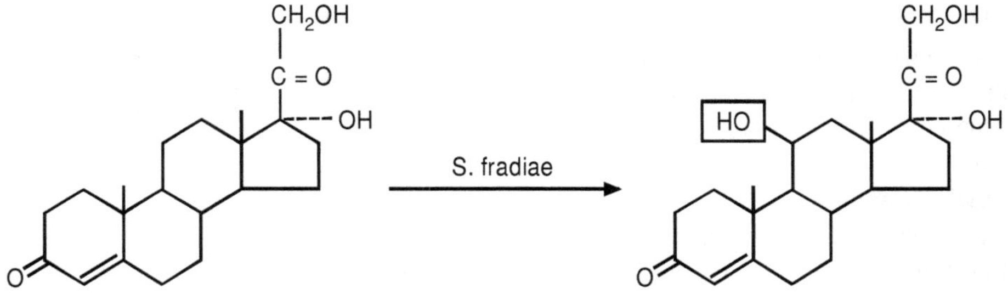

CH_2OH
$C = O$
OH

S. fradiae

HO

CH_2OH
$C = O$
OH

Compound 'S'
(11-Deoxycortisol)

Hydrocortisone

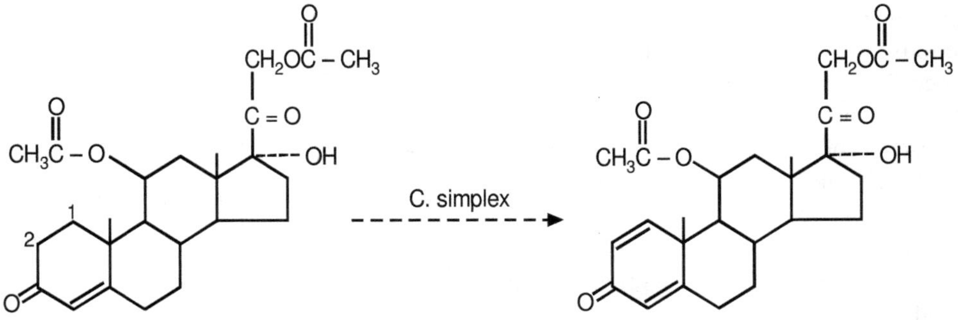

$CH_2O\overset{O}{\overset{||}{C}} - CH_3$
$C = O$
$CH_3\overset{O}{\overset{||}{C}} - O$
OH

C. simplex

$CH_2O\overset{O}{\overset{||}{C}} - CH_3$
$C = O$
$CH_3\overset{O}{\overset{||}{C}} - O$
OH

Hydrocortisone 11, 21 diacetate

1 - dehydrogenated analog

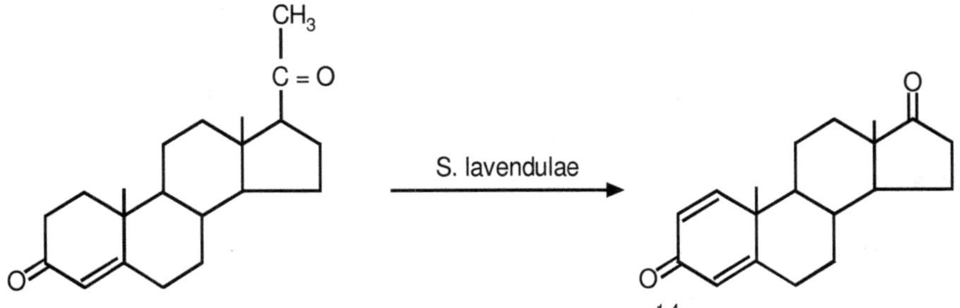

CH_3
$C = O$

S. lavendulae

Progesterone

$\Delta^{1,4}$ - androstadiene - 3, 17 - dione

In 1952, same scientists used Rhizopus nigricans and reported much higher yields of 88-92% at charge level of 3 gm/lit. During the same period, Fried et al, reported the same coversion with Aspergillus niger. This discovery opened a new avenue for the synthesis of steroidal anti-inflammatory agents.

The less common 11β-hydroxylation was first reported by Colingsworth, Brunner and Haines in 1952 with actinomycete (Streptomyces fradiae) with poor yields.

This transformation was carried out at Upjohn company. In 1953, Hanson et came up with same coversion but using Cunninghamella blakesleeana.

(2) Dehydrogenation :

Thus from 1953 onwards, interest in microbial transformations began to develop in various pharmaceutical companies like Merck, Pfizer, Upjohn, Schering, Syntex and so many. Under any investigation work to improve production techniques in 1953, Schering Co. undertook microbial hydrolysis of hydrocortiosone 11, 20-diacetatc ester, by using Corynebacterium simplex culture. But instead of giving cortisol, the major product obtained was an example of 1-dehydrogenation.

Similarly, in 1953, Fried et al reported dehydrogenation of progesterone to $\Delta^{1,4}$-androstadiene 3, 17-dione by using Streptomyces lavendulae.

In all cases of dehydrogenation of pregnane derivatives, it is observed that dehydrogenation is accompanied by removal of side chain at C-17.

Since, most of the potent steroidal anti-inflammatory agents contain 1-dehydro as their structural unit, the fermentation techniques were used widely inspite of many additional route of chemical synthesis e.g. using fermentation techniques the Schering Corporation made Prednisone and prednisolone.

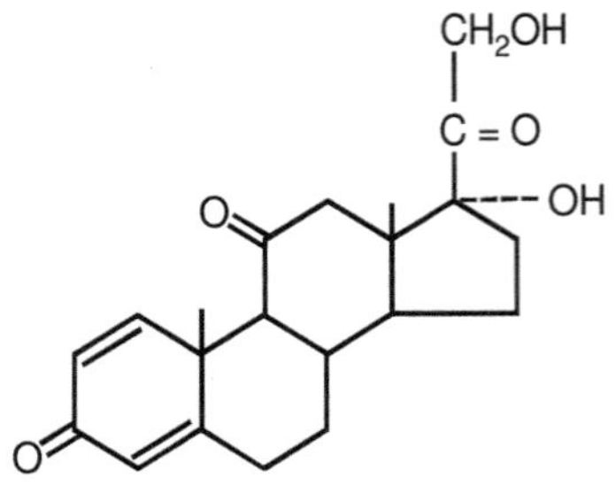

Prednisone

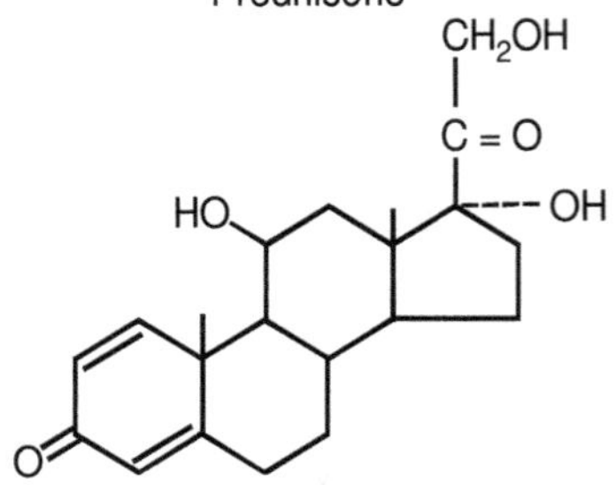

Prednisolone

Bunim et al, 1955 reported an increased anti-inflammatory activity of 1-dehydro analogues of cortisone (prednisone) and cortisol (prednisolone) which stimulated the search for efficient synthetic methods to synthesize these compounds. In 1955, Nobile et al used Corynebacterium simplex and got good yields of prednisone and prednisolone.

Commercial Hydroxylation Processes :

There are three microbial hydroxylations of commercial importance. These include, 11α, 11β and 16α-hydroxylation.

(1) 11α-hydroxylation :

Initially, reported organisms include Rhizopus arrhizus and Aspergillus niger. These were shortly replaced by Rhizopus nigricans ATCC 6227 b.

Besides strain and medium selection, a number of other factors need to be controlled. Growth of organism may be monitored by cell mass and glucose and O_2 consumption, but crucial induction of the 11α-hydroxylase (requiring progesterone at 70.5 g/l) can be followed only by product assay.

Factors such as age of culture and time of addition of substrate are not critical. Contamination by other organisms is not a problem.

A factor of importance in transformation is proper aeration. The mass transfer of O_2 from bulk liquid to mycelium surface and into the cell is crucial for good 11α-hydroxylation and is controlled by rate of delivery of air to the fermentor and the rate of stirring.

(2) 11β-Hydroxylation :

Other 11β-hydroxylating organisms like Streptomyces fradiae and Cunninghamella blakesteeana are not competitive with C. lunata in production.

(3) 16α-Hydroxylation :

Whereas, 11-hydroxylation is essential to all highly active corticosteriod drugs, 16α-hydroxylation is limited to triamcinolone and related fluocinolone.

Thus all important 11-hydroxylating and 16α-hydroxylating micro organisms like Curvularia lunata, Aspergillus ochraceus, Rhizopus nigricans and Streptomyces roseochromogenes can be used satisfactorily for steroid hydroxylations.

(4) Commercial 1-Dehydrogenation :

A large number of bacteria possess 1-dehydrogenating activity free from undesirable degradation activities. Those with superior utility being Arthobacter (Corynebacterium), Simplex ATCC 6946, Bacterium cyclooxydans ATCC 12673, Bacillus lentus ATCC 73805, Bacillus sphaericus ATCC 7055, Mycobacterium globiforme A93, Septomyxa affinis ATCC 6737 and ATCC 13425. Many other organisms including other Mycobacterium and several Nocardia species also appear to have superior 1-dehydrogenation capacities.

Arthrobacter simplex is very versatile and is used in prednisolone and triamcinolone manufacture.

(5) Controlled Multiple Transformations :

Yet better is the possibility of conducting two microbial steps in one fermentation using mixed cultures of hydroxylating and 1-dehydrogenating organisms.

Mixed culture of S. roseochromobenes and A. simplex acting on 9α-flurohydrocortisone gave triamcinolone directly without recovery of intermediates.

4.12 CLASSIFICATION OF MICROBIAL BIOTRANSFORMATIONS

An arbitrary division of the various microbial transformations can be made as follows :

(I) Oxidation :
    (a) Hydroxylation
    (b) Dehydrogenations
    (c) Epoxidation
    (d) Oxidative degradations

(II) Reduction :
    (a) Reduction of C = C bond.
    (b) Reduction of ketones, aldehydes and acids to alcohols.

(III) Esterification, amide formation and hydrolysis.

(IV) Olefinic bond isomerisation.

(V) Miscellaneous.

4.13 OXIDATION

It is the most important reaction amongst the microbial biotransformations. The sub-divisions, hydroxylation and dehydrogenation are the main reactions utilised by research groups due to their technological significance in the synthesis of steroidal anti-inflammatory agents.

(a) Hydroxylation :

Hydroxylation offers an access to otherwise inaccessible sites in the steroid molecule. The steroid ring system has been microbiologically hydroxylated at almost every position, 11 and 16α sites are of great commercial importance. Fungi are the most active hydroxylators. While some bacteria,

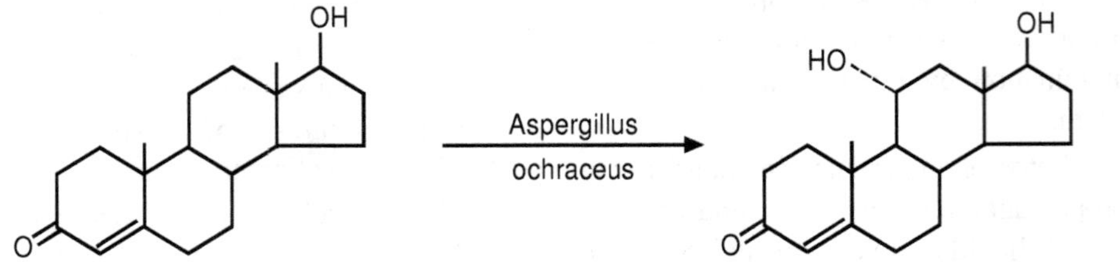

17 β - hydroxyandrost - 4 - ene - 3 - one
→ (Aspergillus ochraceus)

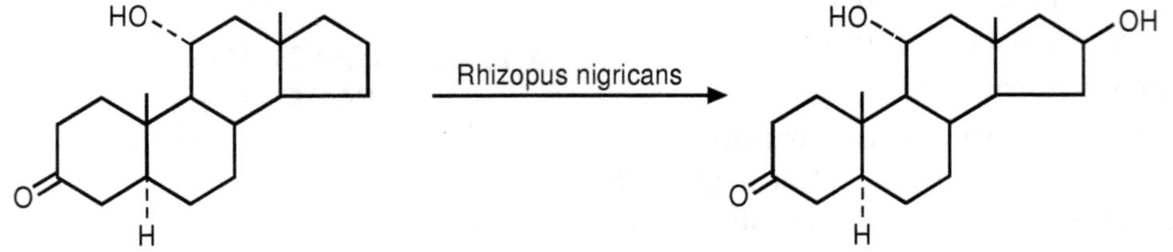

11 α - hydroxy - 5 α - androstan - 3 - one
→ (Rhizopus nigricans)
11 α, 16 β - dihydroxy - 5 α - androstan - 3 - one

particularly the Bacilli (rod shaped), Nocardia and Streptomyces also showed good activity. Each species has its own hydroxylating pattern. Unlike other reactions, hydroxylation depends less directly on the structure of the substrate molecule.

In commercial production, the microbial step is frequently preferred earlier in the synthesis particularly on the starting material progesterone, by using fungi, particularly of the genera Rhizopus, and Aspergillus. A remarkable similarity was observed between microbial and mammalian system in steroid hydroxylations as to positions attacked and mechanism of reaction concerned.

Reaction Mechanisms :

(A) General consideration :

(1) The oxygen function originates from atmospheric oxygen and not from water or any other oxygen containing substrate or the constituent of the media.

(2) The steriochemistry of carbon atom which is hydroxylated is always preserved. The hydroxyl group substitutes directly the H-atom, with a retention of configuration.

(3) Mono-oxygenase (mixed-function oxidases) enzymes participation in mono-hydroxylation is suggested.

(4) The participation of cytochrome P-450 and other electron transport proteins have also been observed (e.g. in the study of intact cells of Bacillus rereus).

(5) In many cases, hydroxylase enzyme was shown to be dependent on NADPH environment.

(6) Beside enolisation (one of the mechanism of hydroxylation) initial epoxidation of the Δ^5-double bond followed by hydration of the epoxide is also postulated.

(B) Proposed reaction mechanisms for hydroxylation :

(1) According to Ringold, hydroxylations at positions 2β, 6β, 10β and 17β, proceed via enolization. The air oxygen is captured by the enzyme to generate OH^+ moiety.

(2) Hayano proposed another mechanism for hydroxylation at sites which cannot be activated by enolisation.

The steps involved in this mechanism are :

1. Oxygen activation
2. Substrate activation followed by oxygen transfer
3. Regeneration of enzyme function.

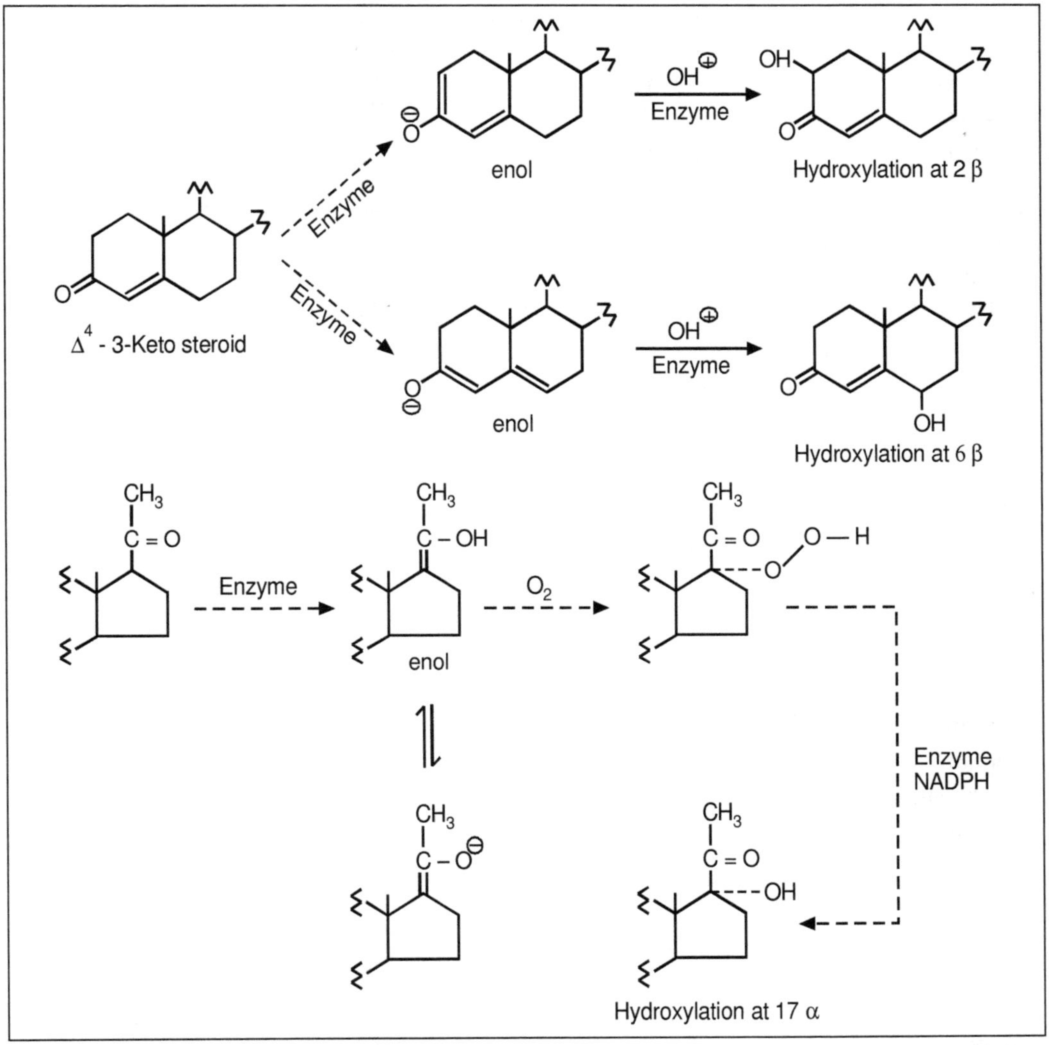

A molecular ratio of 1:1 between the oxygen and NADH was observed to be present during the reaction. The mutual co-operation between oxygen molecule, NADPH and a proton results in the hydroxylation as follow :

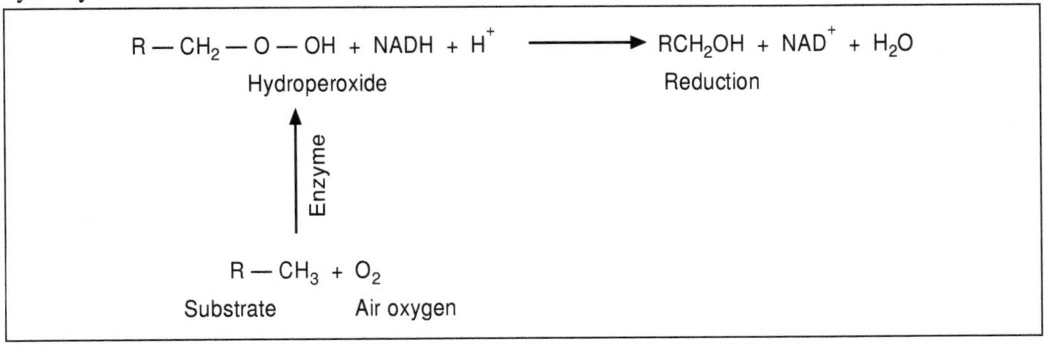

$$R-CH_2-O-OH + NADH + H^+ \longrightarrow RCH_2OH + NAD^+ + H_2O$$

Hydroperoxide   Reduction

Enzyme

$$R-CH_3 + O_2$$

Substrate   Air oxygen

Table 4.1 : Literature Survey- Hydroxylation

Type	Substrate	Microbe species	Product	Yield
1α-Hydroxylation	4-androstene-3, 17-dione 5α-androstene-3, 17-dione 3β Hydroxy -5-andro-stene-l7-one	Penicillium species	1α-hydroxy 1α-hydrosy 1α-hydroxy	24%
1β-Hydroxylation	17α 21-dihydroxy 4-pregnene 3, 20-dione 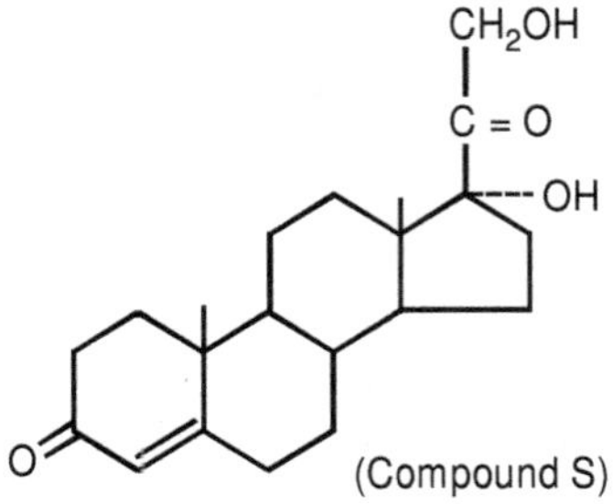 (Compound S)	Rhizoctonia ferrugena	1β-Hydroxylation 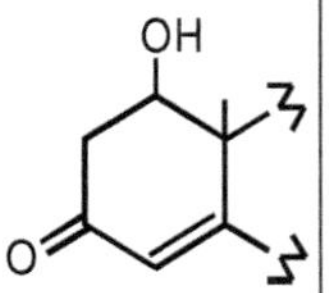	30%
2α-Hydroxylation 17 hydroxy-4-pregn -ene-20-yn-3 one (ethisterone)	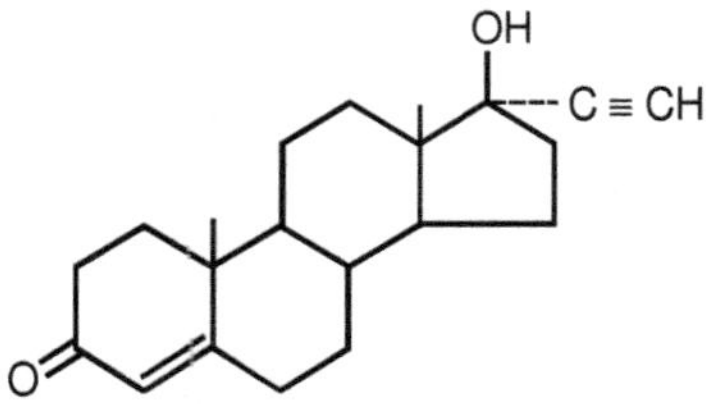	N. corallina	1α and 2α OH derivative	
Compound S or 17α, 21-dihydroxy 4 pregnene, 3, 20-dione. 9α fluoro 11β, 17β dihydroxy 17α methyl-4 androsten-3-one	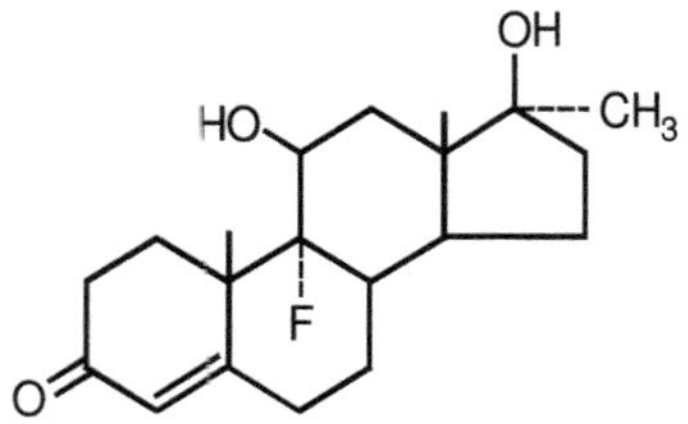	Sclerotina Species N. coralina	2β (side product 11α, 11β derivative) 1α, 2α Hydroxyl derivative	

2β-Hydroxylation		1. Strepto- myces sp. 2. Rhizoctonia ferrugona	2 β derivative	
(1) 17α, 21- dihydroxy 4-pregnene 3, 20 dione (compd.S)	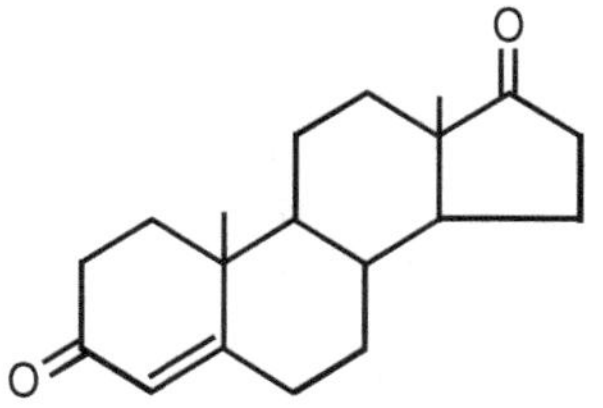			
(2) 4-Androstene 3, 17- dione		Penicillium species	2β hydroxyl derivative	
(3) 17α-Acetoxy 4 Androstene - 3-one (Progesterone)	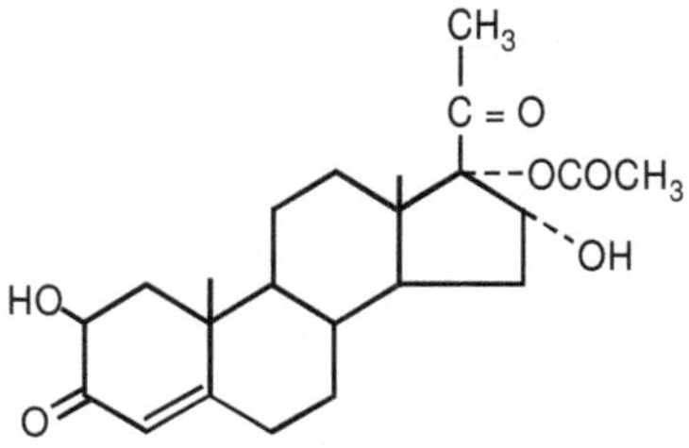	Streptomyces argerteolous MD 2428	2β (and 16α hydroxy simultaneously) i.e. 2β, 16α- dihydroxy 17α-acetoxy, 4-androstene 3-one	
3-Hydroxylation 5-androsten-7-one		Culonectna decora	3-β-12β- dihydroxy 5-androsten- 3-one	
4-Hydroxylation	Nil	Nil	Nil	
5α-Hydroxylation 4-nor-5α- pregnane- 2, 20 dione	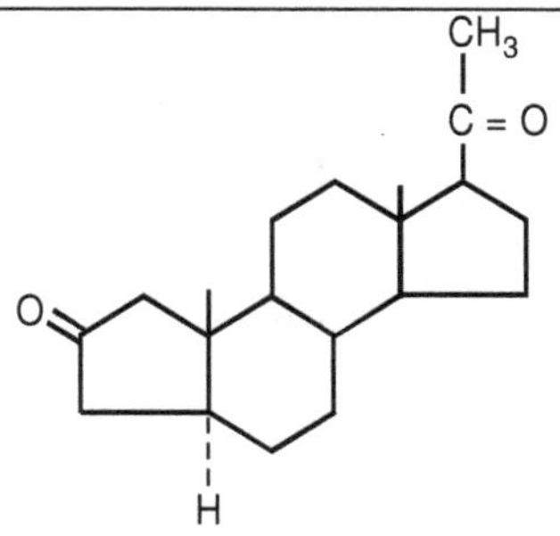	Cokeremyces recurvatus	5α-Hydroxy-4 nor 5α- pregnane-3, 20 -dione 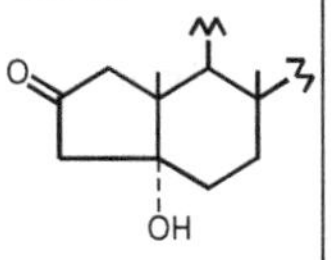	
5β-Hydroxylation Digitoxigenin Cardenolide derivative i.e. 3, 14 dihydroxy, 5-β-cardenolide	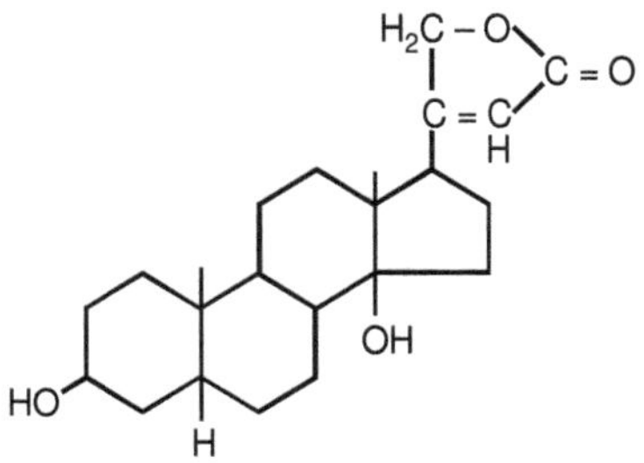	Absedia orchidis	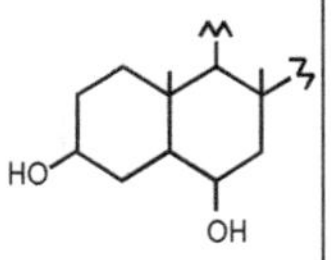	
6α-Hydroxylation	Nil	Nil	Nil	

6β-Hydroxylation (1) 4-androstene- 3, 17-dione		Rhizopus arrhizus	6β 11α	
(2) 17α hydroxy progesterone or 17-α hydroxy- 17-β acetoxy-4 -androstene-3- one 3) Compound. S (11- Deoxycortisol)		M. cornymbifer Aspargillus ochracous Rhizopus arrhizus R. arrhizus	6β + 14α 6β + 11α 6β 6β	
7α-Hydroxylation (1) 17- β acetoxy Δ^4-androst-3- one or progesterone or Δ^4 pregn-3, 20 dione (2) 21-Hydroxy- pregn Δ^4- 3, 20- dione (Deoxycortisone)	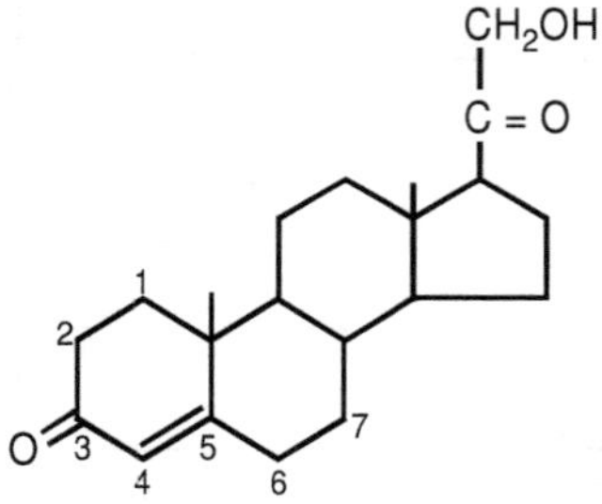	1. Helmintho- sporium Sp. 2.Phycomyces blackesleeana Curvularia species	7α-hydroxy derivative 7-α-hydroxy, 17-acetoxy- Δ4-androst-3- one 7α, 21β- dihydroxy Δ^4 pregn -3-20- dione or 7α- hydroxy, deoxycortisone	18% 4%
7β-Hydroxylation (1) Δ^4 pregn-3, 20 dione (Progesterone) (2) 21-Hydroxy, 5α pregn-3, 20 dione	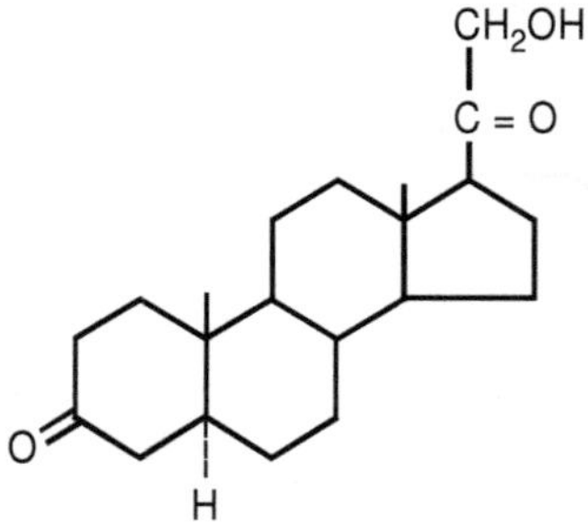	Cladosporium sp. Rhizopus species	7β hydroxy Δ^4 pregn-3, 20 dione 7α hydroxy-5- α-pregn-3, 20- dione	15%
Cholesterol or 3 β hydroxy cholest 5-ene or Δ^5 cholest-3-ol	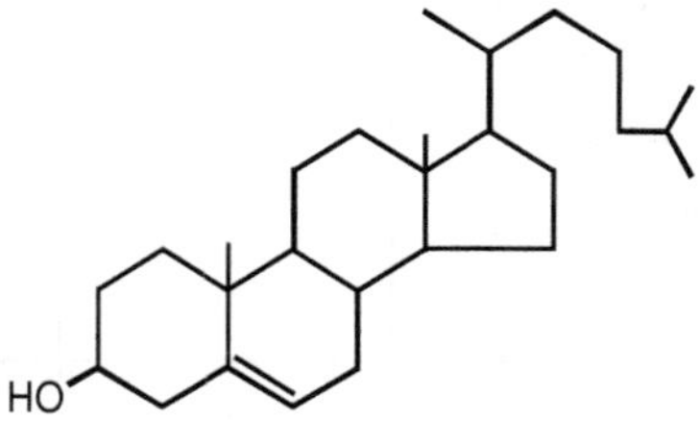	Nocardia reseus	7β-hydroxy Δ^5 cholest-3-ol	

8α-Hydroxylation There is no 8α hydrogen in steroids. With steroids of abnormal nucleus (skeleton) – Reaction remains to be discovered.	–	–	–	–
8β-Hydroxylation Compound S or (17α, 21β-dihydroxy Δ^4 preg-3, 20 - dione)	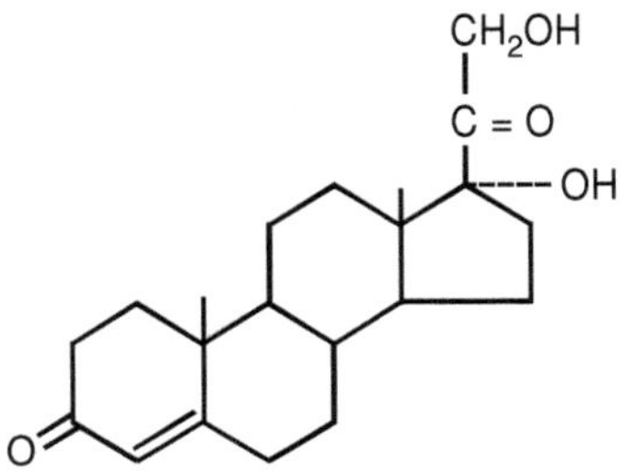 CH$_2$OH C = O ----OH	Cercospor melonis	8β, 17α, 21-trithydroxy Δ^4 pregn-3, 20 dione 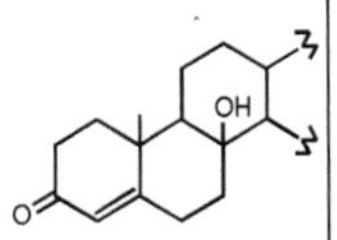	
9α-Hydroxylation (1) 17α, 21-dihydroxy Δ^4 pregn -3, 20 - dione (2) Δ^4 pregn-3, 20 dione (3) Δ^4 pregn-3, 20 dione (4) Δ^4 androst-3, 17 dione (5) $\Delta^{1,4}$ androstra-diene- 3, 17 dione	(compound S) (Progesterone) (Progesterone)	Helicostylum periforme Circinella Species Streptomyces aureofaciens Nocardia species Pseudomonas species	(1) 8β or 9α derivative (2) 9α, OH Δ^4 pregn-3, 20 dione (3) 8 or 9-Hydroxy derivative (4) 9α - OH - Δ^4 androst -3, 17 dione (5) 9α derivative	19% 33%
9β-Hydroxylation Dedrogesterone i.e. Restrosteroid 9β, 10α Δ^4 pregn-3, 20 dione	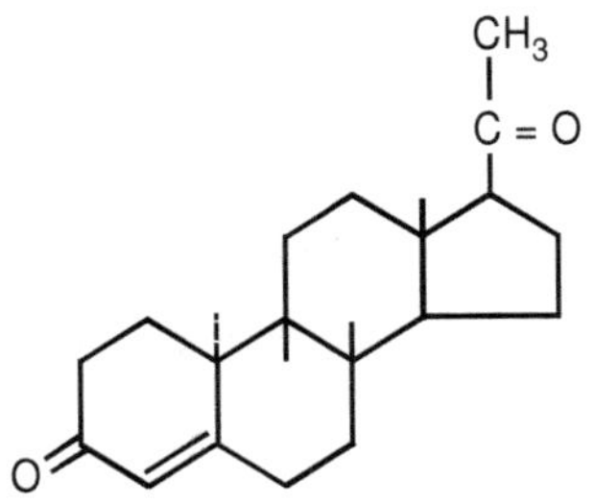 CH$_3$ C = O	No mention of species	Specific 9β Hydroxyl derivative	

10β-Hydroxylation 19-nor-testosterone or 17-hydroxy Δ^4 (10) estrane-3-one		R.nigricans	10β deviative 11α, 17β dihydroxy - 4-estren-3-one	Major product
11α-Hydroxylation (1) Δ^4 pregn-3, 20 dione (or Progesterone)		R. nigricans	11α-hydroxy Δ^4 pregn-3, 20 dione	80-90%
		Aspergillus niger		35%
		Bacillus cereus		
		Aspargillus orchaceus		
		Cephalothecium roseum		
(2) Compound S or 11-deoxycortisol.		Cunninghamella blakesleeana	11α, 11β derivatives	64%
		Absidia glauca	11α 11β	
(3) 17β-Hydroxy $\Delta^{4(10)}$-Estr-3-one (19-nor testosterone)		Rhizopus nigricans	11α	
11 β-Hydroxylation (1) Δ^4 pregn-3, 20 dione (Progesterone)		Curvularia lunata	11 β	
		Streptomyces fradiae	11 β + 21	
(2) Compound S		Cunnighamella blakesleeana	11 β	
		Trichothecium sp.	11 β	
		Pseudomonas sp.	11 β	
		Corticium sasaki	11 β	
		Absidia glauca	11 β	
		Rhodoseptoria sp.	11 β	

12α-Hydroxylation (1) Testosterone or 17α-hydroxy Δ^4-androst-3-one		W. graminis	12α, 17β, dihydroxy-4, 14-andro-stadiene-3-one.
(2) 9 (11)-dehydro-progesterone or $\Delta^{9(11)}$ dehydro, Δ^4 pregn-3, 20 dione		Colletotrichum sp. Thamnidium sp. or Aspargilus nidulans	6β, 12α dihyroxy- 4, 9(11) pregnadiene 3, 20-dione
9α-hydroxy-4-androstene-3, 17 dione		Cercospora melonics	9α, 12α dihydroxylation
12β-Hydroxylation Δ^4 pregn-3, 20 dione	(Progesterone)	Calonectria decora	12β-hydroxy, Δ^4-Pregn - 3, 20 dione
13β-Hydroxylation	Nil	Nil	Nil
14α-Hydroxylation Compound S		Helicostylum piriforme	14 α-hydroxy derivative
Progresterone or (Δ^4 pregn. 3,20 dione) or		Mucor hiemalis	14 α-Hydroxy Δ^4 pregn-3, 20 dione
Deoxycorticosterone		Bacillus cereus Curvularia sp.	same as above same as above	24%
14β-Hydroxylation	Nil	Nil	Nil
15α-Hydroxylation (1) Δ^4 pregn.-3,20 -dione (Progesterone)		Phycomyces blakesteeana Colletotrichum antirrhini	15α-hydroxy Δ^4 pregn-3, 20 dione	24-34%
(2) 21Hydroxy Δ^4 pregn. 3, 20 dione (deoxycortisone)		Giberella baccata	15α, 21β Hydroxy Δ^4-pregn-3, 20-dione
(3) Δ^4 pregn. 3, 20 dione		Lenzites obientina	15α-hydroxy derivative
(4) Δ^4 pregn. 3, 20 dione		Fusarium species	15α-hydroxy derivative	24-34%
(5) Compound S.		Hormodendrum viridae	15α-hydroxy derivative

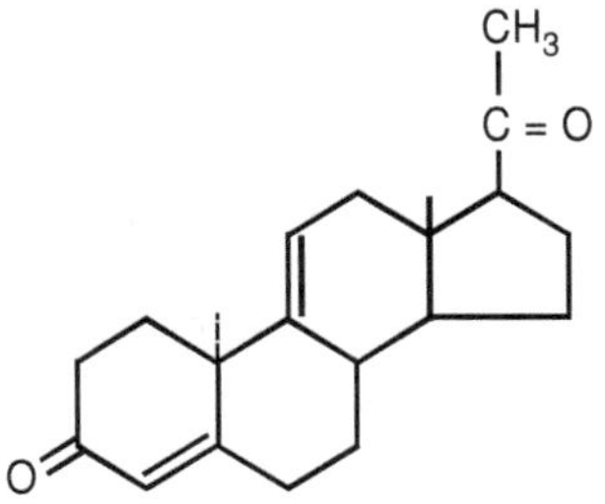

16α Hydroxylation Δ^4 pregn. 3, 20 dione (Progesterone) Testosterone		S.argenteolus S.roseochromo -genus	16α hydroxy- Δ^4 pregn. 3, 20 dione 16α-hydroxy derivative	
16β Hydroxylation Testosterone Androstenedione 3,14-dihydroxy 5 β cardenolide (Digitoxigenin)		Wojnowicia graminis Corticium centrifugum Helicostylum pinforme	16β-hydroxy 16β-hydoxy 3, 14, 16- trihydroxy 5β cardenolides or gitoxigenin	
17α -Hydroxylation Δ^4 pregn. 3, 20- dione (Progesterone)		Trichoderma viridae Cephalothecium roseum Dactylium dendrades	17α hydroxy- Δ^4 pregn- 3, 20 dione 17α derivatives, +11α hydroxy- derivatives 17α + 11α hydroxy- derivatives	
21-Hydroxy Δ^4 pregn-3, 20-dione (Deoxycortisone)		Tri.roseum	17α hydroxy- deoxycortisone	
17β-Hydroxylation	**Nil**	**Nil**	**Nil**	
18-Hydroxylation (1) Δ^4 androst-3, 20 dione		Corynespora meleni	9α, 18 dihydroxy derivative	
(2) 9α hydroxy Δ^4 androst 3, 20 dione		As above	As above	
(3) 11β, 21- dihydroxy Δ^4 pregn-3, 20- dione		Corynespora cassicola	18, 11β, 21 trihydroxy derivative (aldosterone)	

19 Hydroxylation				
(1) Compound S		Corticium sasakii	19 hydroxy Compd. S	
(2) Cholesterol		C. Sasakii	3-hydroxy estra- 1, 3, 5(10)- triene- 17-one (estrone)	

20-Hydroxylation and 22- hydroxylation and beyond :

The 20-position is usually occupied by carbonyl function and thereby not available for reaction. Work with Nocardia sp. on cholesterol shows fission between C_{24} and C_{25}, C_{22} and C_{23} and C_{17} and C_{20}.

21 Hydroxylation 17α-Hydroxy, Δ^4 pregn. 3, 20-dione		O.herpotrichus	17 α, 21β - dihydroxy derivative	

(b) Dehydrogenation :

Dehydrogenation resulting into introduction of a double bond has been reported for all the four rings of steroid nucleus but majority of microbes attack the ring A. Most of the ring A dehydrogenators contain both Δ^1 and Δ^4-dehydrogenating activity and are probably flavoprotein in nature.

Whether dehydrogenation proceeds directly or involves hydroxylation as an intermediate step was a matter of contraversy.

Levy and Talalay in 1957, after an extensive study of the steroid dehydrogenating enzymes of Pseudomonas testosteroni presented a convincing evidence that no intermediate hydroxylation occurs during dehydrogenation reaction. It was also observed that 1α and 2β hydrogen atoms are needed for the microbial dehydrogenation.

Like in mammalian systems, ring A aromatization of the steroid to form estrone structure was reported by Dodson and Muir in 1958 with a Nocardia species.

But unlike mammalian systems, this microbial transformation proceeds via 1-dehydro intermediate.

Stoudt et al in 1958, reported the synthesis of prednisone and prednisolone using Nocardia black wellii.

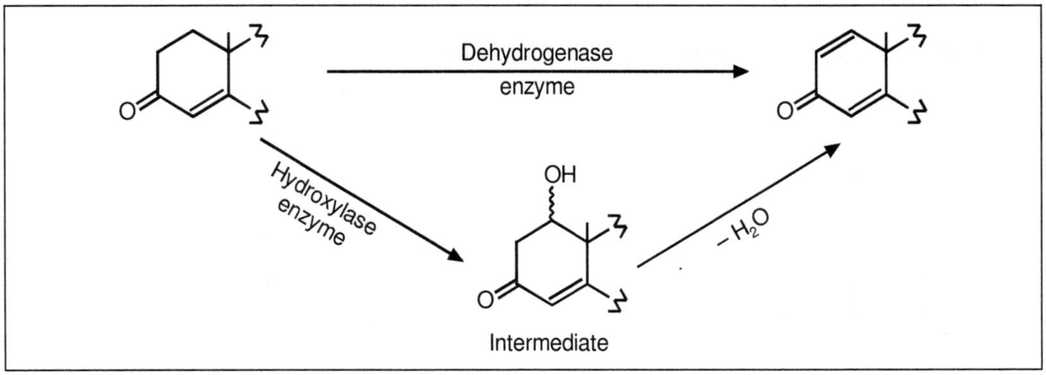

Intermediate

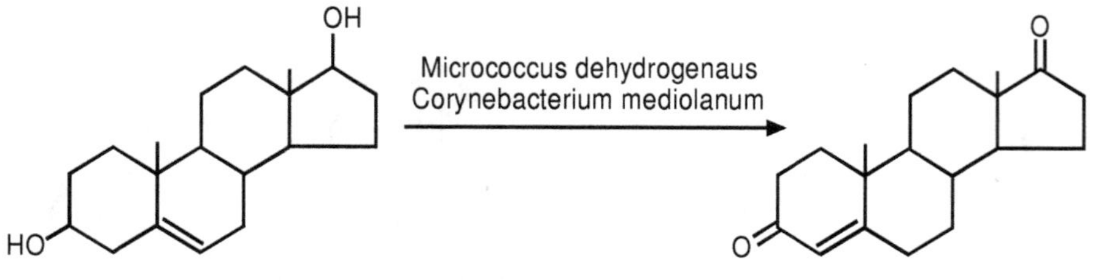

5-androstene-3β, 17β - diol

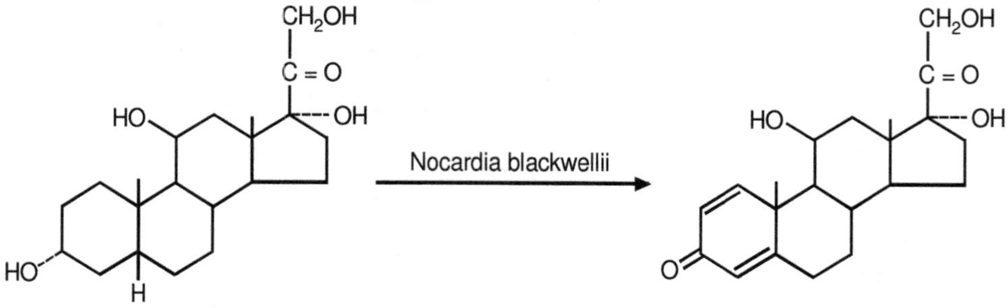

Micrococcus dehydrogenaus
Corynebacterium mediolanum

Pregnane - 3 α, 11 β, 17 α, 21 - tetrol - 2 - one

Nocardia blackwellii

Prednisolone

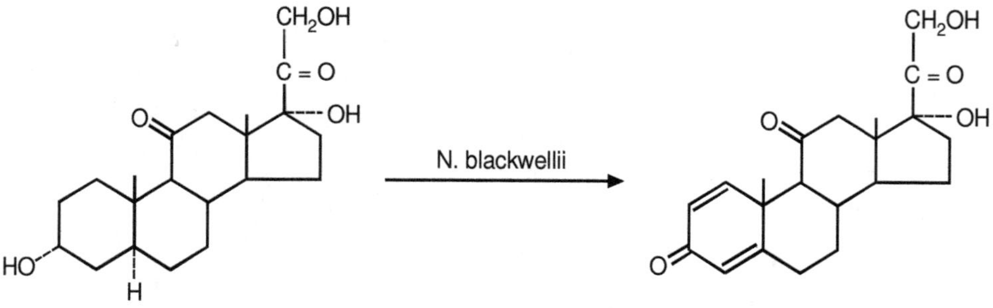

Allopregnene - 3 α, 17 α, 21 - triol - 11, 20 - dione

N. blackwellii

Prednisolone

Laskin and Diassi have reported one example of bromide reduction

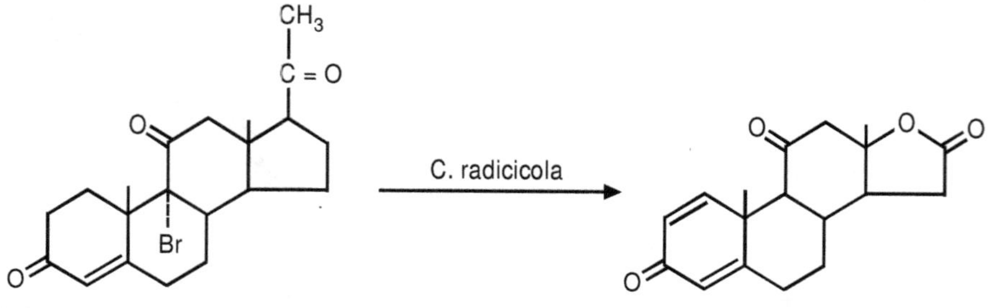

C. radicicola

Reaction mechanism for dehydrogenation :

(1) Vitamin K type quinone structures are essential for dehydrogenation. This fact was supported by the work of Gale et al. Vitamin K type structure may be acting as a cofactor for dehydrogenation reaction in some cases.

(2) Talalay demonstrated with Pseudomonas testosteroni in 1958 that Flavoproteins may be playing coenzymatic role in dehydrogenation reaction.

(3) Ringold, Hayano and Stefanovic proposed that dehydrogenation proceeds via following sequence.

(A) Reaction proceeds via a trans diaxial loss of the 1α, 2β-hydrogens, with the enzyme activating an enolisation of the 3-ketone towards the 2-position.

(B) The step A is followed by the transfer of activated hydride at the 1 position to the coenzyme with the subsequent collapse of the enzyme-substrate complex.

(C) The enzymes involved are of flavin type or some other redox systems. Relatively few vegetative cell cultures possess the oxido-reductases which may operate both dehydrogenation and reduction reactions. The selectivity of reaction depends upon aeration and on the oxidation reduction potential state of the system.

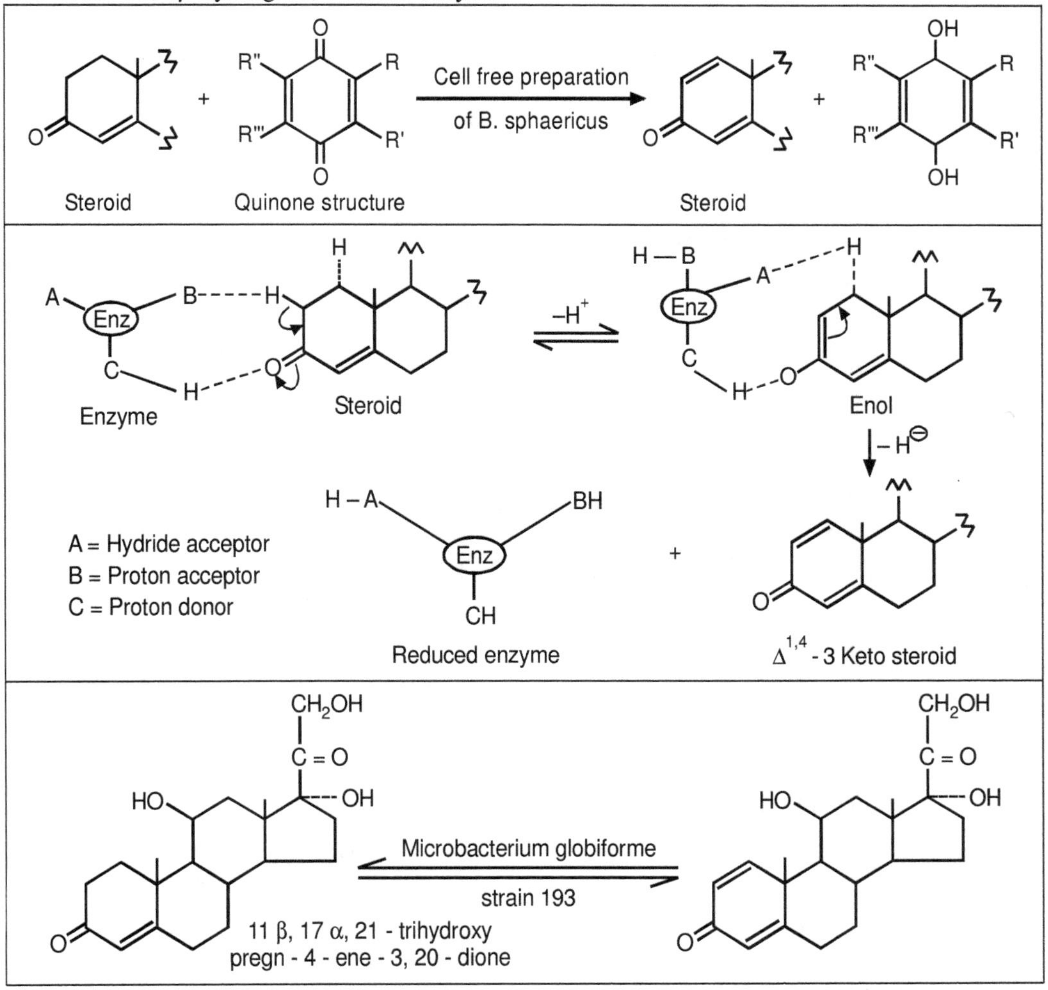

Table 4.2 : Sites of Reaction Dehydrogenation (Double Bond Generation)

Sr. No.	Type substrate	Microbe	Product
Ring Dehydrogenation (Δ 1 Dehydrogenation) :			
(1)	Δ^4 Pregn-3, 20 dione (Progesterone)	(1) Fusarium solani (2) S. lavendulae	(1) $\Delta^{1,4}$ androstadiene -3, 17 dione (2) 1-dehydrotestosterone (17β hydroxy Δ1,4 androst 3-one)
(2)	Compound S $\rightarrow$ 17 α, 21-dihydroxy - Δ^4 - Pregn - 3,20 dione	C. radicicola	D-homo 17 a-oxa, $\Delta^{1,4}$ Androst-3,17 dione 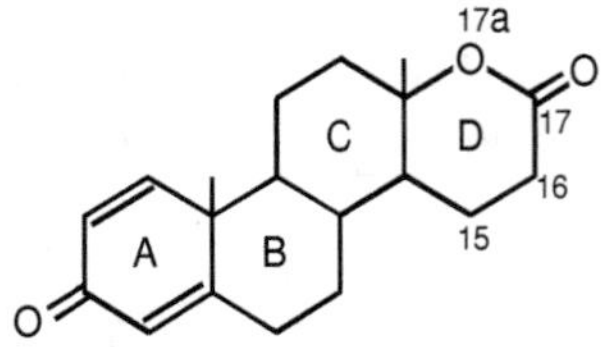
(3)	20, 17 α dihydroxy Δ^4 Pregn-3, 11, 20 trione (cortisone)	Corynebacterium simplex	Prednisone
(4)	21,17α, 11β trihydroxy Δ^4 - Pregn - 3,20 dione (cortisol)	C. simplex	Prednisolone
Δ^4 - Dehydrogenation :			
(1)	Androstane-3, 17-dione	Fusarium sp.	1,4 androstadiene 3, 17 dione
(2)	Allopregnane 3, 20 dione or (5 αH-Preg 3,20 dione)	Fusarium sp.	1,4 androstadiene 3, 17 dione
(3)	Androst 3, 17 dione	Pseudomonas sp.	$\Delta^{1,4}$ androst - 3,17 - dione
(4)	Pregnane 3α, 11β, 17α 21 tetrol-20-one	Nocardia species	Prednisone
Δ^7 Dehydrogenation :			
(1)	Δ5 cholesta 3-ol (cholesterol)	Azobacter sp.	$\Delta^{5,7}$ cholesta-3-ol
Δ^9(11) Dehydrogenation :			
(1)	3 hydroxy $\Delta^{1,3,5(10)}$ estra- 17 one (Estrone)	Glomerella	This course of dehydrogenation accompanied by inversion at 14 position remains to be clarified.

Reports : Regarding dehydrogenation at 14 position with Wojnowicia graminis and 16-dehydrogenation with Tricholhecium roseum are under study.

Table 4.3 : Dehydrogenation of Hydroxyl Group

No.	Substrate	Microbe	Product
(1)	5 pregnene 3 β - ol - 20 one 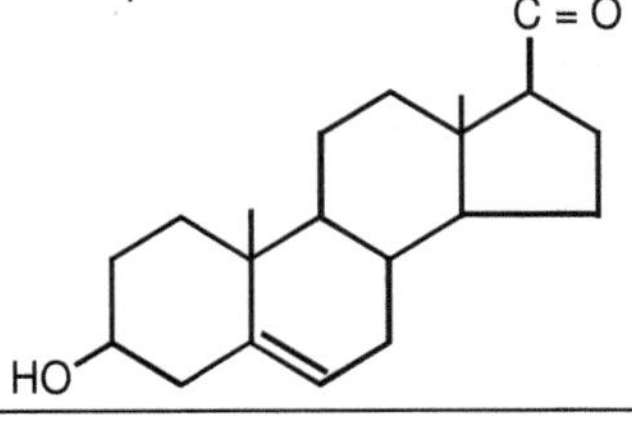	Stretomyces species	Δ^4 preg. 3, 20 dione or Progesterone 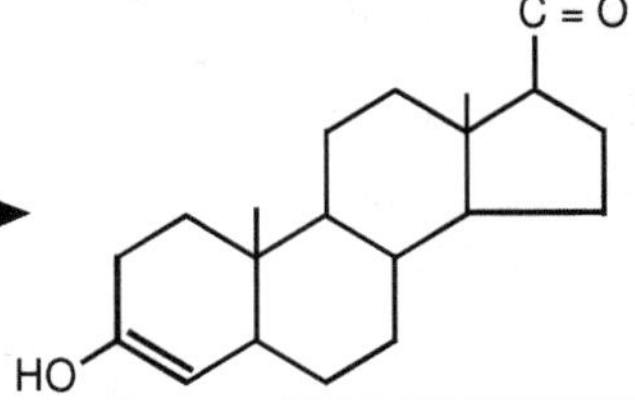
(2)	$\Delta^{1, 3, 5(10)}$ Estr. 3, 17 di-ol (Estradiol) 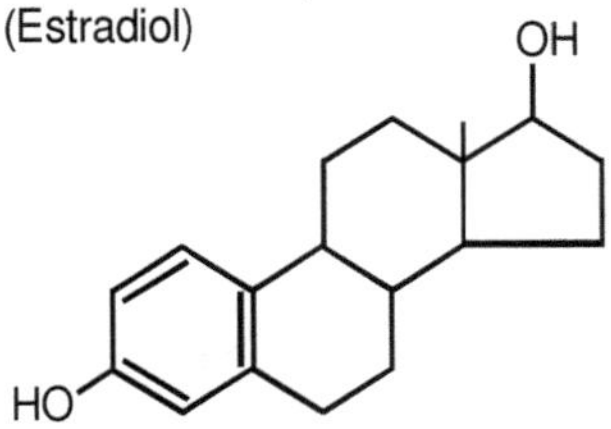	Streptomyces albus	3 - hydroxy, $\Delta^{1, 3, 5 (10)}$ Estr. 17-one 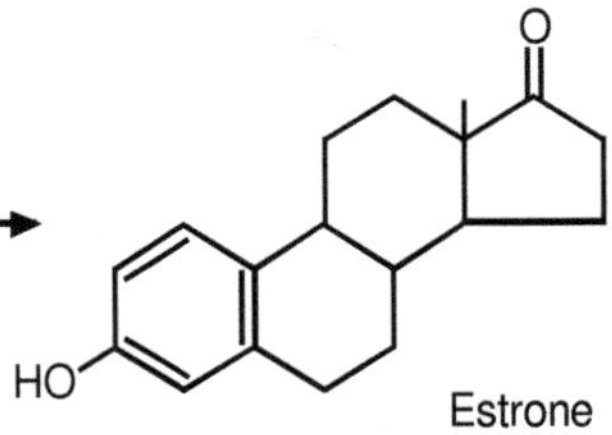 / Estrone
(3)	5 - androstene 3 β, 17 β - diol 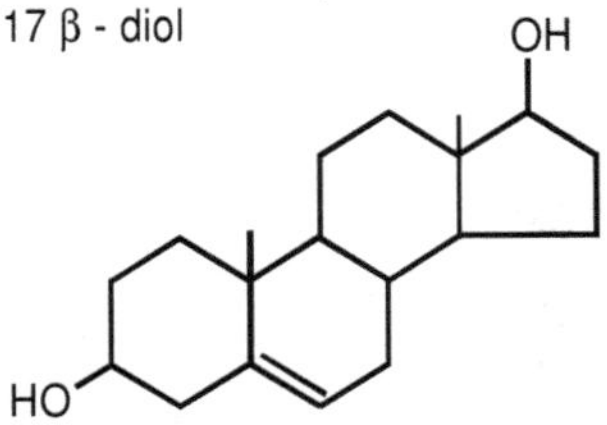	Flavobacterium species	17 hydroxy, Δ^4 Androst - 3 - one (Testosterone) 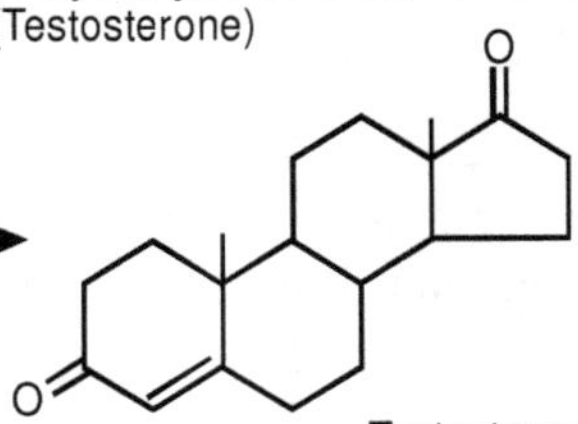 / Testosterone
(4)	Cholic-acid 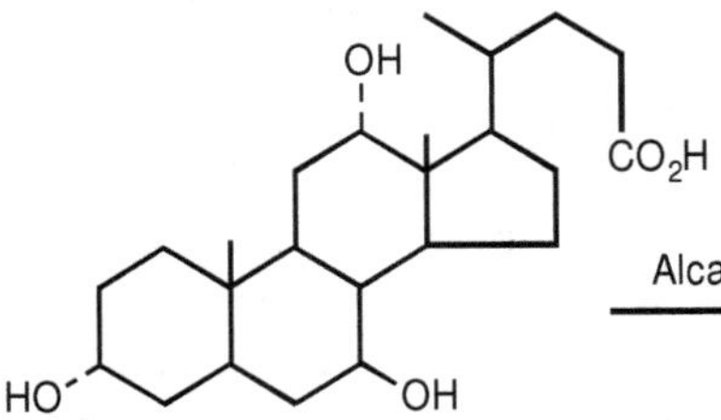	Alcaligenes faecales	3, 7, 12 Triketocholanic acid 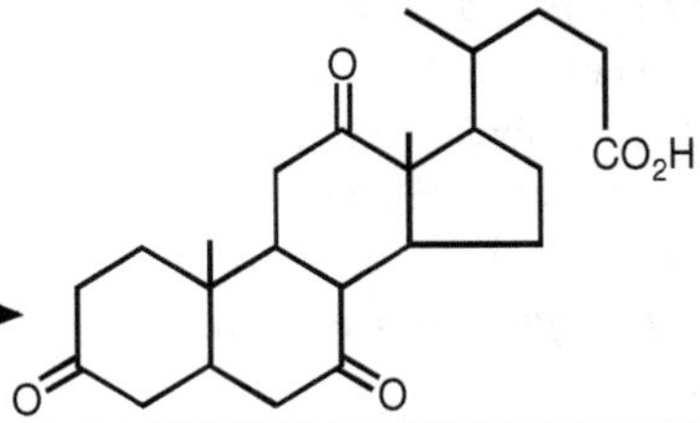
(5)	17 α Methyl 5-Pregnene, 3 β, 7 β, 20 β-triol 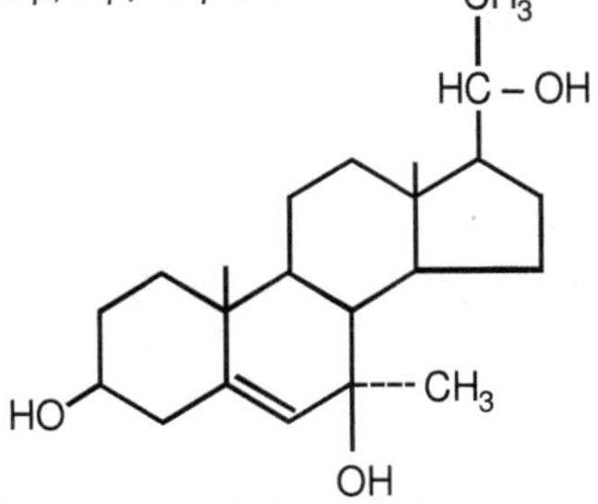	Flavanobacterium dehydrogenase	7 α Methyl - 4 Pregnene, 7 - β - ol - 3, 20 dione 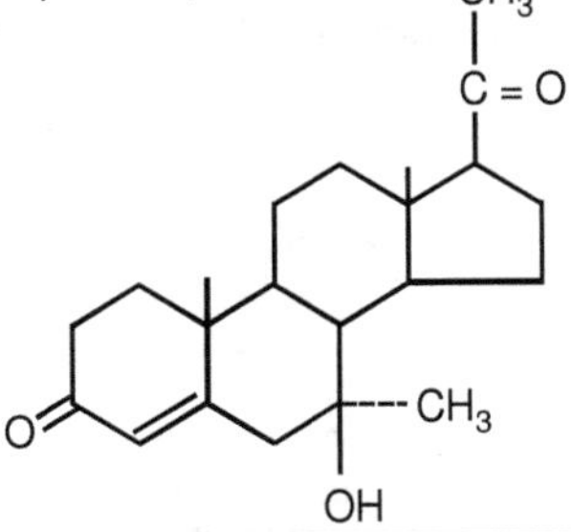

Table 4.4

Sr. No.	Name	Dehydrogenase	Hydroxylase
1.	Nocardia restrictus	Δ^1-dehydrogenase activity	9α-hydroxylase activity
2.	Nocardia corallina	Δ^1-dehydrogenase activity	$1\alpha, 2\alpha$ -dihydroxylase activity
3.	Myobacterium mucasum	Δ^4-dehydrogenase activity	9α-hydroxylase activity

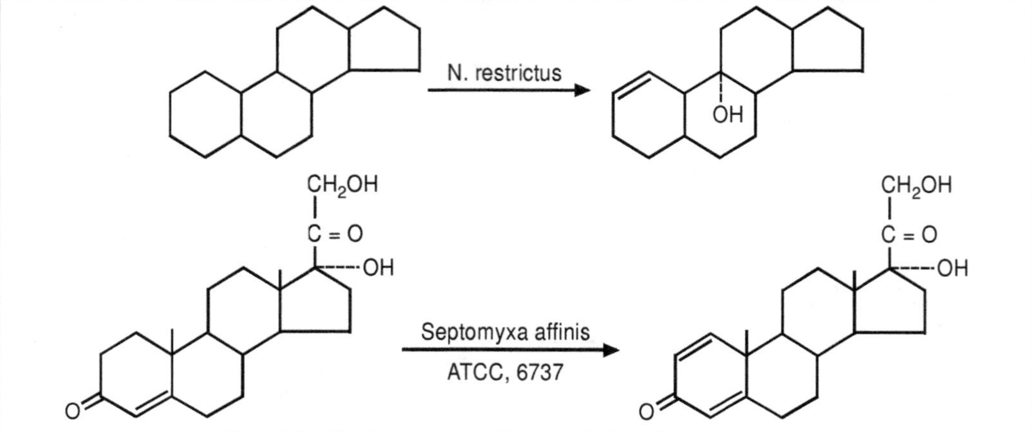

17 α, 21 - dihydroxy pregn - 4 - ene - 3, 20 - dione

These enzymes may function as Δ^1-dehydrogenators under aerobic condition and as Δ^1-reductases under anaerobic condition.

Blending of dehydrogenation and hydroxylase activities :

There are the few but definite examples of the microbial cell culture possessing both dehydrogenase and hydroxylase activities. (See Table 4.4)

Fungal spores and dehydrogenase activities :

Dehydrogenation of certain steroids with the spores of Septomyxa affinis ATCC 6737 and Fusarium solani aroused interest in the line.

(c) Epoxidation :

It is a very rare transformation. Bloom and Shull (1955) proposed that the micro-organisms which normally hydroxylate saturated steroid will epoxidize the unsaturated analog provided that the newly introduced hydroxyl function should be axial in nature. The epoxide oxygen shall have the same conformation (axial) as that of the hydroxyl group which is normally introduced at saturated C-atom. This explains why the initial steps of reaction are same for hydroxylation, and epoxidation although epoxides are not intermediate for hydroxylation.

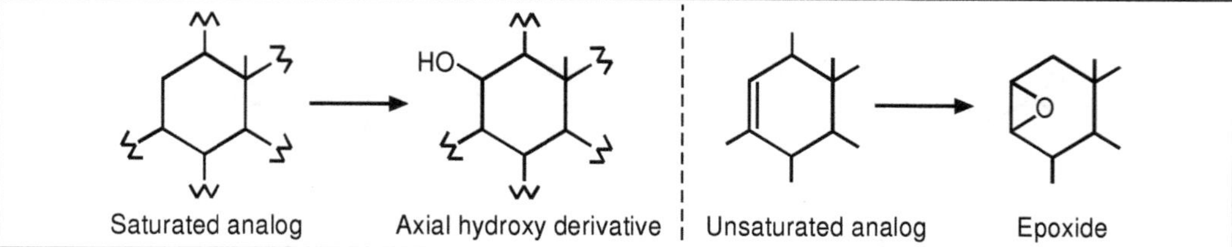

Saturated analog   Axial hydroxy derivative   Unsaturated analog   Epoxide

Bloom and Shull (1955) and Bloom and associates (1956) demonstrated the examples of epoxidation by using :

1) Curvalaria lunata and
2) Cunninghamella blakesleena, as follows.

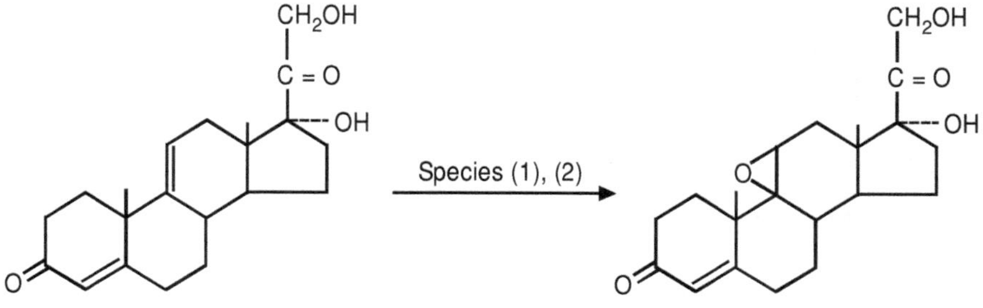

Δ^9 (11) - dehydro compound S → Species (1), (2) → 9β, 11β - epoxido - compound S

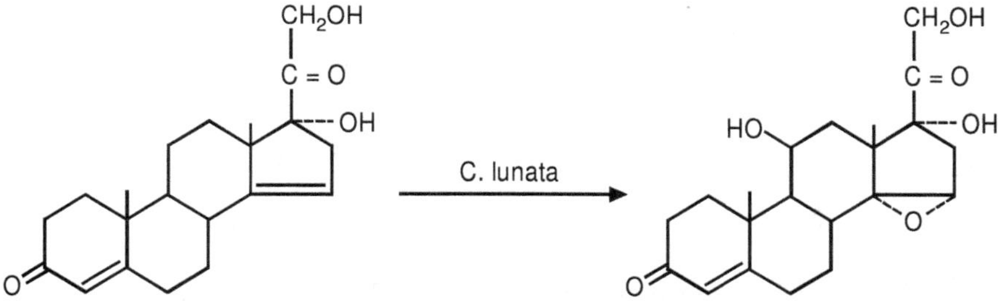

Δ^{14} - dehydro compound S → C. lunata → 14α, 15α - epoxido hydrocortisone

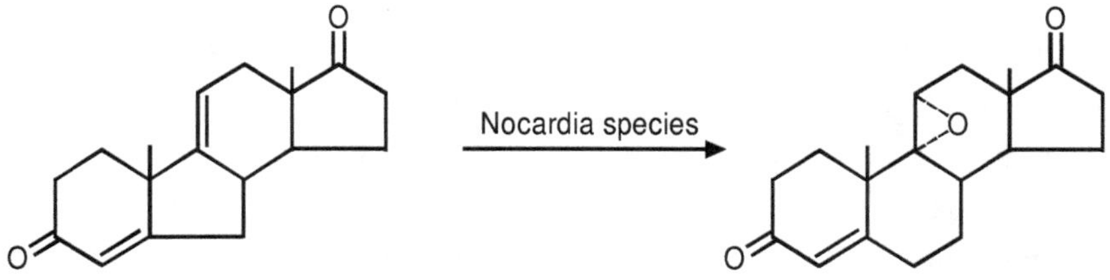

Δ^9 (11) - compound S → Nocardia species → 9α, 11α - epoxide

→ R. nigricans →

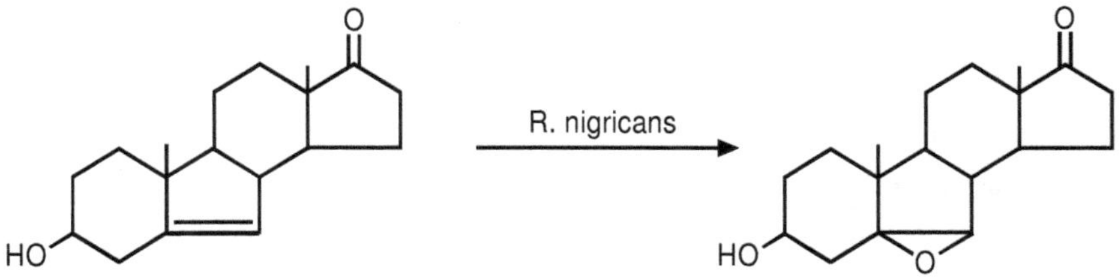

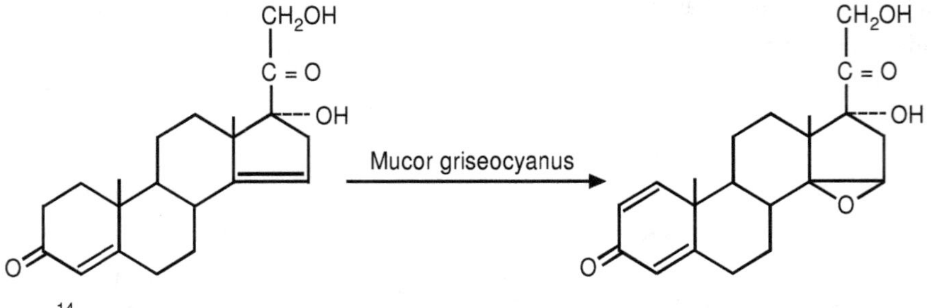

Δ^{14} - dehydro compound S → (Mucor griseocyanus) → 14α, 15α - epoxide compound S

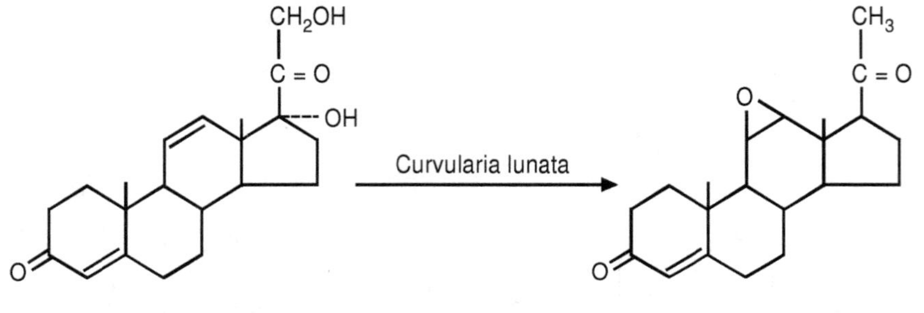

4, 11 - pegn - diene - 3, 20 - dione → (Curvularia lunata) → 11β, 12β - epoxide

Cultures which normally yield the 11α-hydroxy failed to form the 9, 11-epoxide from the corresponding olefin.

(d) Oxidative degradations of steroid :

The oxidative degradation of steroids leading to their conversion into CO_2 and H_2O involves many fundamental reactions. Many microbial genera exhibited their qualifications. Prominant amongst are Corynebacterium, Mycobacterium, Pseudomonas and Nocardia.

The sequential reactions involved may be immarised as follows :

Aromatization with the cleavage of ring B at 9, 10-position is followed by another microbial hydroxylation at C-4 to form a 3,4 dihydroxy-9,10-secophenolic compound.

Further degradation of ring A continues by removal of a fragment which yields pyruvate and propionaldehyde due to aldol type reactions while microbial degradation of remaining portion presents raw material for citric acid cycle.

The steroidal structure (substrate) governs the position (site) of microbial attack. The attack may initiate at the terminal of C-17 side chain or at the steroidal skeleton. In most of the cases, attack at the D-ring and/or in the A/B ring is recognized. A ring aromatization and associated B ring scission are regularly encountered in degradation reactions. But scission of the ring A without aromatization or scission of B ring alone has also been reported.

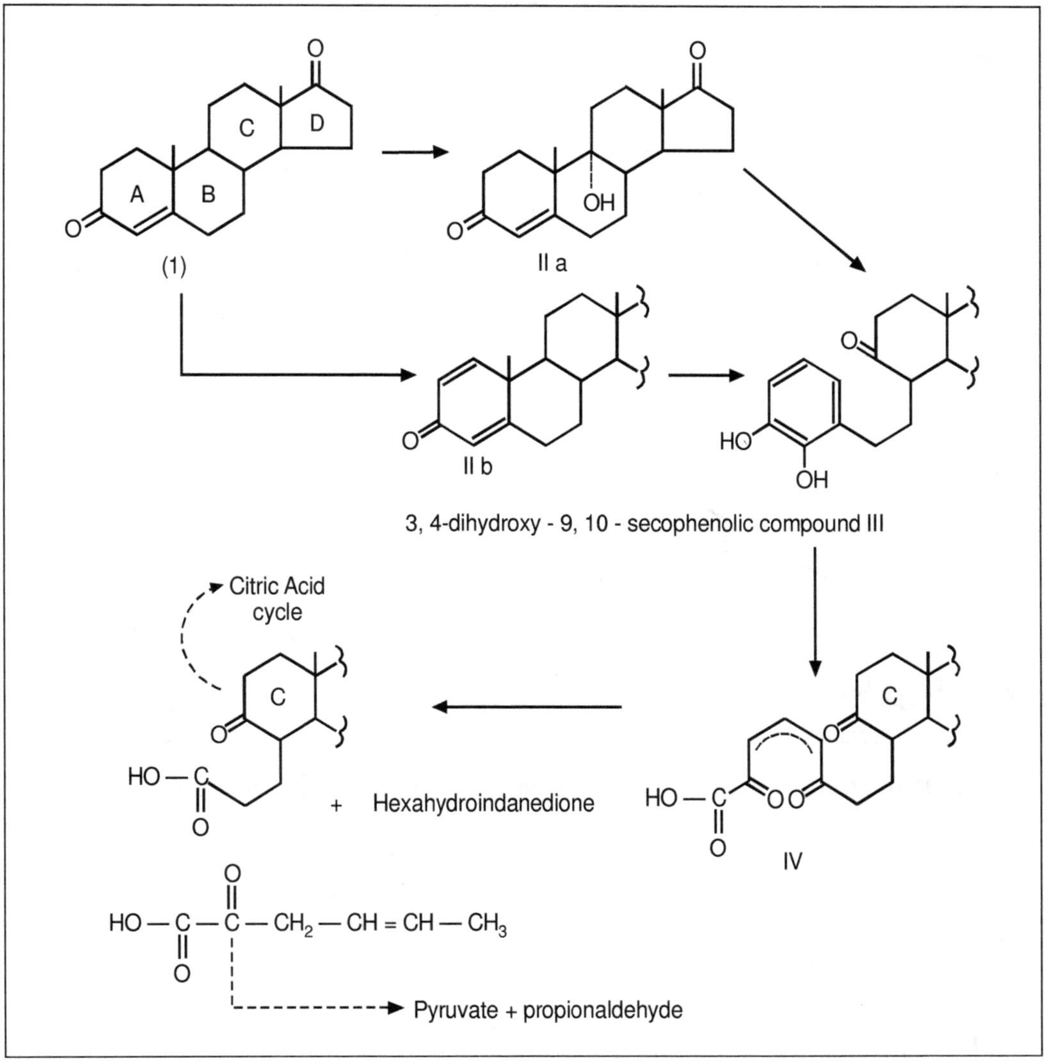

O
C
D
A
B
(1)
O
OH
II a
II b
HO
OH
3, 4-dihydroxy - 9, 10 - secophenolic compound III
Citric Acid cycle
C
HO — C
O
+ Hexahydroindanedione
HO — C
IV
HO — C — C — CH₂ — CH = CH — CH₃
Pyruvate + propionaldehyde

In another degradative study, the initial sequence is not found to be retained. The sequence of reactions is as follows :

(1) 19-hydroxylation

(2) Δ^1 -dehydrogenation

(3) Clevage of C-19 carbon atom.

(4) Aromatization of ring A → 9, 10-seco steroid.

In the degradation, where attack first initiated at side chain of steroid substrate, cleavage of one side-chain is effected by 26-hydroxylation, leading to the formation of 17-ketone.

Turfit in 1948, showed that pro-actinomyces was capable of degrading the side chain of 4-cholestenone to 3-Keto-4 etiocholenic acid.

Blending of activities :

Side-chain oxidation and Δ^1-dehydrogenation : The examples are shown in next table :

e.g. (1) Peterson et al (1953)

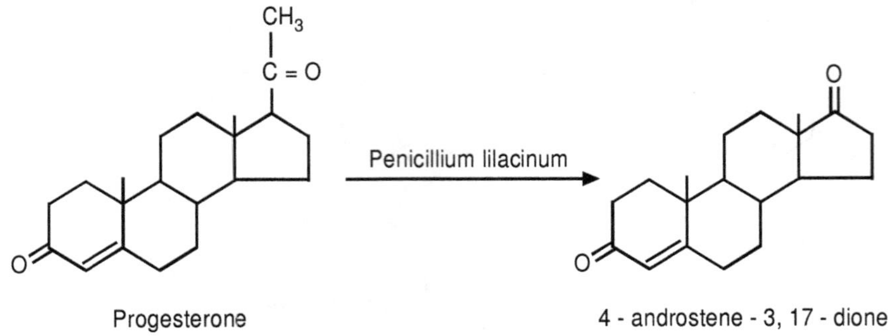

Progesterone →(Penicillium lilacinum)→ 4 - androstene - 3, 17 - dione

(2) Ciba group

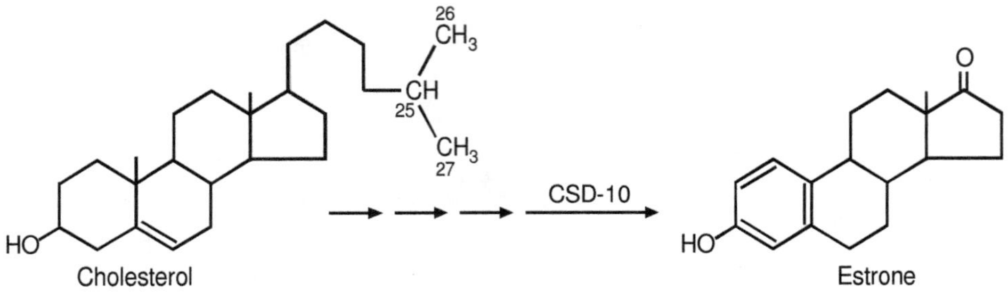

Cholesterol →→→(CSD-10)→ Estrone

CSD 10 : Culture isolated from soil using cholesterol as a sole source of carbon

(3)

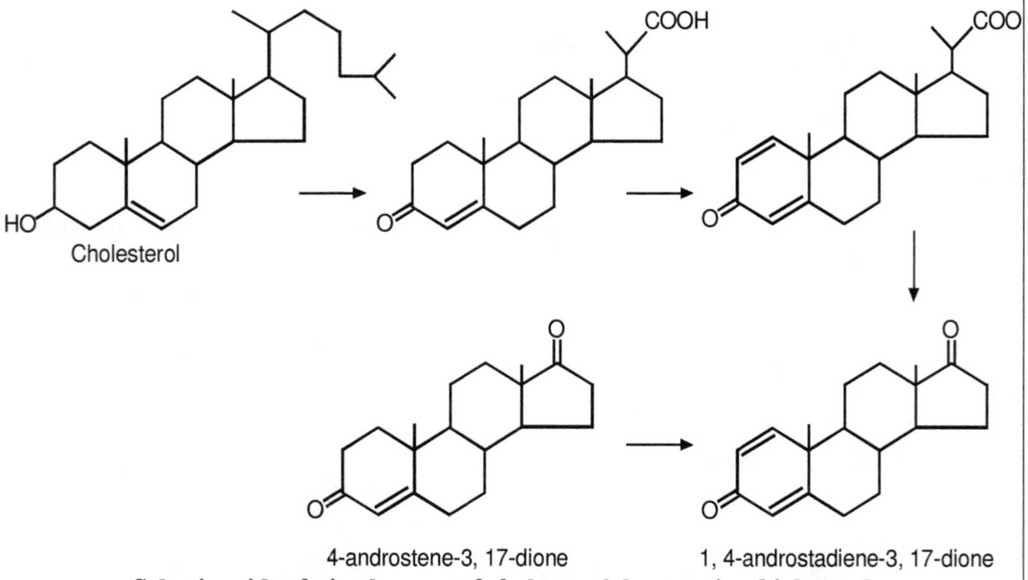

Cholesterol → → →

4-androstene-3, 17-dione → 1, 4-androstadiene-3, 17-dione

Selective side-chain cleavage of cholesterol due to microbial attack

(4)

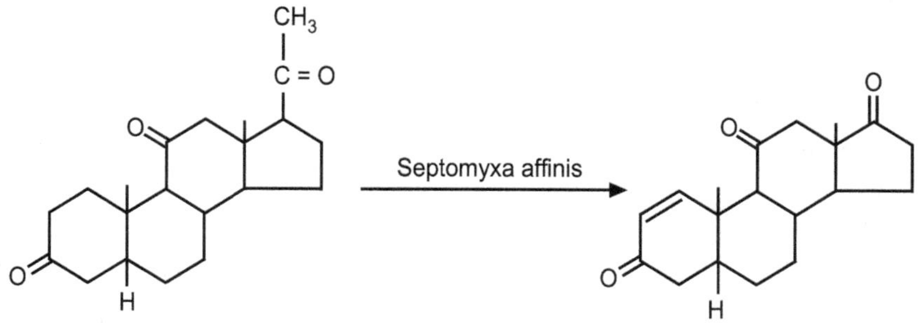

5βPregnane - 3, 11, 20 trione
(Allopregnane structure) → Septomyxa affinis → High yields

(5) Side-chain oxidation and hydroxylation : Peterson et al. 1953

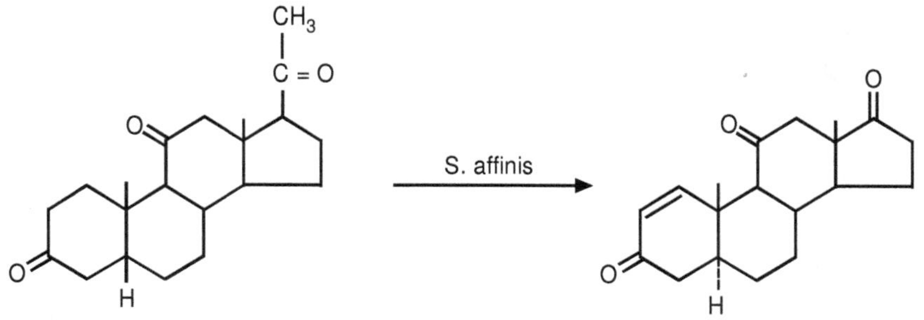

Pregnane - 3, 11, 20 trione → S. affinis → Low yields

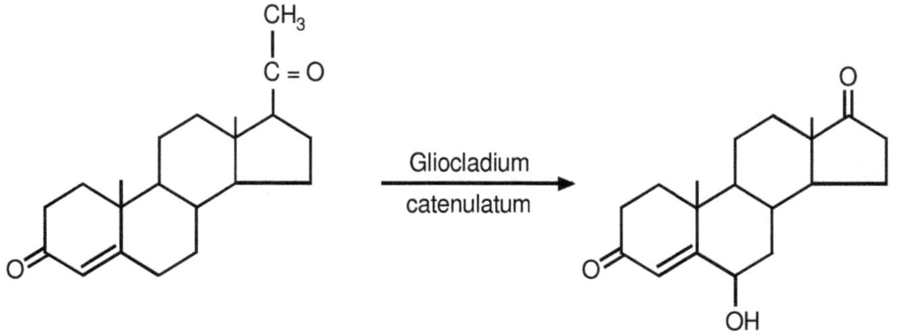

Progesterone → Gliocladium catenulatum → 4-androstene - 6β - ol - 3, 17-dione

4.14 REDUCTION

(a) Reduction of – C = C – (double bond) :

The reduction of C-C double bond or hydrogenation can be reviewed under following heads.

1. Reduction of ring double bonds.
2. Reduction of side chain double-bonds.

The enzymes are oxido-reductases which may catalyze both dehydrogenation and reduction reactions.

Decreased aeration or addition of ethanol to the fermentation increased the amount of reduced product.

Δ^1 Hydrogenation, Herzog et al 1959 :

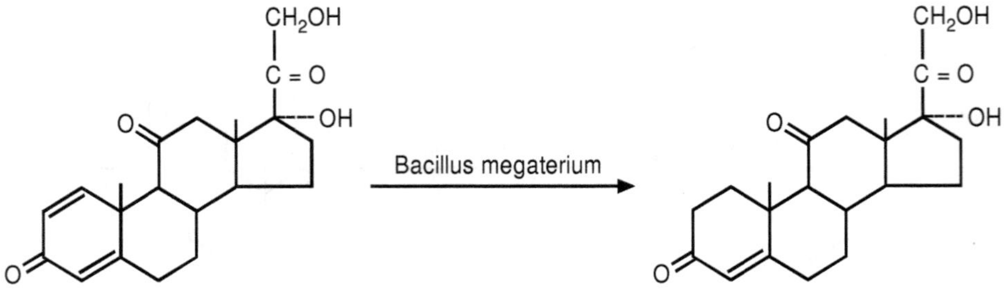

$$CH_2OH$$
$$C = O$$

Bacillus megaterium →

Prednisone

Cortisone

Δ^4 Hydrogenation, Mamoli et al 1939 :

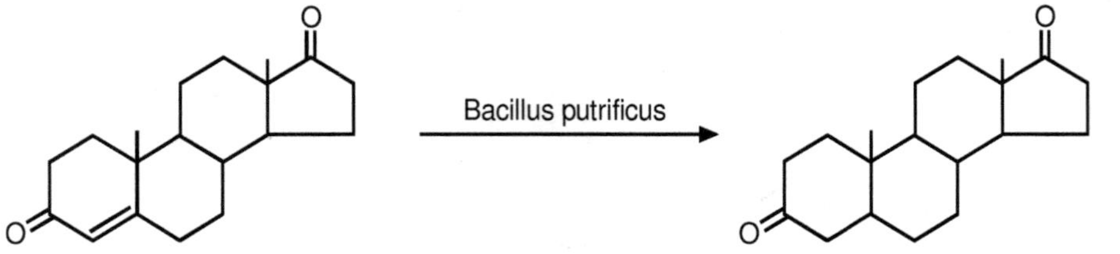

Bacillus putrificus →

4 - androstene - 3, 17 - dione

Androst - 3, 17 - dione

Δ^{16} Hydrogenation, Meister et al 1953 :

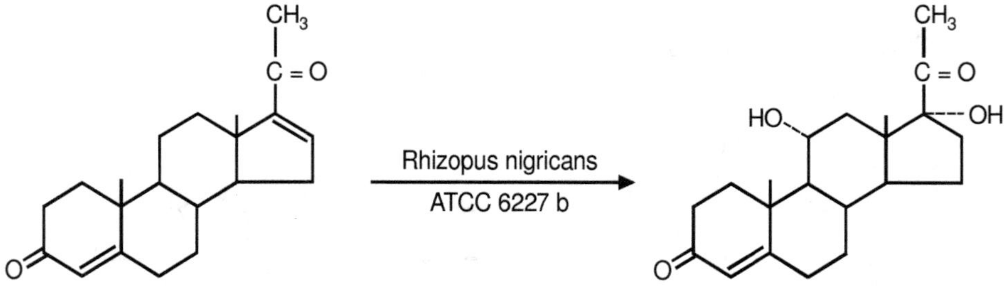

$$CH_3$$
$$C = O$$

Rhizopus nigricans
ATCC 6227 b →

Δ^{16} - Progesterone

11α - hydroxy - 17α - hydroxy - progesterone

Δ^1 - Hydrogenation alongwith 3 - Keto reduction

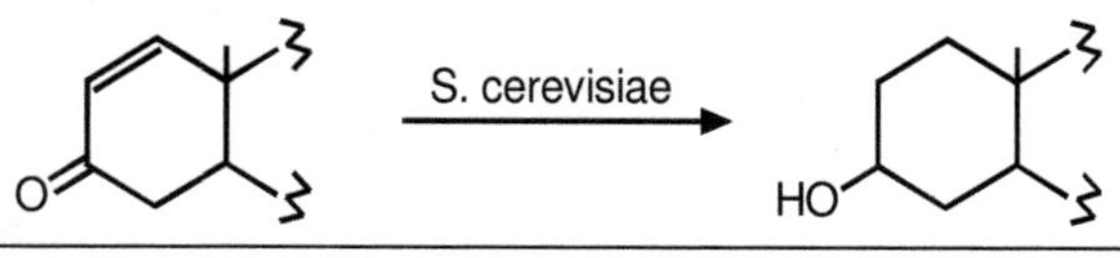

S. cerevisiae →

Selective Δ^4 - Hydrogenation

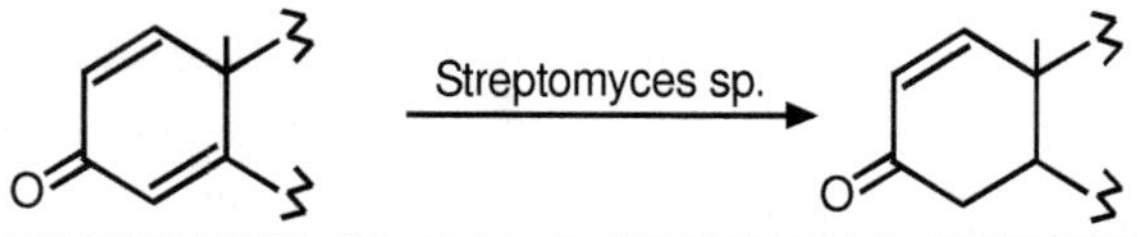

Streptomyces sp. →

Reduction of functional group in side-chain

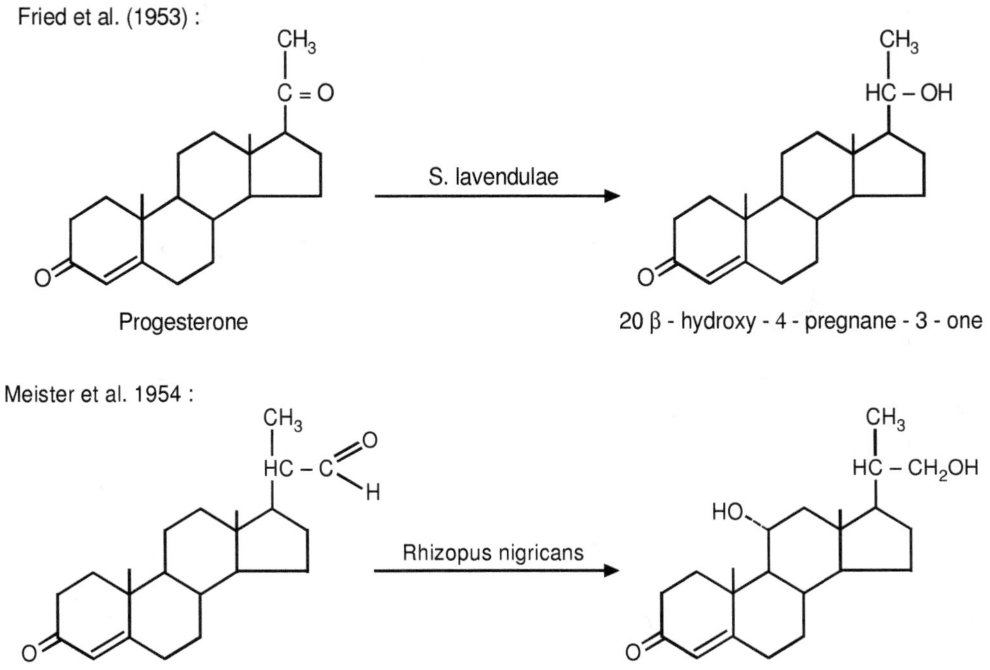

Fried et al. (1953) :
CH3
C = O
S. lavendulae
CH3
HC – OH
O
O
Progesterone
20 β - hydroxy - 4 - pregnane - 3 - one
Meister et al. 1954 :
CH3
HC – C
O
H
Rhizopus nigricans
CH3
HC – CH2OH
HO
O
O

(b) Reduction of ketones, aldehydes and acids :

Hydroxy to the oxy interconversion reactions require NAD^+ as a cofactor.

$$R_2C = O + NADH + H^+ \underset{}{\overset{\text{Enzyme}}{\rightleftharpoons}} R_2CHOH + NAD^+$$

The enzymes are generally termed as hydroxy steroid : NAD oxidoreductases regardless of whether they are utilised in forward reaction (reduction) or in backward (dehydrogenation) reaction.

Generally, the enzymes from Gram positive bacteria need NADP as a cofactor whereas that from Gram negative bacteria require NAD.

In the kinetic study of the 20-oxo-steroid reduction process, hydrogen transfer from the β-side of the pyridine ring of the cofactor NADH to the 20-oxo function so as to affect its reduction to alcholic function has been reported.

Generally, the hydroxyl groups at C_6, C_{11} and C_{17}, α-methyl group at C_{16} and Δ^1 unsaturation lead to decrease in reduction rate. The presence of electron withdrawing groups at the C-6 in 3 Keto-Δ^4 substrate, shift the direction from oxidation to reduction. Thus electron density on carbonyl carbon is important in determining equilibrium.

Table 4.5 : Reduction of Ketone Function to Hydroxyl

S. N.	Substrate	Product
1.	5α - pregn-3, 11, 20-trione 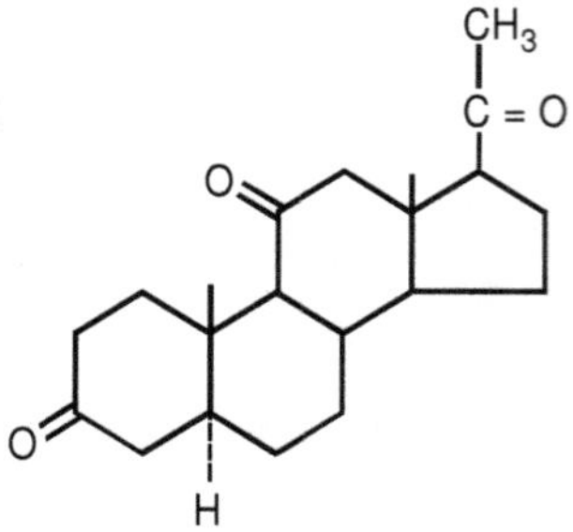	3 α OH derivative 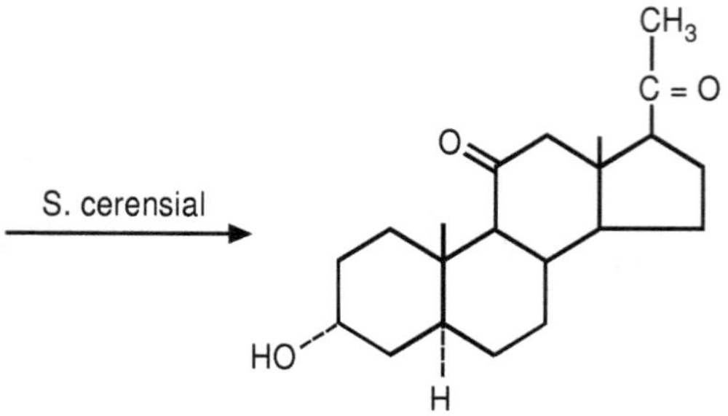
2.	5β - pregn-3, 11, 20-trione 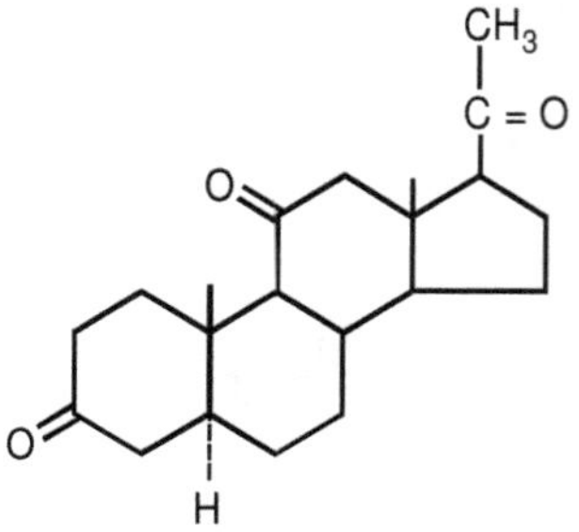	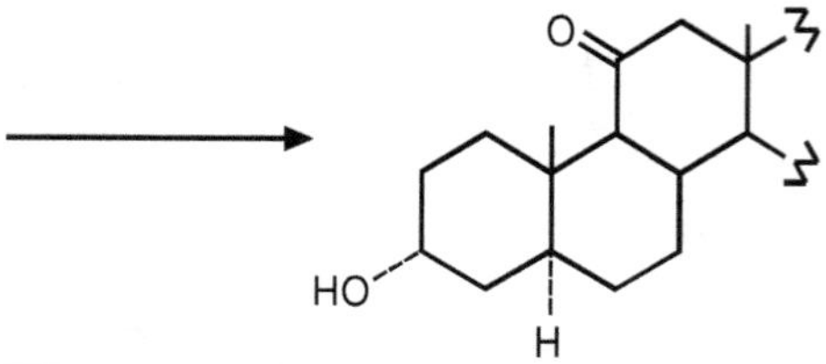
3.	5α Hydrogen, 11α hydroxy pregn-3, 20-dione 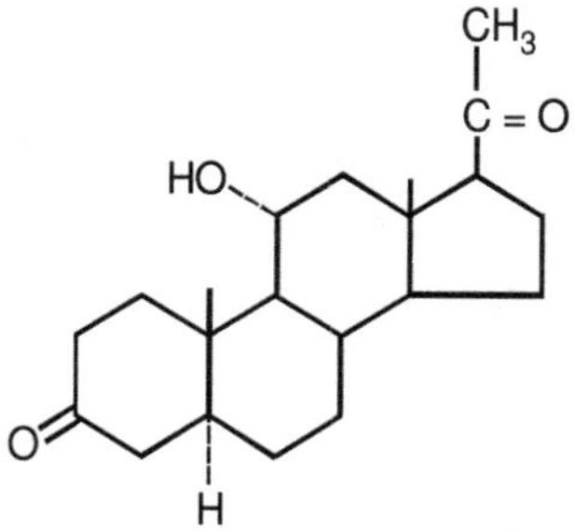	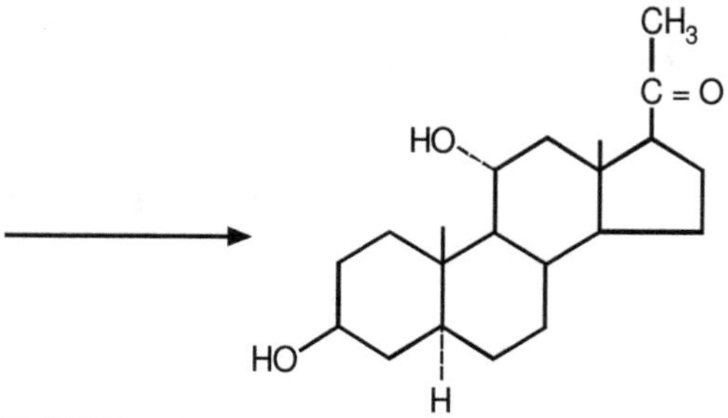
4.	5α, 1-androsten-3, 17-dione 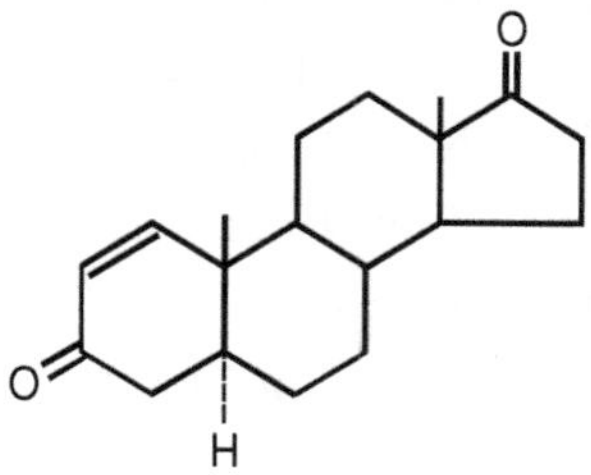	5α androst-3β, 17β-dione 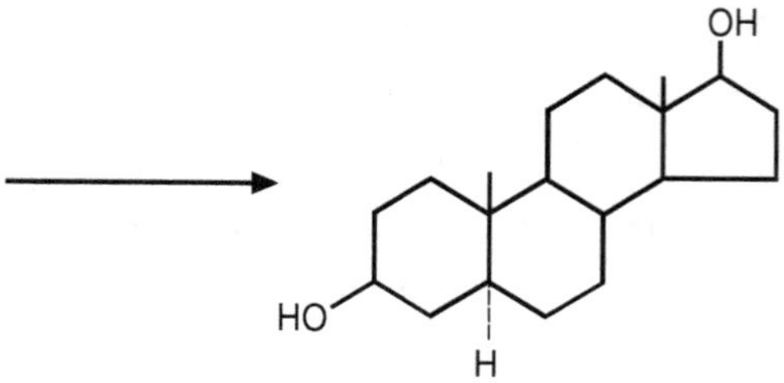

5.		Selective steriospecific reduction of only one Ketone group →
6.	19 - hydroxy - 4 androstene - 3, 17 - dione	Nocardia sp. → Estrone
7.	Progesterone	S. lavendulae →

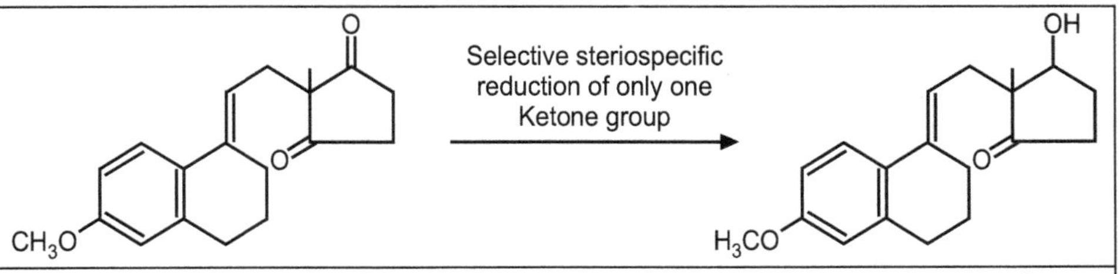

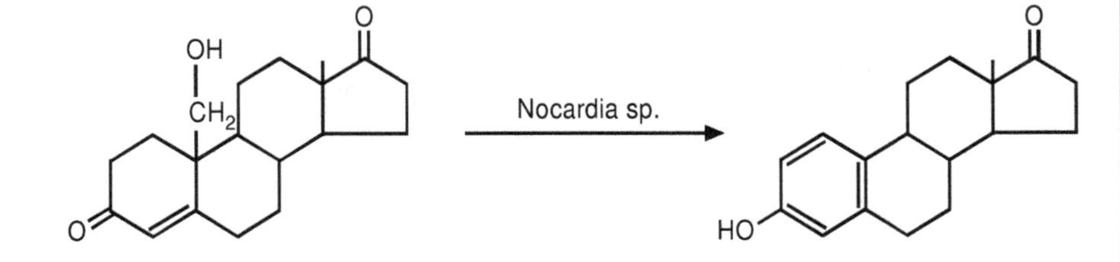

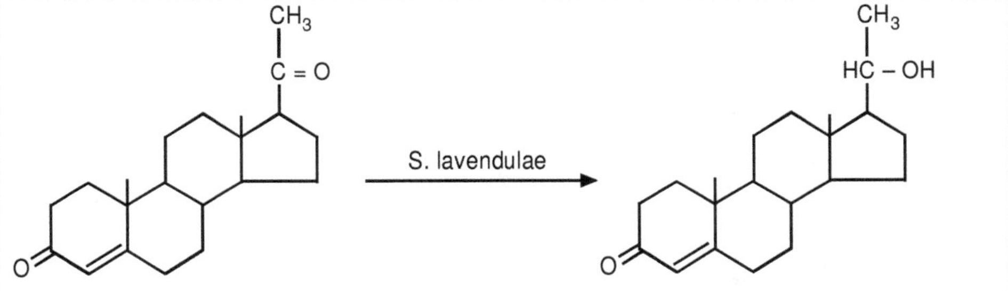

Ringold and his associates showed that Pseudomonas testosteroni reduces the 3-keto group of testosterone only when the latter is either florinated at 2α, 4, 6α, or 6β position or chlorinated at C-4.

Reduction of 7-ketone to 7α-hydroxyl has been reported with Streptomyces gelaticus and Corynebacterium species. Similarly, the reduction of C-20 ketone function is also reported.

4.15 ESTERIFICATION, AMIDE FORMATION AND HYDROLYSIS

(a) Esterification :

Unlike other transformations, esterification is a reaction rarely witnessed and reported in literature. The first report is from Holmlund and associates.

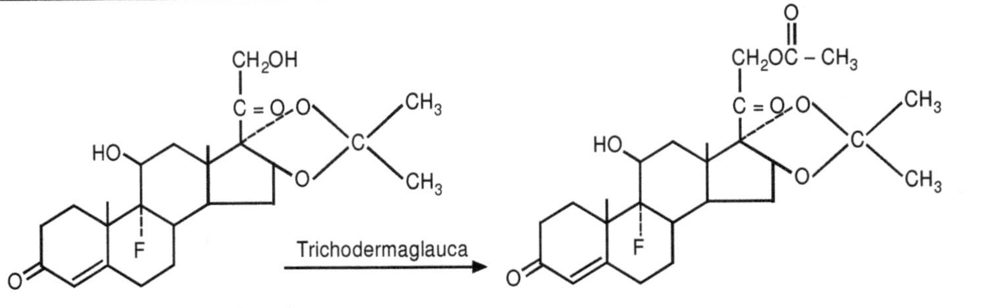

16, 17 - acetonide of 9 α - fluoro - 16 α hydroxy hydrocortisone

Trichodermaglauca →

In another report, esterification was effected by using strains of Sacchromyces fragilis.

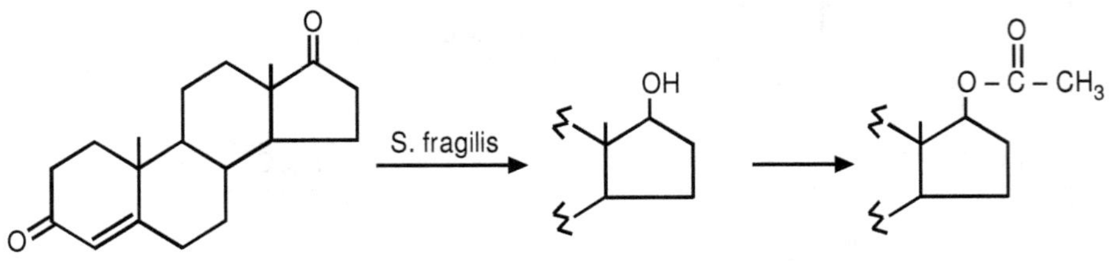

4 - androsten - 3, 17 - dione   Intermediate (Testosterone)   Testosterone acetate

Oxidation of ketone to ester is also documented by Fried, Thoma and Klingsberg.

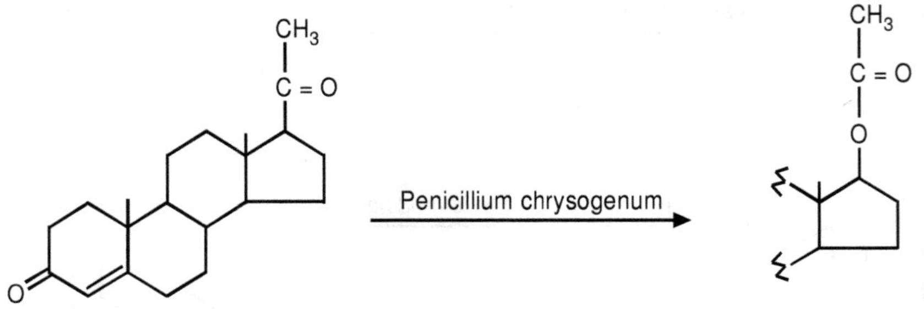

Progesterone

(b) Amide formation :

It is relatively rare microbial transformation e.g. by smith and coworkers.

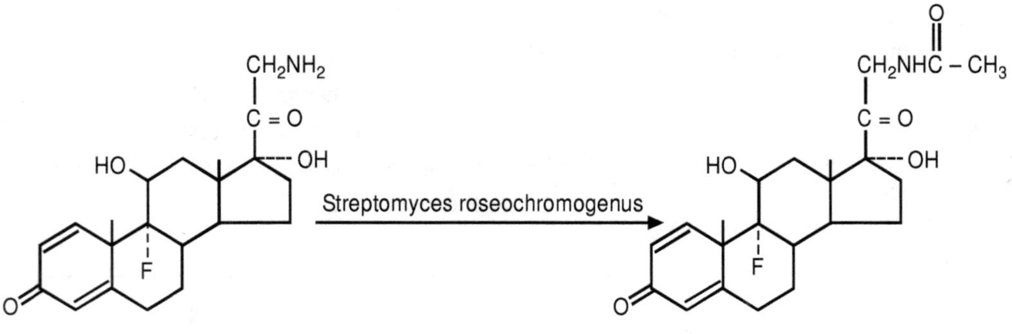

21 - amino - 9α - fluoro -
11 β, 17α - dihydroxy -
1, 4 - pregnadiene - 3, 20 - dione

(c) Hydrolysis :

The wide spread occurrence of esterases capable of hydrolysing steroid esters is evidenced by the fact that 3 and 21-acetates are generally hydrolyzed prior to hydroxylation or dehydrogenation. Ester hydrolysis is also frequently accompanied by Δ^1-dehydrogenation.

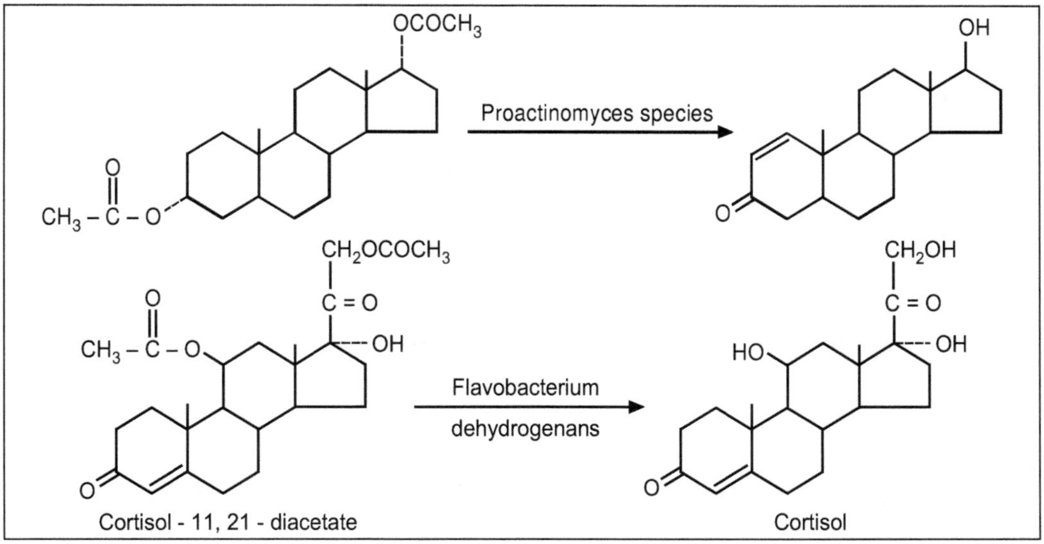

Mechanism of Reaction :

The mechanism of microbial hydrolysis of steroid ester was proposed by Blender and Kezdy which has a close resemblance with the mechanism of hydrolysis of acetylcholine by cholinestrase enzymes in human.

The proposed mechanism can be presented as :

(1) The enzyme surface provides required imidazole moiety and a hydroxyl group.

(2) Water participates in
  (a) Cleavage of steroid ester linkage, and
  (b) Regeneration of the enzyme hydroxyl site.

Unlike esters, the epoxides are relatively resistant to esterase enzymes. In 1959, Camerino and Schiaky reported an epoxide hydrolysis with fermenting yeast.

An attempt to study the hydrolysis of steroid glycosides was made by Brack, Renz and coworkers by using fungi-Aspergillus and Penicillium sp.

It is a matter of doubt whether to call this reaction as hydrolysis or transglycosylation.

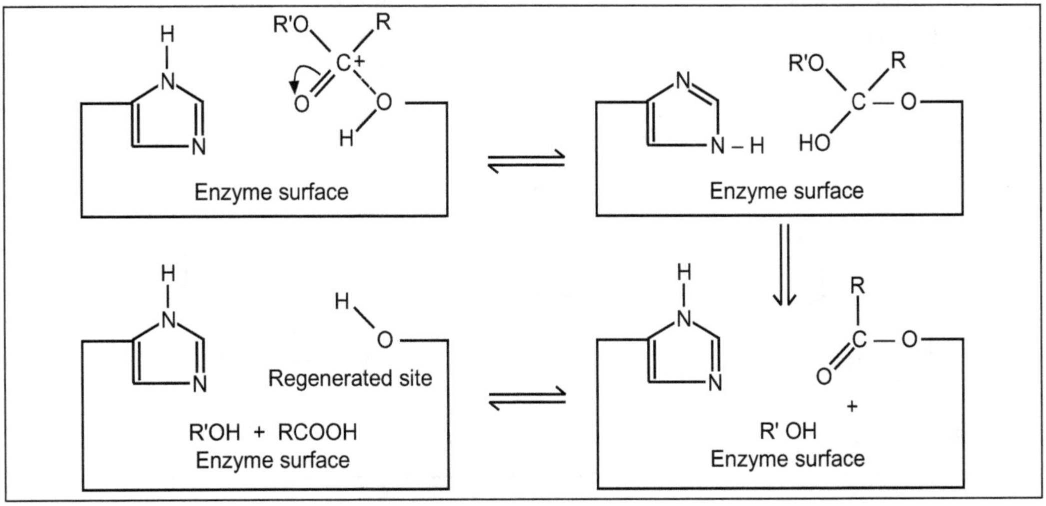

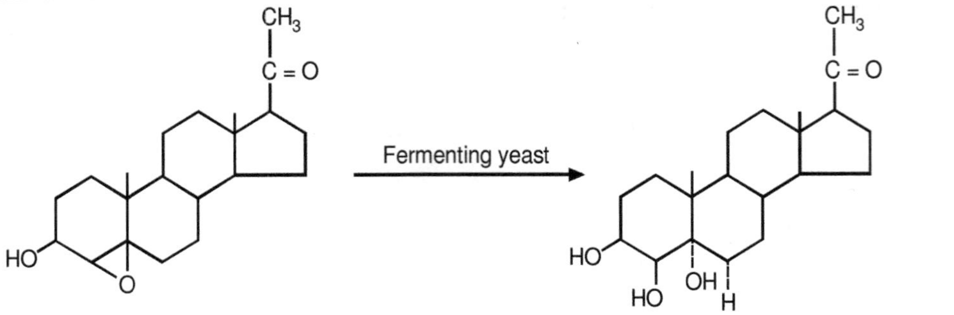

4β - 5 - epoxyprogesterone

Allopregnane - 3α 4β, 5α - triol - 20 - one

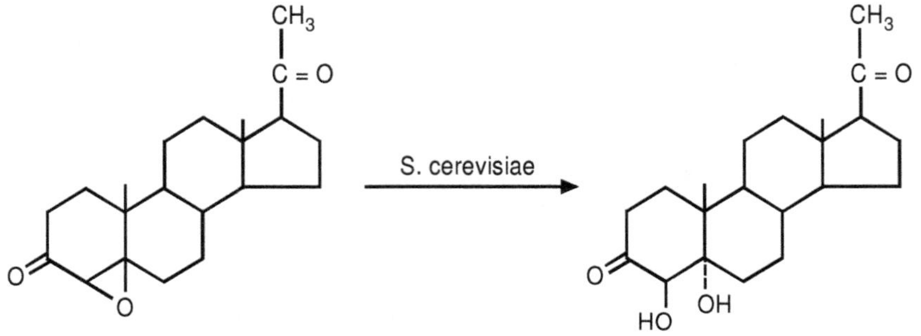

S. cerevisiae

Glycol with diaxial opening

4.16 OLEFINIC BOND ISOMERISATION

Although isomerisation of the double bond From Δ^5 to Δ^4 as among the reactions first recognised by Mamoli with Corynebacterium mediolanum, isomerase enzyme from Pseudomonas testosteroni ATCC 11996 has been extensively studied.

In these and other similar reactions although the A^5-double bond isomerisation is a separate reaction from the hydroxy steroid dehydrogenation, isomerization generally accompanies dehydrogenation of the 3-alcohol resulting into corresponding Δ^4-3 oxo-steroid.

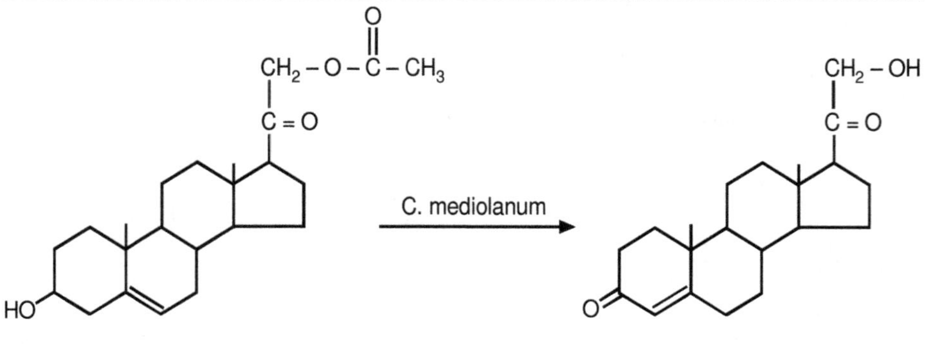

3β, 21 - dihydroxy - 5 - Pregnen - 20 - one - 21 - acetate

Deoxycorticosterone

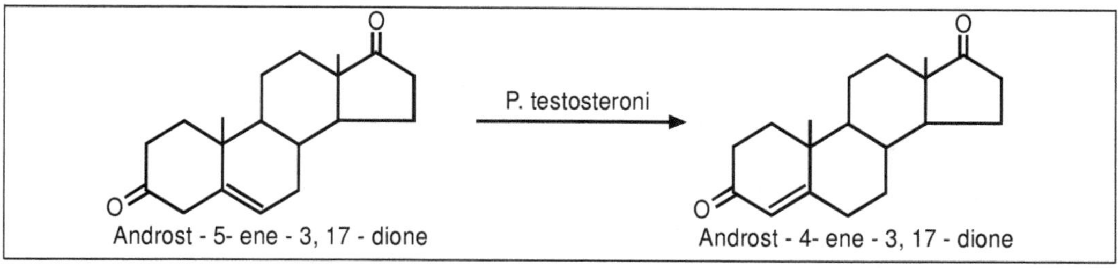

Androst - 5- ene - 3, 17 - dione → (P. testosteroni) → Androst - 4- ene - 3, 17 - dione

The isolated Δ^5-isomerases from P. testosteroni found to exist as a trimer of identical subunits containing about 125 amino acid residues. The sequence is well in order and has a very high percentage of β-structure as a pleated sheets.

Estradiol, 17β-dehydroequilenin, 19-nortestosterone, vinca and ergot alkaloids and some deoxyribonucleoside analogues are found to inhibit isomerase activity of P. testosteroni.

Reaction mechanism :

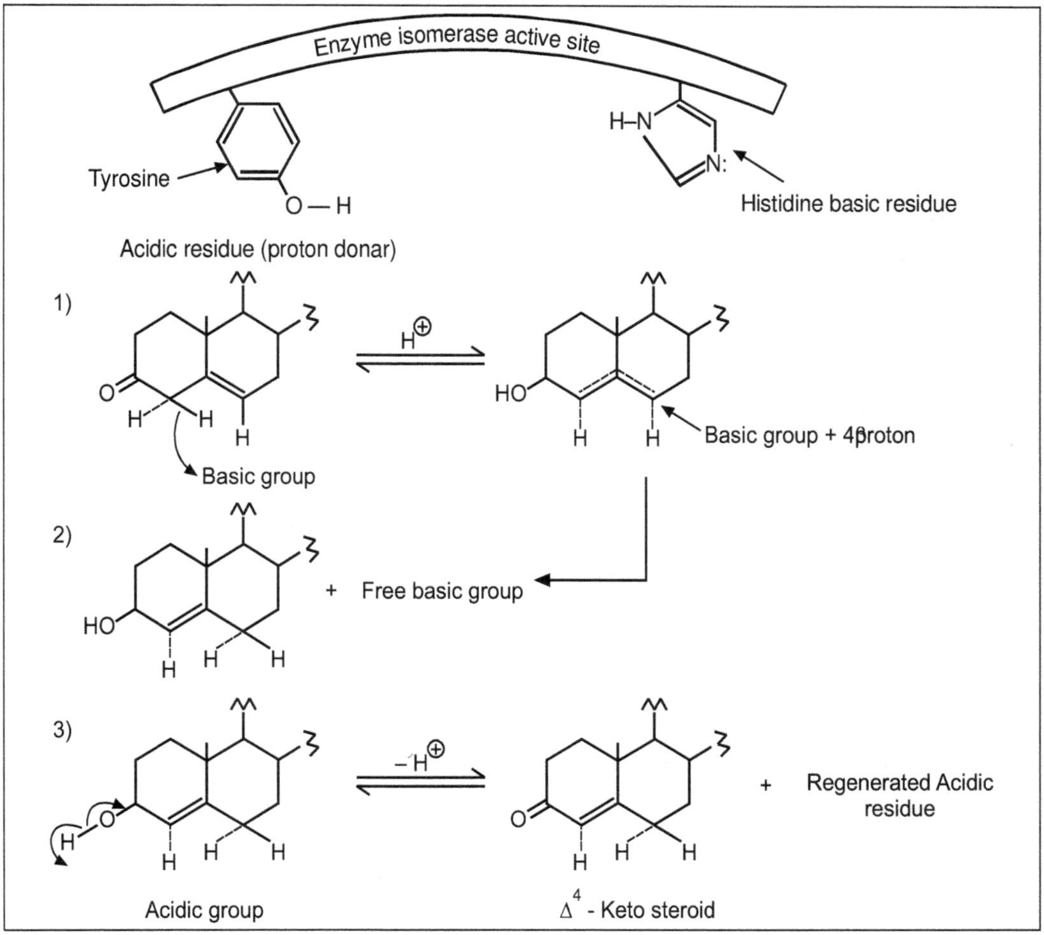

The enzyme surface possesses an acidic residue (proton-donor) tyrosine and a basic residue-probably a histidine moiety. The reaction sequence starts with an enolization of

the 3-keto function with specific transfer of the 4β-hydrogen to the 6β-position. Enolization is affected by protonation of the 3-keto group by a proton donar, followed by loss of the 4β proton at the 6β-position.

In the last step, 3-keto group is regenerated by deprotonation whereby the acidic residue receives back its proton.

If the concentration of organic solvent in the aqueous medium is increased, the affinity of the substrate for the enzyme decreases. Thus it bears a inversely proportional relationship.

4.17 MISCELLANEOUS REACTIONS

(a) Aromatization :

Like in mammalian systems microbial aromatization had also been reported in 1958 by Dodson and Muir.

Aromatization with cleavage of side chain :

In 1957, Levy and Talalay examplified aromatization by using Pseudomonas testosteroni. Generally, Pseudomonal sp. ATCC 6737, Nocardia sp. (N. restrictus), Septomyxa affinis and Corynebacterium simplex are the most commonly used cultures.

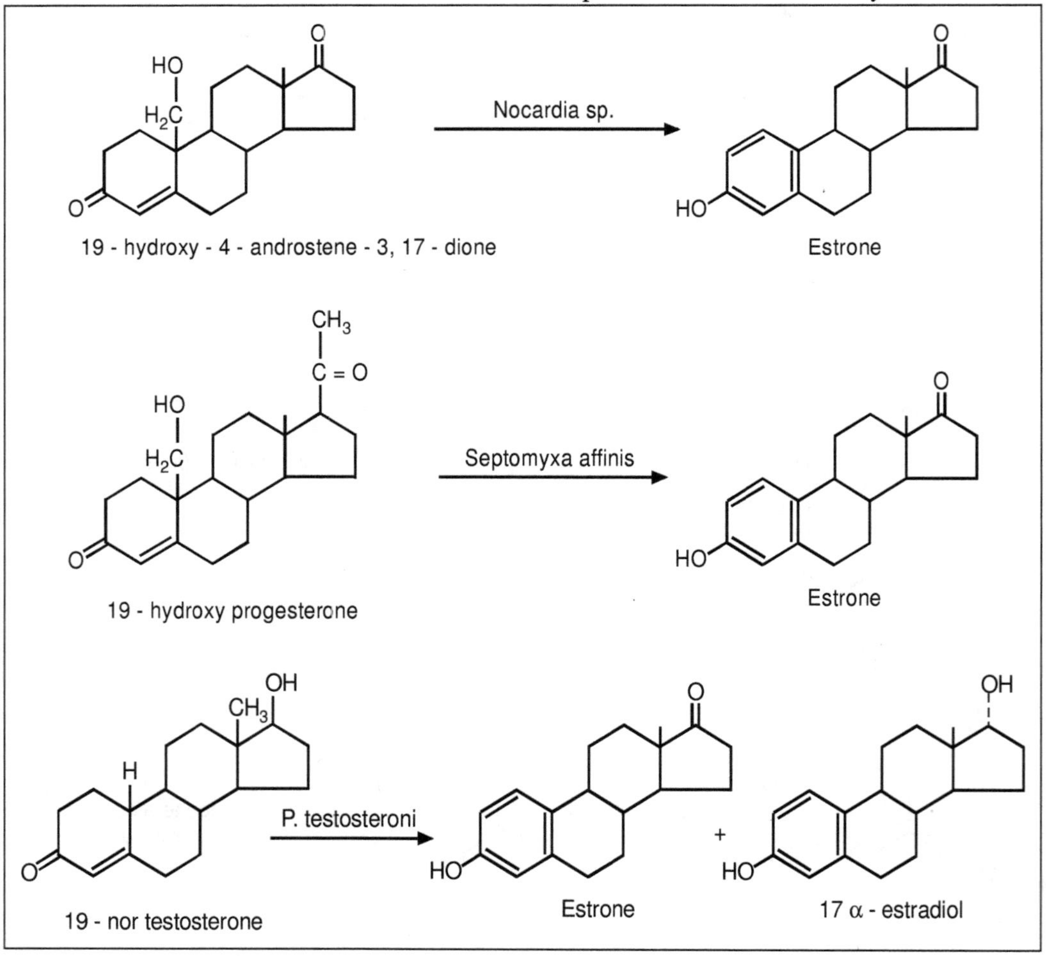

19 - hydroxy - 4 - androstene - 3, 17 - dione → Nocardia sp. → Estrone

19 - hydroxy progesterone → Septomyxa affinis → Estrone

19 - nor testosterone → P. testosteroni → Estrone + 17 α - estradiol

(b) Halogenation :

Haloperoxidase enzymes from Caldariomyces fumago catalyze the halogenation reactions of steroid.

Reaction is carried out at pH 3 and incubating at 25°C.

An important feature of this transformation is, it can neither be categorised under oxidation nor under reduction.

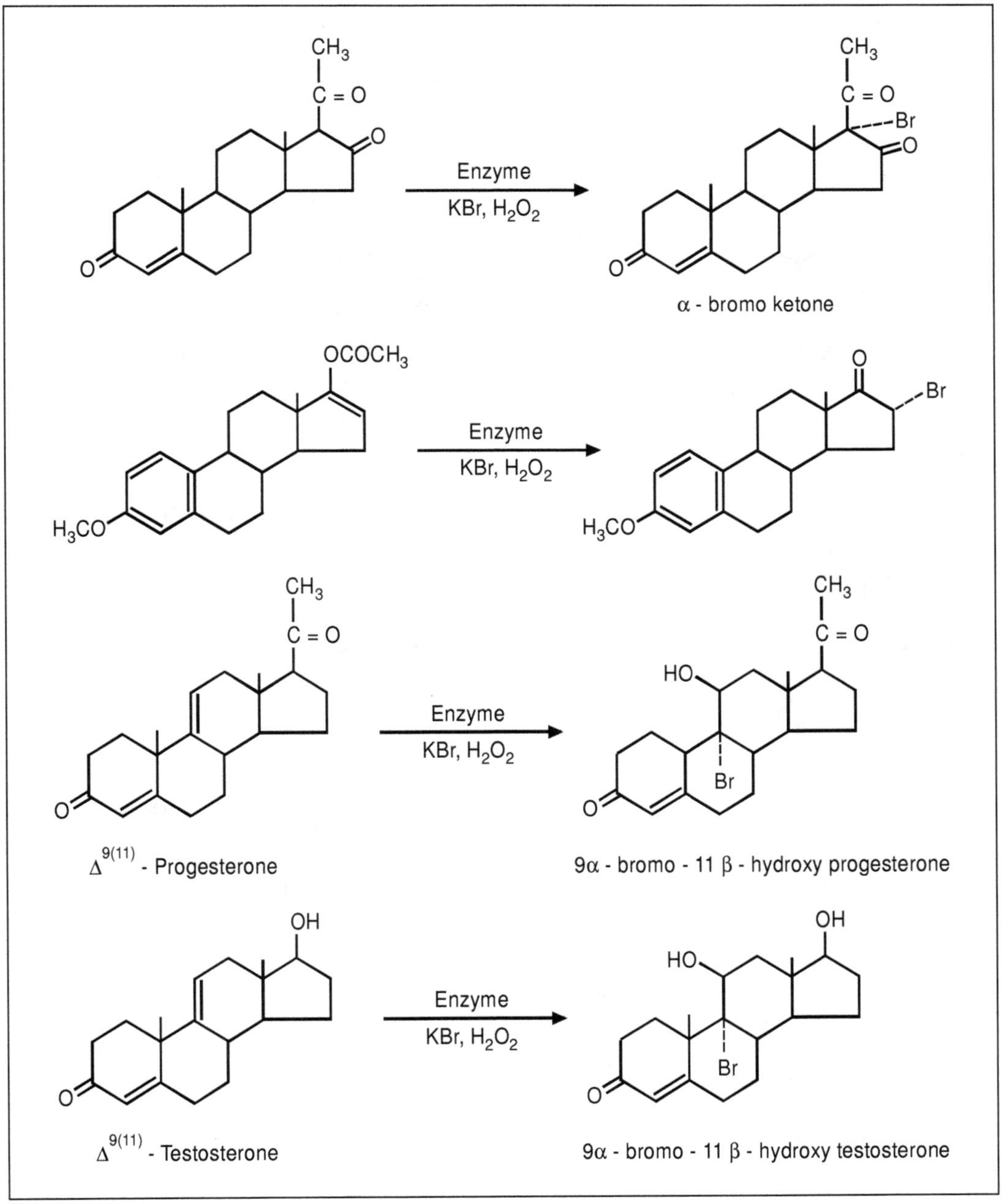

Summary :

The remarkable similarity of microbial and mammalian systems in steroid metabolism gave birth to microbial coversions of steroidal compounds. Microbiology and sterodial chemistry had been moulded together to search out valuable adjunct to a chemical synthesis of the complex steroid hormones and their analogues. On the basis of cost benefits if pharmaceutical industries are keen to adopt microbial processes, the latter should show high conversion efficiencies in the presence of large substrate concentration and also site specificity. Enzyme inhibitors or mutagenic treatment are but only some of the tools employed to achieve this goal.

Microbiology employed in the synthesis of steroid hormones :

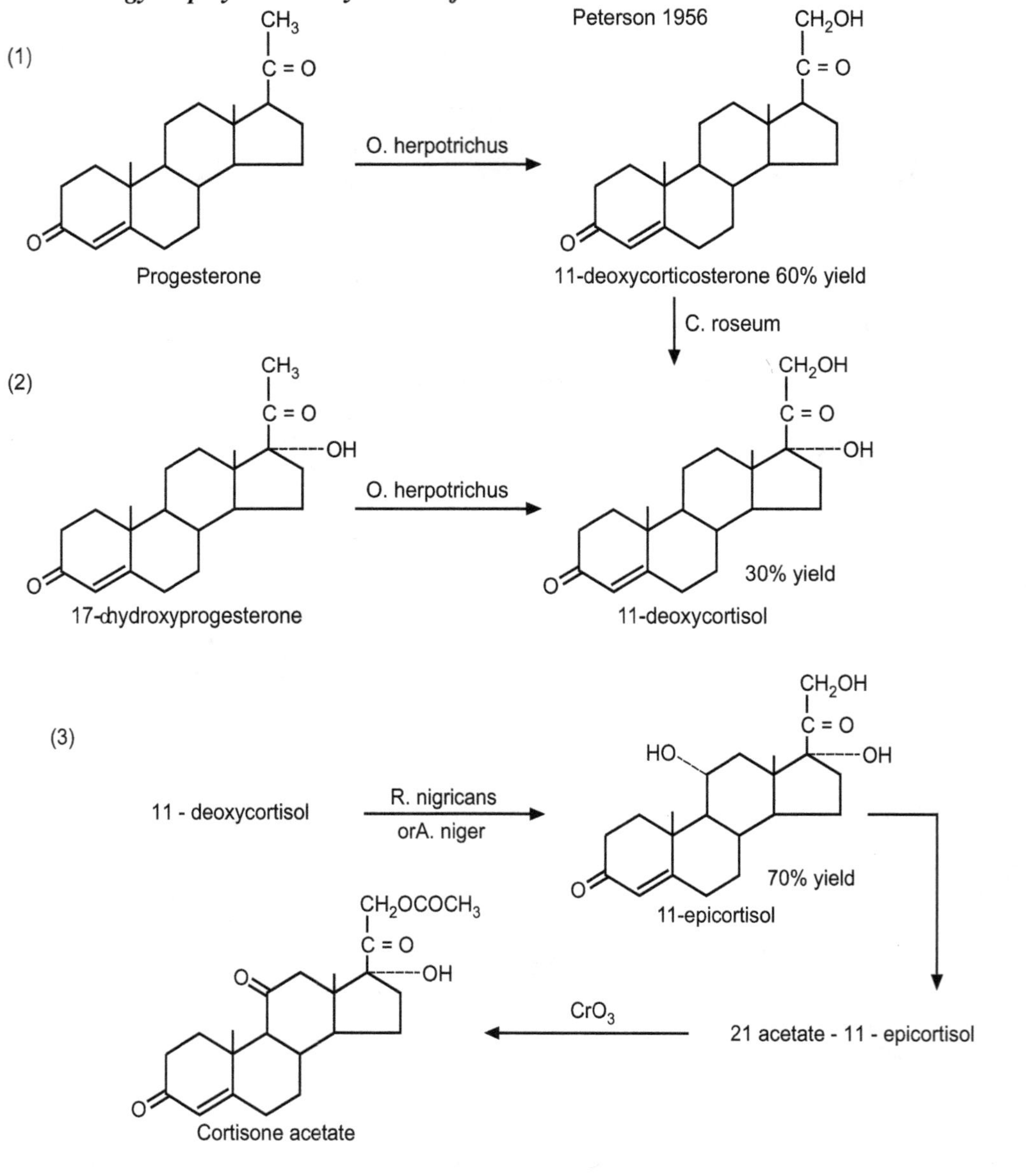

(1) Progesterone → O. herpotrichus → 11-deoxycorticosterone 60% yield (Peterson 1956)

↓ C. roseum

(2) 17-αhydroxyprogesterone → O. herpotrichus → 11-deoxycortisol 30% yield

(3) 11 - deoxycortisol → R. nigricans orA. niger → 11-epicortisol 70% yield → 21 acetate - 11 - epicortisol → CrO$_3$ → Cortisone acetate

Drug Design · 4.47 · *Microbial Bioconversions in Steroids*

(4) 11 - deoxycortisol $\xrightarrow{\text{C. blakesleeana}}$ Cortisol (60 - 70% yield)

(5) 11 - deoxycorticosterone $\xrightarrow{\text{C. blakesleeana}}$ Corticosterone (45% yield)

(6) Progesterone $\xrightarrow{\text{F. solani}}$ $\xrightarrow{\text{Yeast}}$ Testosterone

(7) 19 - hydroxy androstenedione $\xrightarrow{\text{N. restrictus}}$ Estrone

❖ ❖ ❖

5

MICROBIAL BIOCONVERSIONS IN PROSTAGLANDIN

(A) MICROBIAL BIOCONVERSION IN PROSTAGLANDINS

5.1 INTRODUCTION

In 1933, Maurice Goldblatt and Von Euler independently found that a humoral principle present in the human seminal fluid leads to both smooth muscle contraction and vaso-constriction. Euler (1935) identified the lipid soluble nature of that component and gave the name, prostaglandin to these substances in the belief that the biologically active substance found in the human semen was a secretion of the prostate gland. He defined prostaglandin as a "lipid soluble smooth muscle stimulating and blood pressure lowering factor with acidic properties in human seminal fluid and some accessory genital glands of man and sheep".

The work on the identification of prostaglandins was commenced by Bergstrom (1949). He recognized the presence of more than one unsaturated hydroxy fatty acid in partially purified prostaglandin extracts. The isolation in pure crystalline form from sheep vesicular glands of the first two prostaglndins, now called prostaglandin E_1 (PGE_1) and prostaglandin $F_{1\alpha}$ ($PGF_{1\alpha}$) was reported by Bergstrom and Sjovall in 1957. Later, additional compounds having related structures were isolated from different organs. The natural prostaglandins are hydroxylated C_{20}-polyunsaturated fatty acids having extensive and varied activities in mammalian system, such as :

(a) stimulating or relaxing uterine smooth muscles,

(b) constriction of bronchi,

(c) lowering or raising blood pressure,

(d) inhibiting gastric secretions,

(c) mediating inflammation,

(f) promoting sodium ion excretion, and

(g) inducing labour.

Thus, they qualify to be called as local hormones.

Occurrence :

Although prostaglandins were first discovered in seminal plasma and in vesicular glands, their distribution is not restricted to the male accessory genital glands and their secretions. Prostaglandins are known to be distributed widely in mammals. They can be extracted from most animal tissues. The total prostaglandin production in the adult human is 1 to 2 mg per day. Human seminal fluid contains the highest concentration and greatest number of Prostaglandins (about 31 prostaglandins). Similarly, sheep prostate contains PGE_1, PGE_2, PGE_3 and $PGF_{1\alpha}$. The following Table 5.1 shows some of the tissues and fluids in which prostaglandins are present.

Table 5.1 : Prostaglandins Present in Human Tissues

	Source	Prostaglandins
1.	Bronchi	PGE_2, $PGF_{2\alpha}$
2.	Cardiac muscle	PGE_2
3.	Cervical sympathetic nerve	PGE_2, $PGF_{2\alpha}$
4.	Endometrium (lung)	PGE_2, $PGF_{2\alpha}$
5.	Maternal venous blood during labour	PGE_2, $PGF_{2\alpha}$
6.	Menstrual fluid	PGE_2, $PGF_{2\alpha}$
7.	Placental blood vessels	PGE_1, PGE_2, $PGF_{1\alpha}$, $PGF_{2\alpha}$
8.	Semen	PGA_1, PGA_2, PGB_1, PGB_2, PGE_1, PGE_2, PGE_3 $PGF_{1\alpha}$, $PGF_{2\alpha}$
9.	Stomach mucosa	PGE_2
10.	Vagus nerve	PGE_2, $PGF_{2\alpha}$

5.2 NOMENCLATURE AND CHEMISTRY OF PROSTAGLANDINS

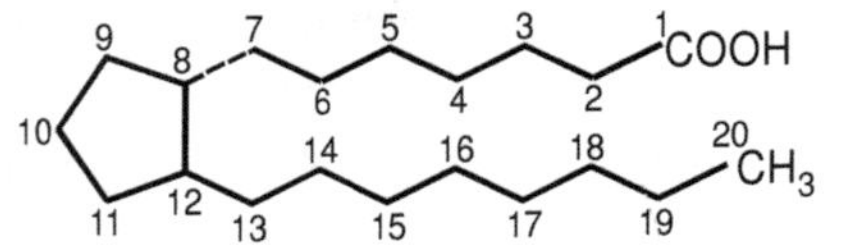

Prostanoic acid

Structurally, prostaglandins are derivatives of prostanoic acid and have a cyclopentane ring with two side-chains attached to adjacent carbon atoms. Systematic nomenclature of prostaglandins is based upon the hypothetical parent 'prostanoic acid' numbered as shown. With the increasing number and types of prostaglandins coming out, it became virtually essential to define the norms of nomenclature and classification of prostaglandins.

The present classification is based upon the nature of :

(a) Cyclopentane ring,

(b) Two adjacent side chains, and

(c) Configuration of newly introduced functional group.

(a) Nature of the cyclopentane ring :

Depending upon the nature of functional groups present, the cyclopentane ring may be categorised into :

(i) A-type cyclopentane ring contains 10, 11 - unsaturated 9 - ketone function.

(ii) B-type cyclopentane ring contains 8, 12 - unsaturated 9 - ketone function.

(iii) C-type cyclopentane ring contains 11, 12 - unsaturated 9 - ketone function.

(iv) E-type cyclopentane ring contains β-hydroxy ketone system.

(v) F-type cyclopentane ring contains 1, 3 - diol system.

PGA and PGB were so called because of their stability in acids and bases respectively. The names of other prostaglandins were based on the separation procedures, i.e. PGE partitioned into ether and PGF into phosphate (Fosfat in Swedish) buffer. Other types like PGC, PGD, PGG and PGH have also been described.

(b) Nature of adjacent side-chains :

Two side-chains are attached to the cyclopentane ring at carbon atom 8 and 12. The upper side-chain having carboxyl (–COOH) group at its terminal, is termed as carboxylhexyl or α-side chain while the lower side-chain (attached to C_{12}) having hydroxyl at C_{15} is called as hydroxyoctyl (ω) side chain. Compounds in these groups, are further characterised by a subscript 1, 2 or 3 depending on the number of double bonds in the side-chains. The side-chains may contain as many as 3 to 4 double bonds.

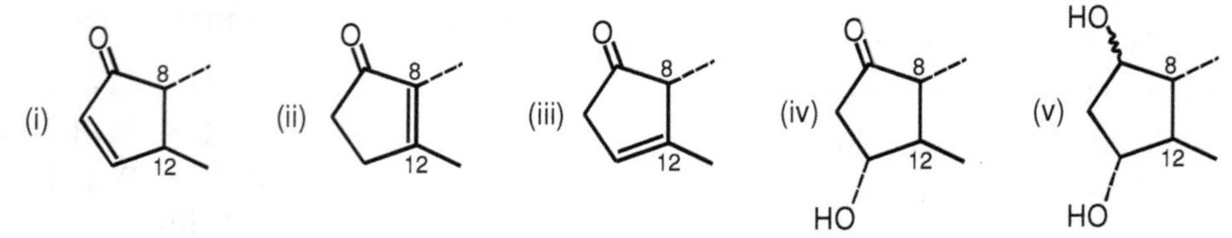

(i) A - type	(ii) B - type	(iii) C - type (unstable)	(iv) E - type	(v) F - type

For example,

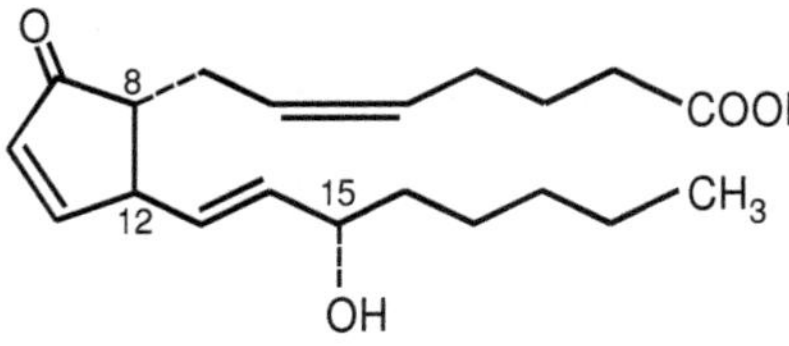

(I)

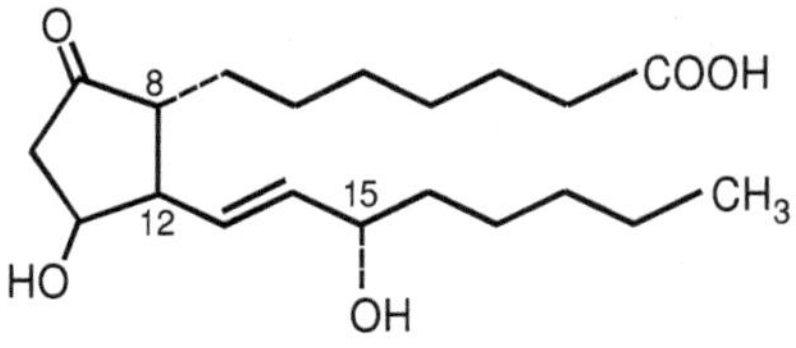

(II)

In the above structures, (I) contains cyclopentane ring of type A and two double bonds in the side-chains. Hence, the name will be PGA$_2$. While, the structure (II) contains the cyclopentane ring of the type E and only one double bond in the side-chain. Hence, it can be named as PGE$_1$.

In all the natural prostaglandins, the upper side-chain is attached to the cyclopentane ring through an α-bond (i.e., projecting behind the plane of the ring) and is shown by a dotted line. Similarly the naturally occuring prostaglandins possess an α-hydroxyl group at C$_{15}$-atom. Any change in this configuration must be specified by adding epi- as a prefix to the name alongwith the number of carbon atom at which this change has occurred.

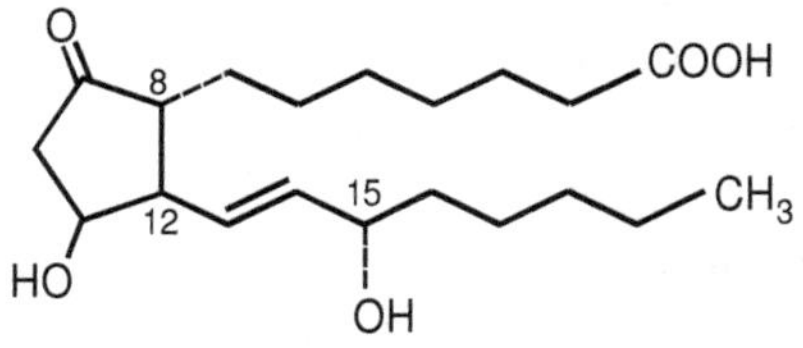

15 - epi PGE$_1$

(II)

(c) Nature of the configuration :

This parameter is needed to define the configuration of newly introduced functional group in the molecule. The literature prior to 1968 was extended by Anderson (1969) to designate further possible isomers and the optical antipodes. For example, PGE can be converted to PGF by reducing the C$_9$-ketone to a hydroxyl group. Thus, the PGF group can be further divided into PGF$_\alpha$ and PGF$_\beta$ types, depending on whether the hydroxyl at C$_9$ is behind the plane (α) or above the plane (β) of the ring.

The generic name, eicosanoids is given to a class containing prostaglandins, leukotrienes and related compounds because the basic skeleton is of 20-carbon fatty acid containing 3, 4 or 5 double bonds. In man, arachidonic acid (precursor of prostaglandins) is either derived from dietary linoleic acid or is ingested as a dietary constituent. Thromboxanes (TX) contain a six member oxane ring instead of the cyclopentane ring of prostaglandins. While prostacyclin (PGI$_2$) has a double-ring structure in addition to a cyclopentane ring.

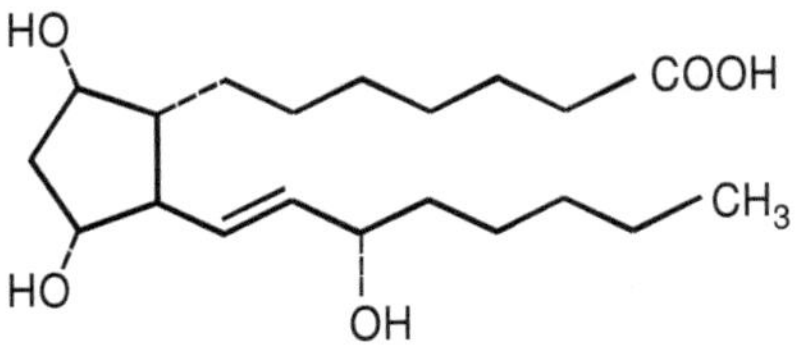

PGF$_{1\alpha}$

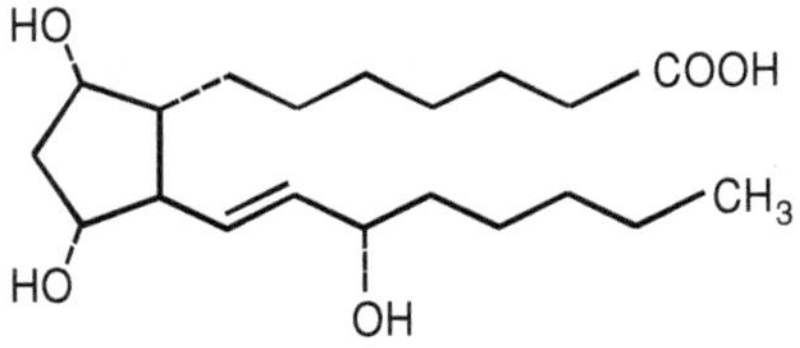

PGF$_{1\beta}$

Hydroperoxyeicosatetraenoic acids (HPETEs) are obtained from arachidonic acid by the attack of lipooxygenase enzymes. The HPETEs are unstable intermediates and are further metabolised by a variety of enzymes. All HPETEs may be converted to their corresponding hydroxy fatty acid (HETE) either by a peroxidase or non-enzymatically. Similarly, leukocytes convert 15-HPETE to trihydroxylated metabolites called lipoxins.

5.3 BIOSYNTHESIS AND METABOLISM OF PROSTAGLANDINS

Prostaglandins are synthesized enzymatically from certain open chain C_{20}-unsantrated fatty acids which include -

(a) 8, 11, 14 eicosatrienoic acid (dihomo-7-linolenic acid)

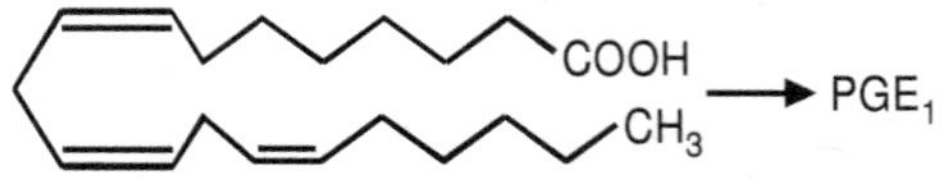

(b) 5, 8, 11, 14-eicosatetraenoic acid or arachidonic acid

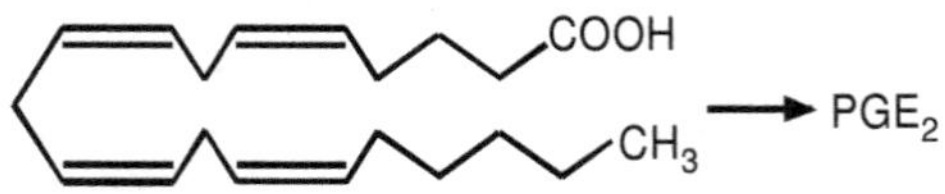

(c) 5, 8, 11, 14, 17-eicosapentaenoic acid

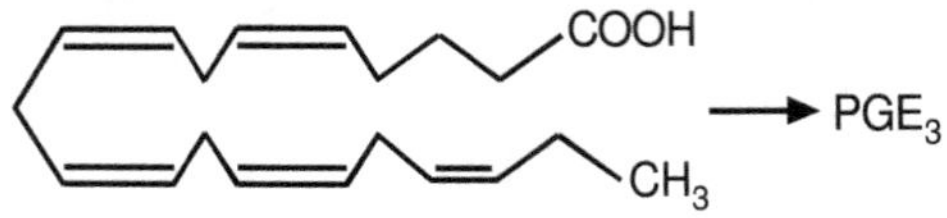

These acids are precursors of the in-vivo prostaglandin synthesis. The overall sequence of reactions include,

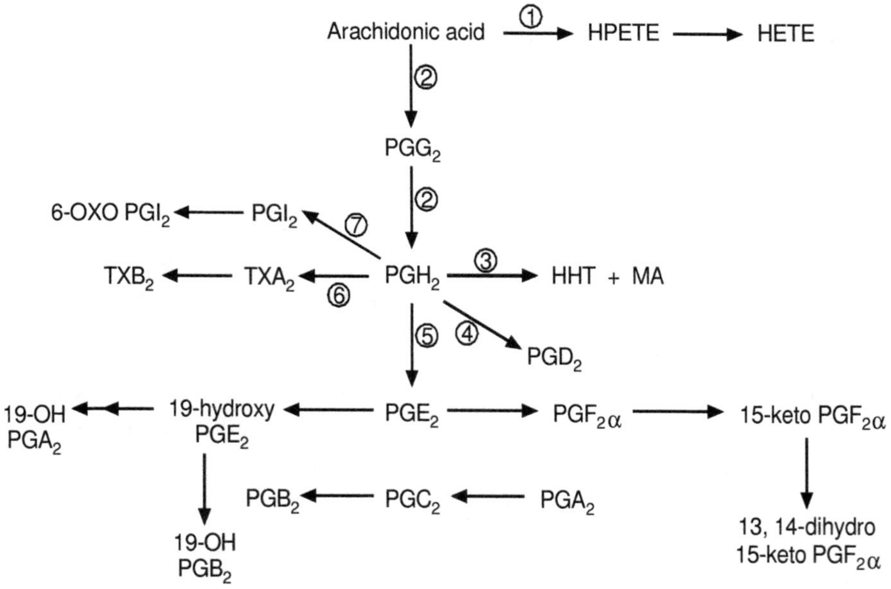

Fig. 5.1 : Biosynthesis of Various Prostaglandins

where,

HHT : 12 - L - hydroxy - 5, 8, 11 - heptadecatrienoic acid

MA : Malondialdehyde

HETE : 12 - L - hydroxy - 5, 8, 10, 14 - eicosatetraenoic acid

HPETE : 12 - L - hydroperoxide analogue

Enzymes involved in the biosynthesis of prostaglandins :

(1) lipo-oxygenase
(2) cyclo-oxygenase (PG-endoperoxide synthetase)
(3) serum albumin glutathione -s- transferase
(4) PG-endoperoxide reductase
(5) PG-endoperoxide-E- isomerase
(6) PG-endo-thromboxane A isomerase (thromboxane A_2 synthetase)
(7) PG - endoperoxide I isomerase.

5.4 PHARMACOLOGICAL ACTIONS OF PROSTAGLANDINS

Prostaglandins have been extensively studied because of their profound effects on physiological processes. All such important biological effects of prostaglandins include :

(a) Gastrointestinal system :

Prostaglandins are found to exert following actions on GIT system :

(i) decrease the gastric acid secretion
(ii) increase the non-acid secretion in rats
(iii) induce contraction of smooth muscles.

(b) Urinary system :

Specifically PGE_2 and $PGF_{2\alpha}$ increase bladder activity and help to maintain blood flow.

(c) Bronchial and tracheal smooth muscles :

Some prostaglandins (e.g. PGA, PGE_1, PGE_2) relax the bronchial smooth muscles while PGF induces bronchoconstriction.

(d) Reproductive system :

Prostaglandins increase the rate of synthesis and release of testosterone. Hence, PG - deficiency in male may lead to infertility. They stimulate myometrial smooth muscles that leads to uterine contraction (e.g. $PGF_{2\alpha}$). Hence, clinically it may be used to induce abortion.

(e) Cardiovascular system :

Prostaglandin endoperoxide and TXA_2 cause platelet aggregation and vasoconstriction. While PGI_2 (prostacyclin) decreases platelet aggregation and leads to vasodilation. Similarly PGE_2 and PGA_2 produce peripheral vasodilation and they may be used in the treatment of hypertension.

(f) Nervous system :

Prostaglandins affect mood, behaviour, brain excitability and EEG-pattern. The CNS-effects vary from CNS-depression to excitation. However they do not influence A.N.S. functioning.

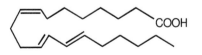

8, 12, 14 - eicosatrienoic acid

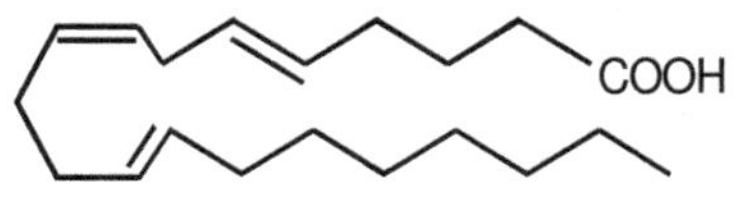

5, 8, 12, 14 - eicosatranoic acid

5.5 METABOLISM OF PROSTAGLANDINS

Gastric tissuse easily metabolise Prostaglandins, as shown in the rat. Only about 0.1 % of prostaglandins in the lumen reaches the serosal surface unaltered but it is not known which metabolites are formed. Besides this, other possible sites of PG-metabolism include liver, kidney, lungs, adrenal glands and uterus. For example, in the lungs the 15-hydroxyl group of prostaglandins E_1, E_2, A_2 and $F_{2\alpha}$ is metabolised by means of an enzyme system thought to involve 15-hydroxy prostaglandin dehydrogenase. The 15-keto compound is then reduced to the 13, 14-dihydro derivative, a reaction catalyzed by prostaglandin Δ^{13}-reductase. Subsequent steps involve β and ω, oxidation of the side-chains of the prostaglandins, giving rise to a polar dicarboxylic acid, which is excreted in the urine.

5.6 PROSTAGLANDIN ANTAGONISTS

The receptor sites at which prostaglandins act in isolated segments of gastrointestinal muscle have been investigated mainly by the use of selective pharmacological antagonists. It was found that PGE_1 and PGE_2 inhibit the circular muscle of the human, guinea pig and rat gut by acting at sites on the muscle which are different from α- and β-adrenoceptors. The excitatory receptors appear to differ from receptors for acetylcholine, 5-hydroxytryptamine and histamine. The excitatory (longitudinal muscle) and inhibitory, (circular muscle) PGE receptors therefore appear to be different. The prostaglandin antagonists SC-19220 and polyphloretin phosphate antagonize the excitatory effects of PGE and PGF compounds but not the inhibitory (circular muscle) effects of PGE compounds.

Certain compounds inhibit prostaglandin synthesis by competitive antagonism. This ability is due to their structural resemblance with prostaglandin precursors. These include.
(1) 8, 12, 14 - eicosatrienoic acid and
(2) 5, 8, 12, 14 - eicosatetrenoic acid.

Besides these, gold, silver, zinc, cupric ion inhibit the prostaglandin synthesis. Non-steroidal anti-inflammatory drugs inhibit the cycloxygenas enzymes.

Other important prostaglandin-antagonists include

(a)

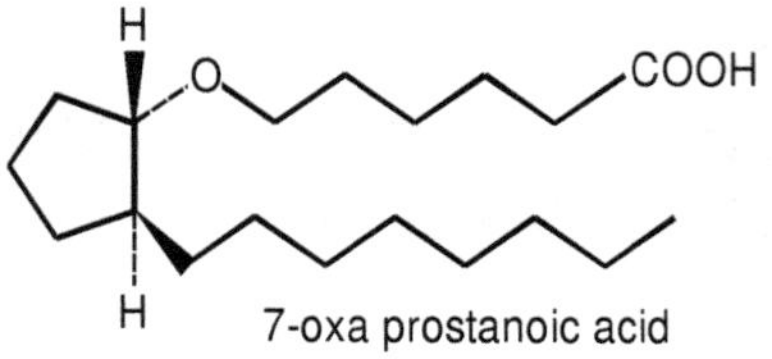

7-oxa prostanoic acid

(b)

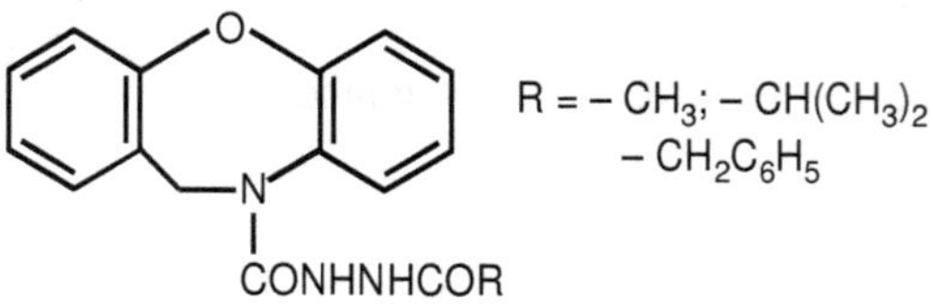

$R = - CH_3; - CH(CH_3)_2 - CH_2C_6H_5$

Bibenzoxazepine hydrazide derivatives

(c)

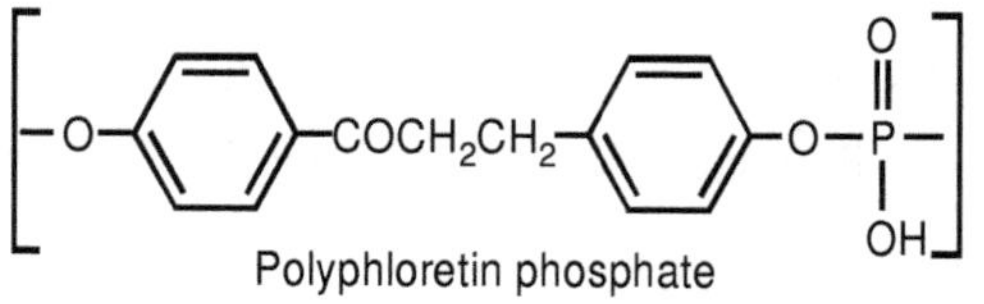

Polyphloretin phosphate

(d) Other drugs like morphine, quinidine and procaine were also reported to have antagonistic actions.

5.7 CLINICALLY USED PROSTAGLANDIN ANALOGS

These have been based on modification of the structure of natural prostaglandins (mainly PGE_1 and PGE_2), to increase resistance to metabolism or achieve a lower incidence of side effects at therapeutic doses. For example : enprostil has relatively long half-life. The main prostaglandin analogues are listed below :

(a) Arbaprostil :

It is an analogue of 15-methyl PGE_2. It is rapidly absorbed and eliminated with a short half-life. Doses of approximately 2 µg/kg produce more than 60% inhibition of basal and stimulated acid output in humans. Antisecretory doses of arbaprostil (150 µg, 4 times a day) heal duodenal ulcers but the lower cytoprotective doses (10 µg to 25 µg about 4 times a day) are ineffective. Arbaprostil may inhibit gastrin release and has been shown to protect against asprin induced gastric injury in doses of 0.6 µg/kg/day.

(b) Trimoprostil :

It is 11-methyl analogue of PGE_2 which is well absorbed. Doses in the range 7.5-10 µg/kg reduce the basal acid secretion while doses upto 40 µg/kg inhibit meal stimulated acid secretions for upto 3 hours. Doses in the anti-secretory range (2 mg/day and upward) reduce asprin injury. Trimoprostil stimulates gastric bicarbonate secretion. When given, 750 µg 4 times daily, it is less effective at healing duodenal ulcers and gastric ulcers than cimetidine, 200 mg 3 times daily or 400 mg at night.

(c) Misoprostol :

Both ulcer healing and pain relief effects of misoprostol are dose dependent in the doses of 100 mg 4 times daily or more. Misoprostol 200 µg 4 times daily, was of similar efficacy to cimetidine 300 mg 3 times daily, in healing duodenal ulcers and gastric ulcers over 4 weeks.

Misoprostol is a methyl ester of 15-methyl PGE_1. It is rapidly absorbed after oral administration. It is rapidly de-esterified to free acid, binds to albumin and is concentrated in gastroinstestinal, hepatic and renal tissues. It is rapidly oxidized and eliminated with a half-life of about 1.5 hours. It has been shown to inhibit basal, daytime and overnight acid secretion and that stimulated by histamine, betazole, pentagastrin, tetragastrin and caffeine. It helps to reduce alcohol injury in man and produces a substantial dose-dependent rise in duodenal bicarbonate secretion.

(d) Rioprostil :

This is a methyl PGE_1 derivative, orally well absorbed with a short half-life. Doses of 300 to 600 µg reduced basal and stimulated acid secretion and pepsin output. It also prevents gastric bleeding and promotes healing rate. With this dosing regimen, diarrrhoea and abdominal pain were said to be infrequent.

(e) MDL-646 :

This is a PGE_1 - derivative which has local protective effects on gastric mucosa. Single doses of MDL in the range of 800-1200 µg reduced basal acidity but had much less effect on stimulated acid output.

(f) Enprostil :

About 35-140 µg per day of enprostil heals duodenal ulcers and gastric ulcers. However, daily doses of 70 µg are less effective than ranitidine 300 mg in healing duodenal ulcers. Maintenance treatment with enprostil 35 µg at night is less effective in duodenal ulcer patients than ranitidine 150 mg.

(g) Prostacyclin :

It caused a reduction in duodenal ulcer size in a dose of 5 µg/kg/hr. infused for 5 hours per day over 6 days. It also increases gastric bicarbonate secretion but does not affect pentagastrin stimulated acid secretion.

Table 5.2 : Some Prostaglandin Analogues

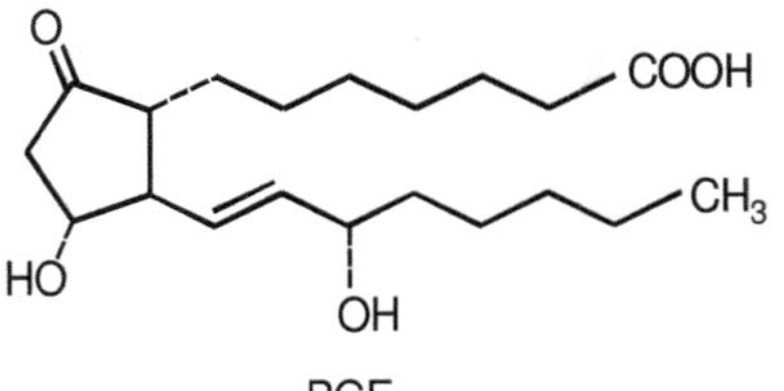

PGE₁

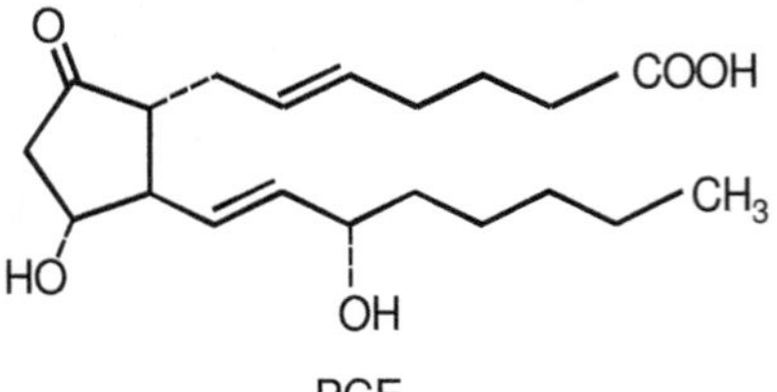

PGE₂

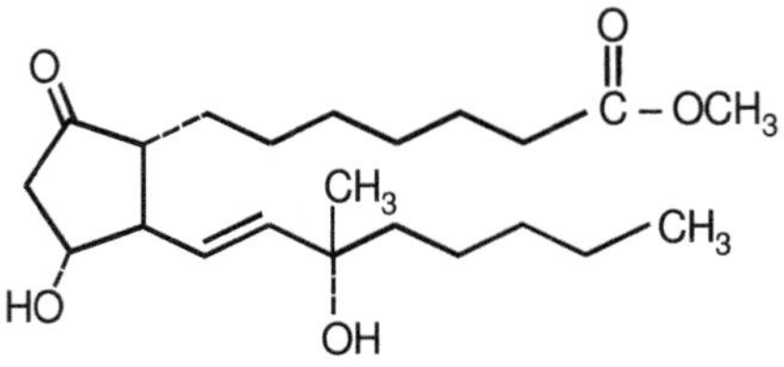

(±) Misoprostol

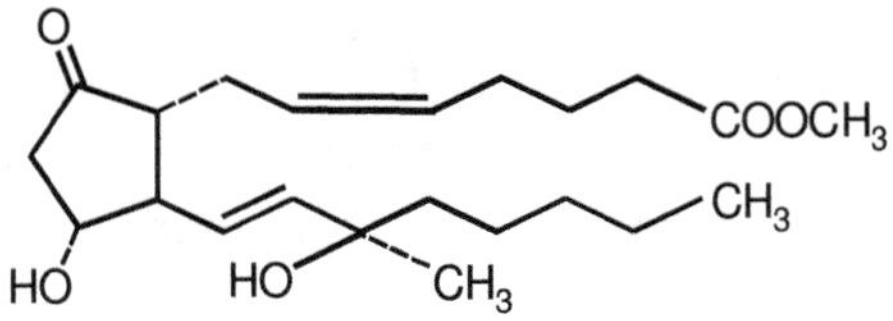

Arbaprostil

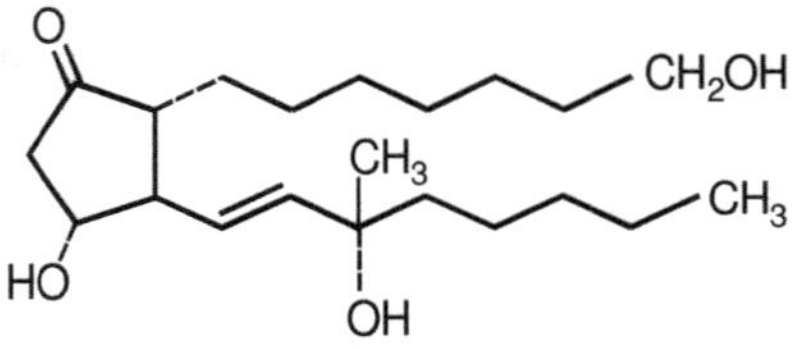

Rioprostil

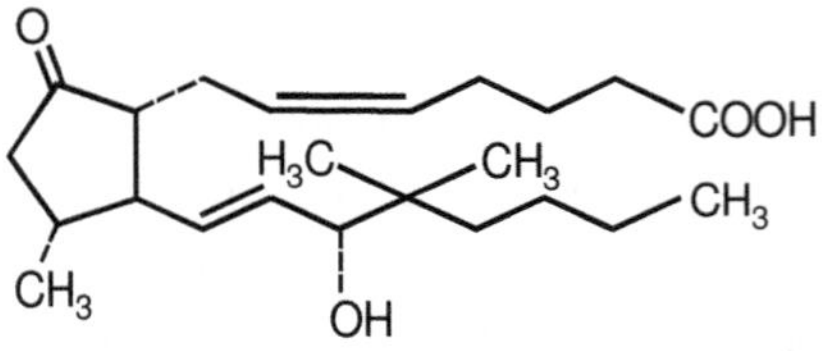

Trimoprostil

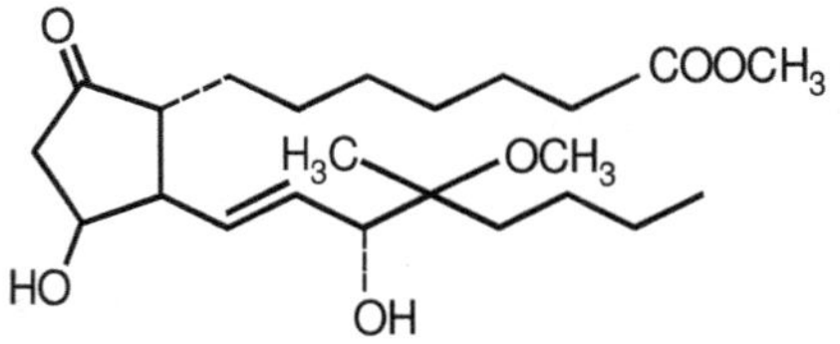

MDL 646

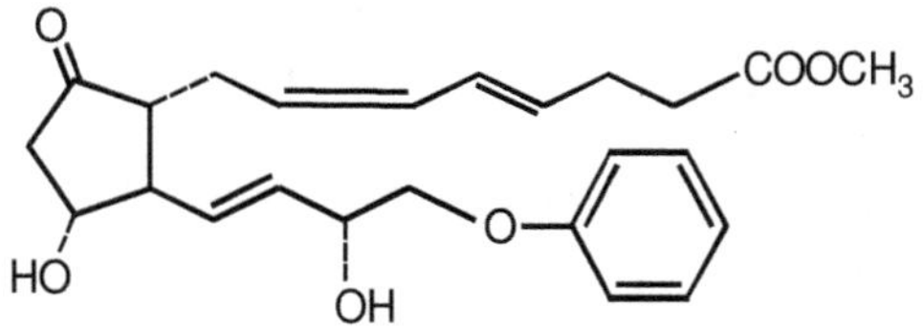

Enprostil

(h) FCE 20700 :

This is a new PGE₂ derivative (11-deoxy-13, 14 - dehydro -16 (S) - methyl PGE₂ methyl ester) in doses of 1 and 2 mg produces a small but significant dose related inhibition of acid secretion.

Many of the available ulcer healing drugs (sucralfate, carbenoxolone, bismuth chelate etc.), which do not affect acid are able to enhance prostaglandin level. Other prostaglandin analogues include carboprost, cloprostenol sodium, dinoprost (prostin F_2), dinoprostane (prostine E_2), epoprostenol sodium (prostacyclin), fluprostenol sodium, prostalene and sulprostone.

5.8 ADVERSE EFFECTS OF PROSTAGLANDIN ANALOGUES

Acid inhibition by available prostaglandin analogues is moderate. Comparative studies are few but there are no analogues where it is clearly established that clinically useful doses are more effective than cimetidine. All available analogues are characterized by diarrhoea to varying degree. There are also chances that the motility of the pregnant female uterus be increased to induce abortion.

Dinoprostone :

It is marketed in the form of vaginal suppositories containing 20 mg of PGE_2. It is used to induce abortion and to treat benign hydatidiform mole. While carboprost tromethamine is a solution containing 0.25 mg of carboprost (15-methyl $PGF_{2\alpha}$) per ml. It may be used intramuscularly to induce abortion or to treat postpartum hemorrhage owing to uterine atony.

5.9 SAR-STUDIES OF PROSTAGLANDINS

(1) Expansion or contraction of the cyclopentane ring or its replacement by heteroaromatic rings results in decrease in the activity in the E_2 and F_2 series.

(2) Replacement of hydroxyl group in the ring gives more stable analogues. For example, thio-PGI_2 (I) possesses platelet aggregation inhibiting activity with vasodilatory effect. Similarly, the aromatic pyridazo derivative (II) is an excellent vasodilator.

(3) Modification of the carboxylic acid side-chain has also been reported. For example, the phenoxy derivative (III) is about 10 times more active than PGE as an inihibitor of platelet aggregation while the sulfonamide derivative (IV) is 15-30 times more potent than PGE_2 as an antifertility agent and possesses less side effects.

(4) While the 7-oxo and 7-thio analogues were found to show an antagonistic activity on isolated smooth-muscles.

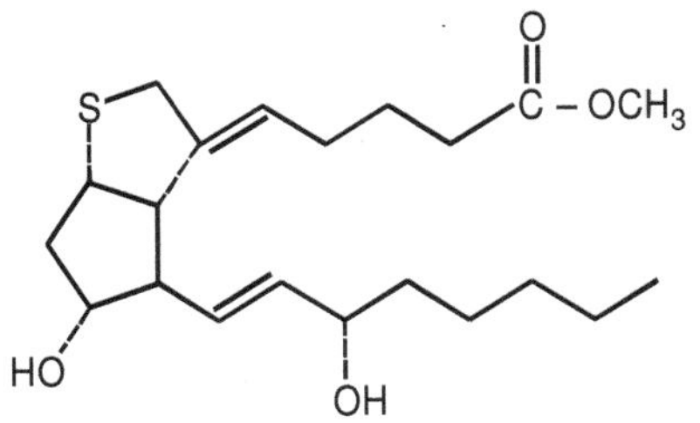

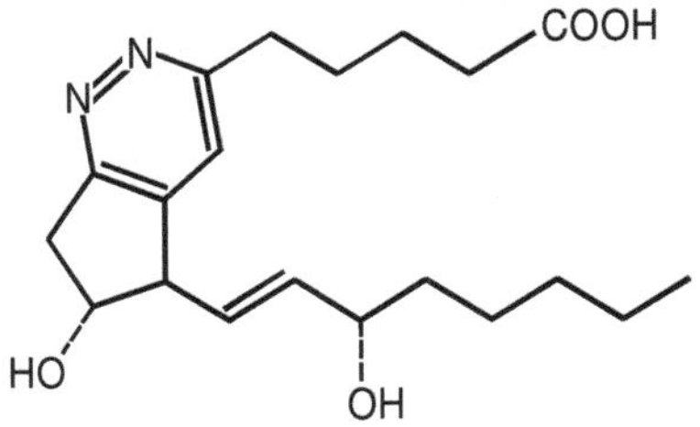

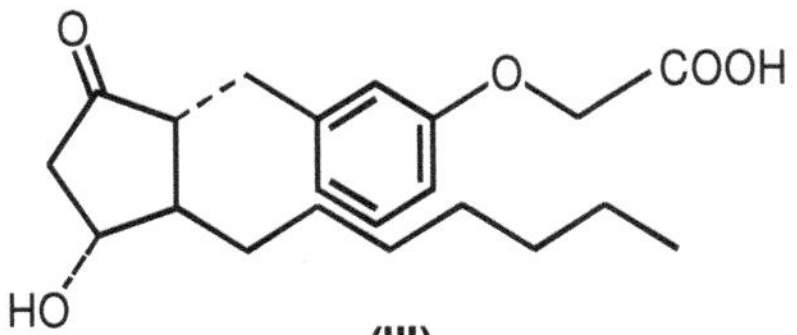

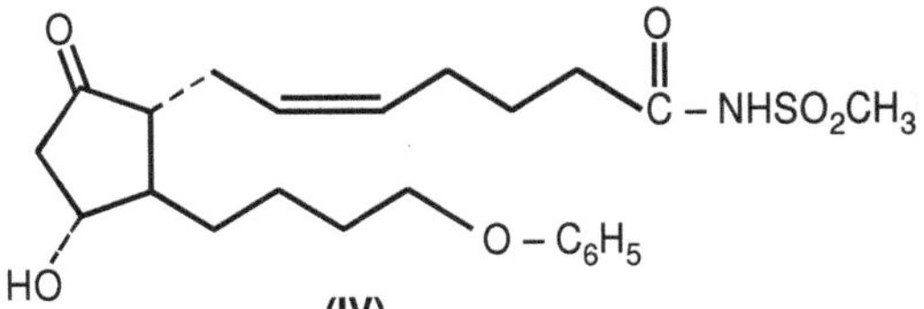

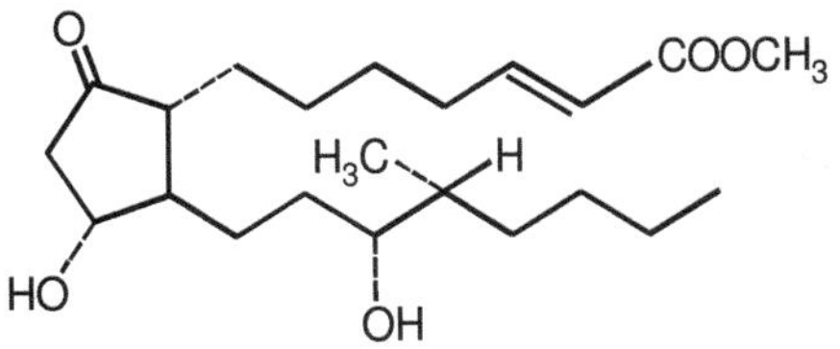

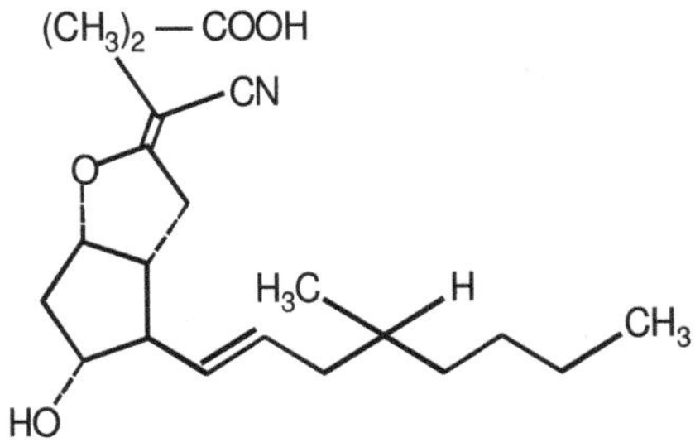

(5) Incorporation of a methyl group in the lower side-chain leads to an increase in uterotonic activity. For example, carboprost and compound (V) are used to induce abortions while nileprost (VI) is an experimental antiulcer agent. They [carboprost and compound (V)] probably inhibit the dehydrase enzyme that inactivates prostaglandins by removing the 15-hydroxyl group.

5.10 MICROBIAL BIOTRANSFORMATIONS OF PROSTAGLANDINS

Micro-organisms are known to possess a diversed range of enzyme systems which can catalyze most of the common reaction types involved in organic synthesis like, oxidation, reduction, hydrolysis and condensation. More often, a comparison is made between the microbial transformation and metabolic pattern of drugs in mammalion system. The microbial system presents both, the reaction specificity and site specificity. Other points of advantages are listed below.

(1) Ease of handling due to mild physiological conditions.

(2) In cases, where the synthesis of key intermediates needs several steps and consume many chemicals, extra labour, time and money and yet release poor yield.

Table 5.3 : Biosynthesis of Prostaglandins from Arachidonic Acid

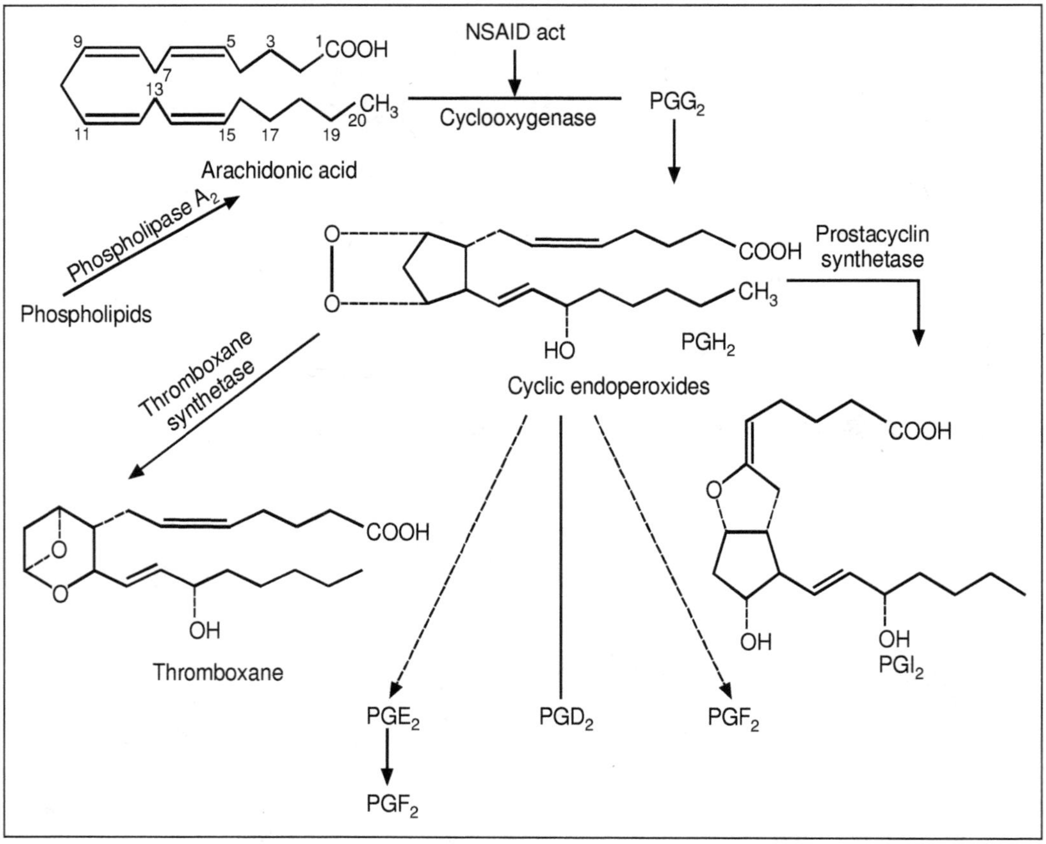

(3) Efficiency with which the common transformations (e.g. oxidation, reduction, hydrolysis and condensation) are carried out.

(4) Prostaglandin molecule can have as many five asymmetric centers. Chemical synthesis of natural prostaglandins usually provides a racemic mixture of dl-epimers which upon resolution may theoretically yield about 50% of product. The microbial enzyme, on other hand, due to their substrate specificity and sterioselectivity are well suited to obtain a desired sterioisomer in proportionately higher yields.

5.11 BIOLOGY OF PROSTAGLANDINS

Prostaglandins have been extensively studied because of their profound effects on physiological processes. The precursors of prostaglandins are C-20 essential fatty acids present in the cell-wall of the tissue cells. In human, arachidonic acid serves as a precursor for the biosynthesis of prostaglandins. Non-steroidal (NSAID) anti-inflammatory drugs inhibit prostaglandin biosynthesis but do not influence the action of exogenous prostaglandins or inflammatory response.

5.12 MICROBIAL TRANSFORMATIONS

Considerable volume of work on microbial bioconversions of prostaglandins had been published. Conveniently, the work can be classified, depending upon the type of transformation involved, as follows :

(A) Oxidation :
- (i) Hydroxylation
- (ii) Dehydration in the cyclopentane ring.
- (iii) Dehydrogenation of the C-15 hydroxyl group to the corresponding ketone function.

(B) Reduction :
- (i) Reductions of the 13, 14-double bond.
- (ii) Reductions of C-9 ketone function.
- (iii) Reduction of C-15 ketone function.

(C) Isomerization :
Isomerization of the ring 10, 11 - double bond (PGA) to the 12-position (PGB).

(D) Hydrolysis

(E) Cyclization.

(A) Oxidation :

(I) Hydroxylation :

Although probably a very common reaction, micro-organism have the capacity to hydroxylate the prostaglandin mostly at C-18, C-19 and C-20 positions only. Fungi in general are noted for their versatile hydroxylation at non-activated carbons in a variety of substrates like steroids, alkaloids and hydrocarbons. In all instances hydroxylation of prostaglandin side-chains is supposed to be an initiation of the oxidative degradation of prostaglandins. Several species of Streptomyces were found to be useful for hydroxylation but S. ruber was more efficient. For example, incubation of 15-acetoxy PGA_2 methyl ester (I) with S.ruber yielded the 17, 18 and 19 hydroxylated derivatives.

It means the complete hydrolysis of the diester (I) through all intermediate (II) gives a mixture of C-17, C-18 hydroxylated analogues. The part of the starting material undergoes partial hydrolysis to give structure (III) which upon hydroxylation yields only (IV). Hydroxylation is accompanied by reduction of 10, 11-double bond, in the above reaction.

Strains of bacteria and fungi useful in hydroxylation :

Screening of Streptomyces sp. for their hydroxylation capacity on prostaglandins showed that Streptomyces sp. CBS 479.48, Streptomyces sp. CBS 188.74, Streptomyces sp. CBS 190.74 and Streptomyces aureofaciens were holding good capacity to introduce 17, 18 or 19 hydroxyl groups. The predominance of the product type was found to be substrate and culture dependent. Fungi also rank at the top to introduce 18 and 19 hydroxyl functions. e.g. Thazetellopsis tocklaie CBS 378.58 and Ophiobolus graminis ATCC 12761. When PGA_2 or PGB_2 incubated with Aspergillus niger 9142 or Stemphyliun solani, give C-20 hydroxylated derivatives.

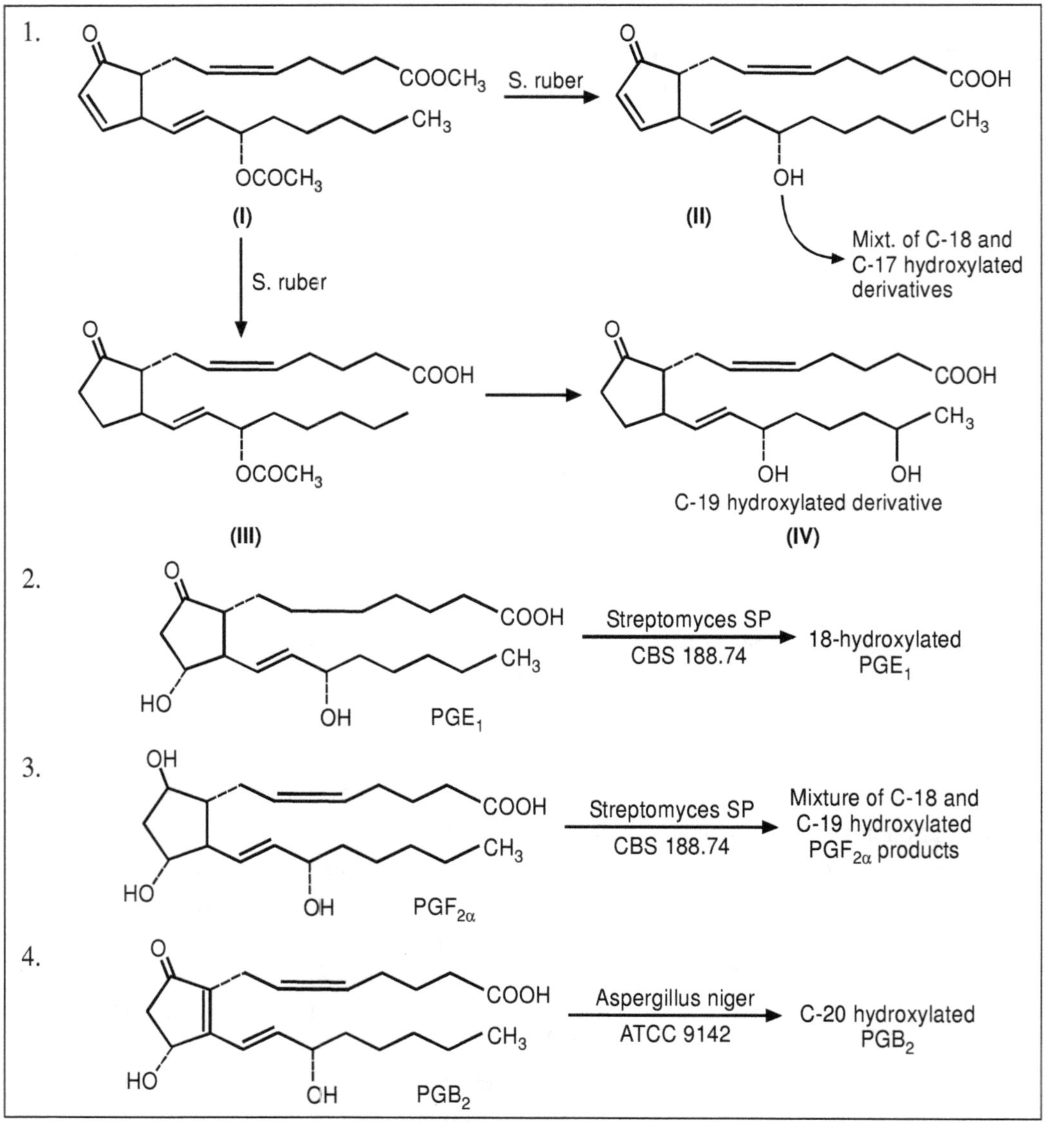

5. Prostaglandin intermediate → 11-hydroxylated analog

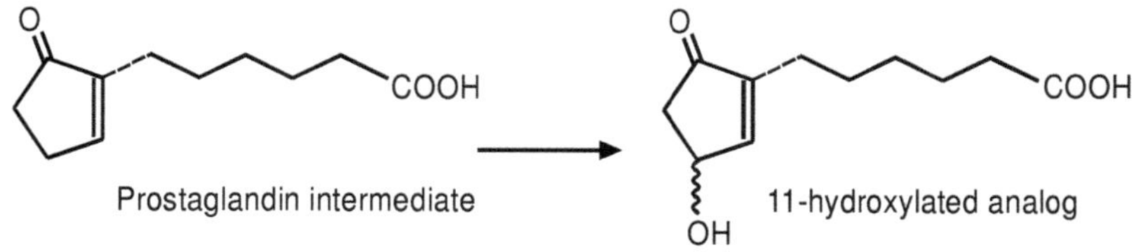

6. PGA₂ → Cunninghamella blakesleeana (ATCC 9245) → 10, 11 - dihydro - 18 hydroxy PGA₂

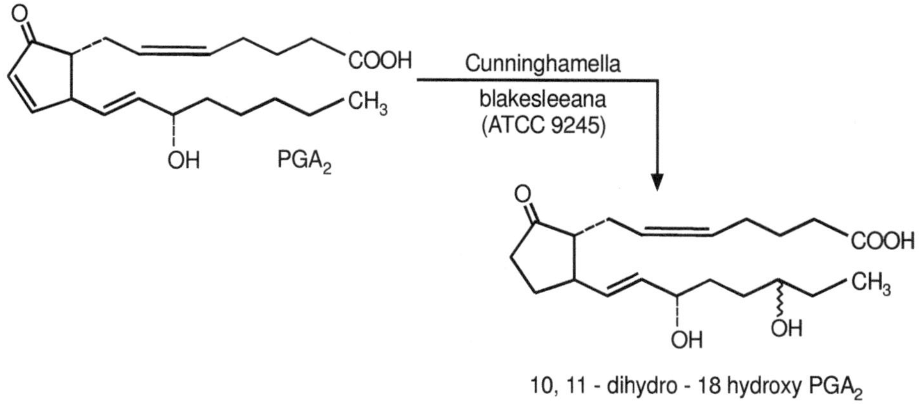

(II) Dehydration in the cyclopentane ring :

This type of transformation is very rare, not because it is very difficult to occur but this transformation occurs very rapidly if the pH of the medium is slightly changed even in the absence of micro-organism. For example, the E-type prostaglandin is very labile towards both acidic or basic conditions resulting into dehydration to A-type compounds.

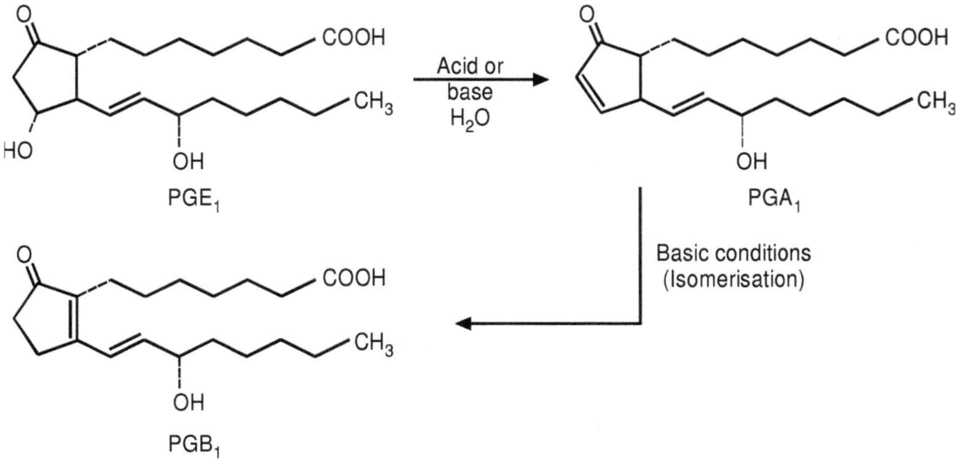

PGE₁ → Acid or base H_2O → PGA₁ → Basic conditions (Isomerisation) → PGB₁

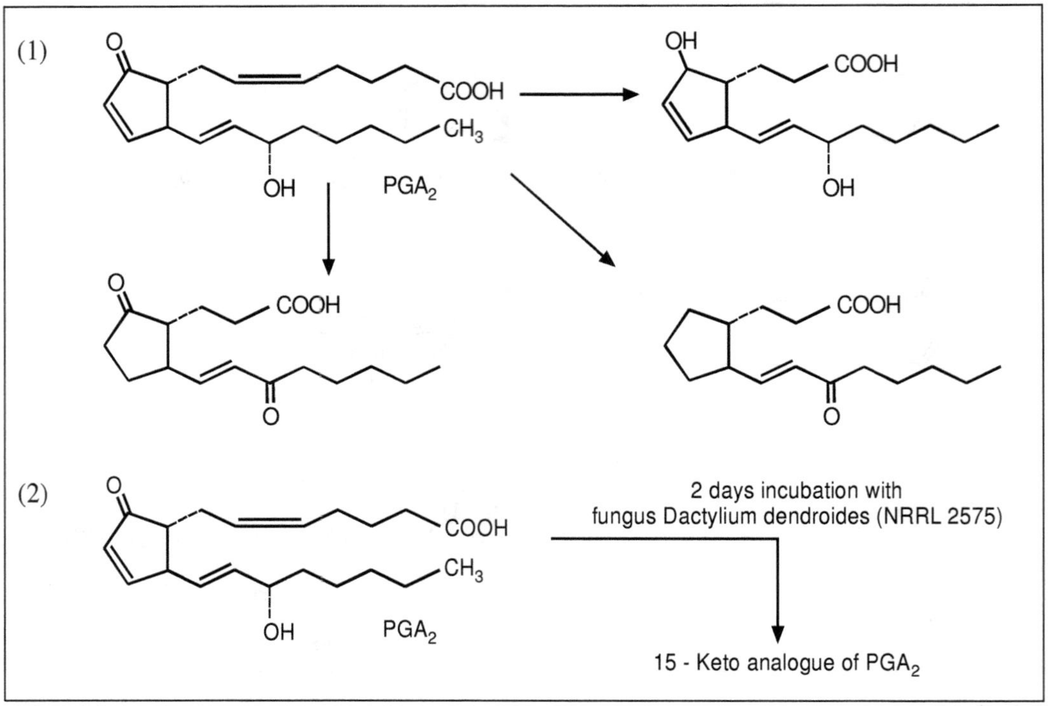

(III) Dehydrogenation of the C-15 hydroxyl group to the corresponding ketone function :

This is again a rare transformation. Thus, in the β oxidation of PGA_2 by Aureobasiduim pullulans, some of metabolites possess dehydrogenated C-15 hydroxyl group.

(B) Reduction :

A number of synthetic routes to a natural and synthetic prostaglandins have been reported in the literature which involve reduction as an important step.

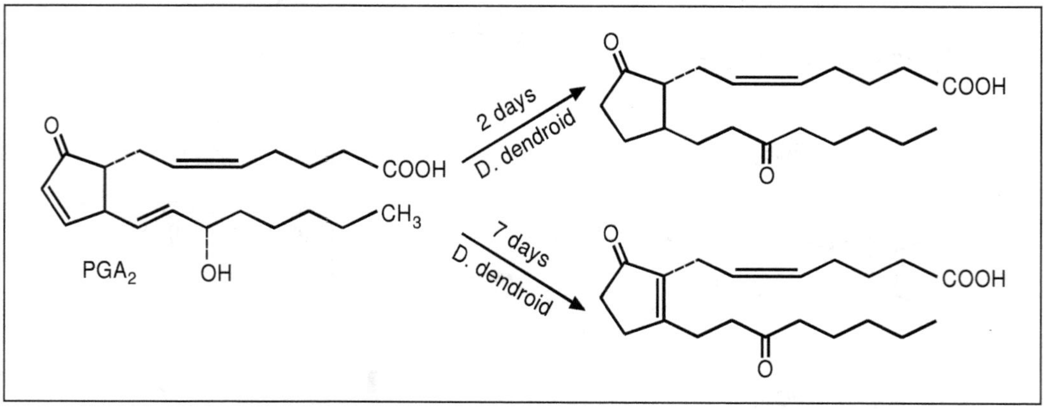

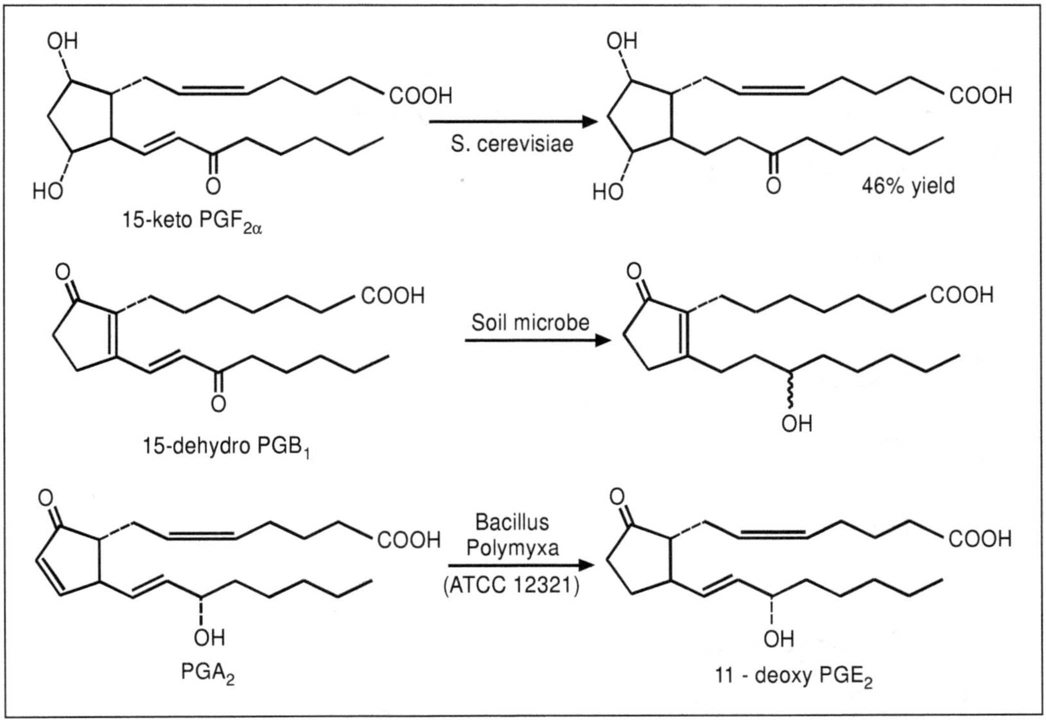

This microbial bioconversion can be conveniently categorised and studied under the following heads.

(i) Reduction of 13-14 double bond :

Wide variety of micro-organisms display double bond reduction capacity as a side reaction. For example the fungus, Aureobasidium pullulans can perform dehydrogenation of C-15 and C-9 ketone groups alongwith the reduction of the 10, 11 and 13, 14 double bonds. Similarly, Dactylium denroides (NRRL 2575) reduces the 10, 11 and 13, 14 - double bond and dehydrogenates 15α hydroxyl group to 15 ketone moiety.

In 15 keto $PCF_{2\alpha}$ the 13 (14) double bond is reduced when Sacchromyces cerevisiae is used.

Above reaction is also found to be catalysed by a Cephalosporium species (NRRL 5605), Streptomyces griseus and by organisms of the genera Pseudomonas and Corynebacterium.

(ii) Reduction of C-9 ketone function :

Reduction of C-9 ketone to the hydroxyl function is an important reaction in the conversion of PGE to PGF. The chemical methods usually result into a mixture of enantiomers. Hence, microbial system can be used for sterioselective introduction of secondary alcoholic group. Schneider and Murray employed yeast to reduce E-prostaglandins to F-type prostaglandins.

(iii) Reduction of C-15 ketone function :

In an attempt of sterioselective reduction and optical resolution of racemic $\Delta 8(12)$ 15-dehydro PGE_1, Marsheck and Miyano used, Flavobacterium species.

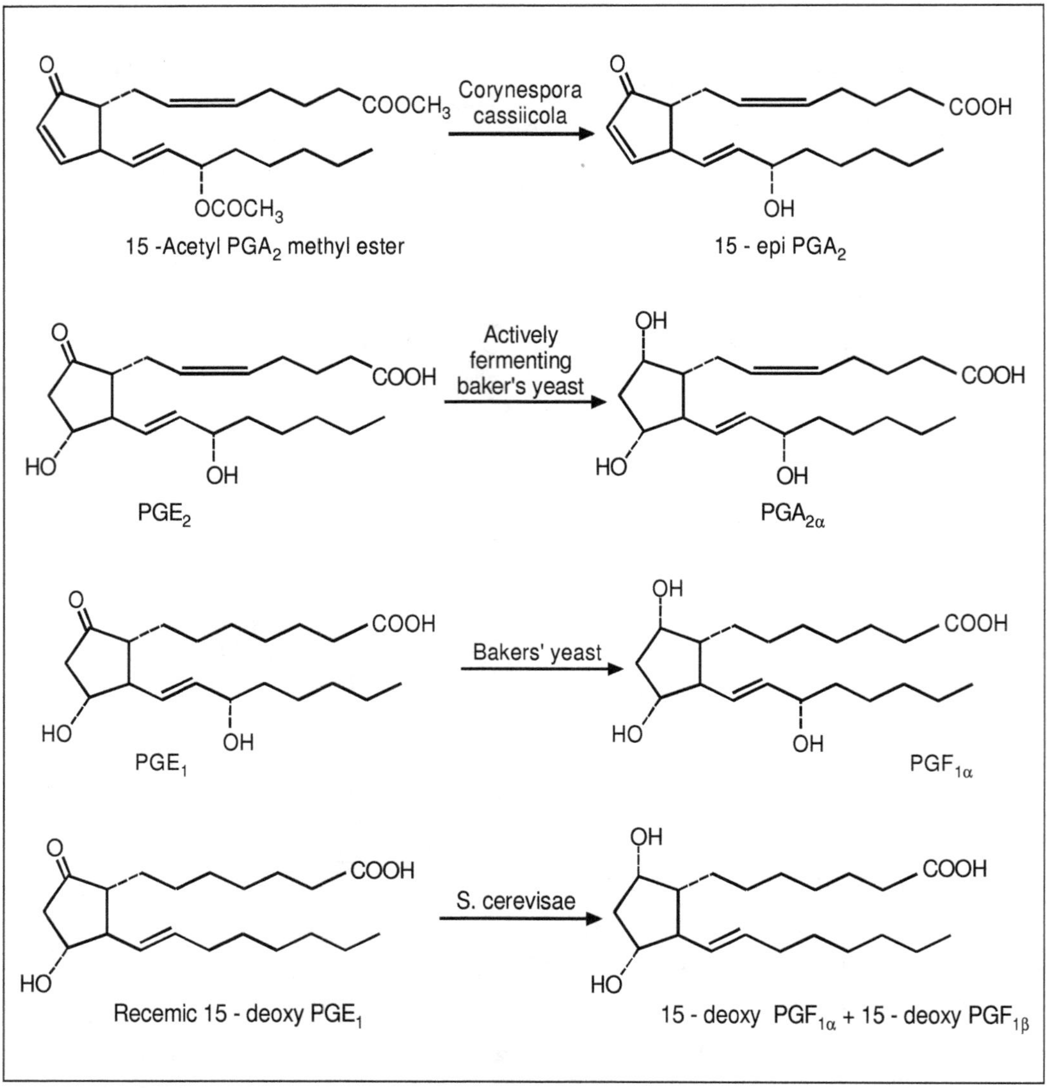

(C) Isomerization of the ring 10, 11 double bond (PGA) to the 8, 12 position (PCB) :

Literature survey of the microbial biotransformations of prostaglandins revealed no clearcut examples of isomerization. But under basic conditions, PAGs are found to get converted into PGBs without the aid of micro-organism.

Hence, whenever a microbial bioconversion of PGA type is desired, careful pH monitoring of the medium is generally advised.

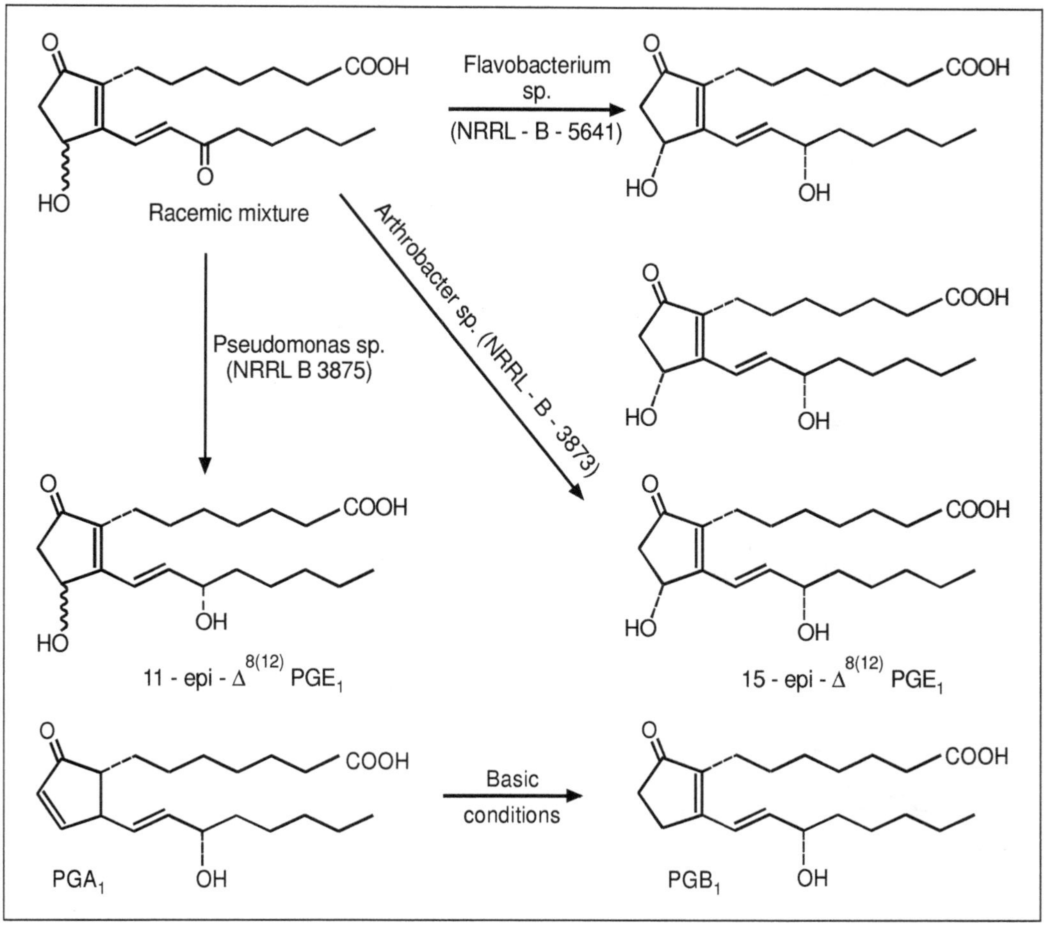

(D) Hydrolysis :

The sterioselective hydrolytic cleavage of prostaglandin esters has been demonstrated by using microbial enzyme systems. These enzyme systems have proved to be of great synthetic potential for the optical resolution of recemic mixtures of dl-isomers. In addition to sterioselectivity, extremely mild reaction conditions they present, adds to their qualification as efficient resolving agents. The examples of microbial hydrolysis were spread over the area other than steroids and prostaglandins. To avoid the possibility of generation of degradation products, generally the process is carried out using mild conditions, even under a N_2 atmosphere.

A number of bacteria and fungi contain enzymes having esterase activity, e.g. Rhizopus oryzae or baker's yeast. Saccharomyces sp. (1375 - 143), Saccharomyces sp. (NRRL Y 7342), Cladosporium resinae (ATCC 274) and many others.

Resolution Alongwith Reduction :

Cell-free extracts of Cladosporium resinae (ATCC 274) have been used to hydrolyze PGE methyl-esters.

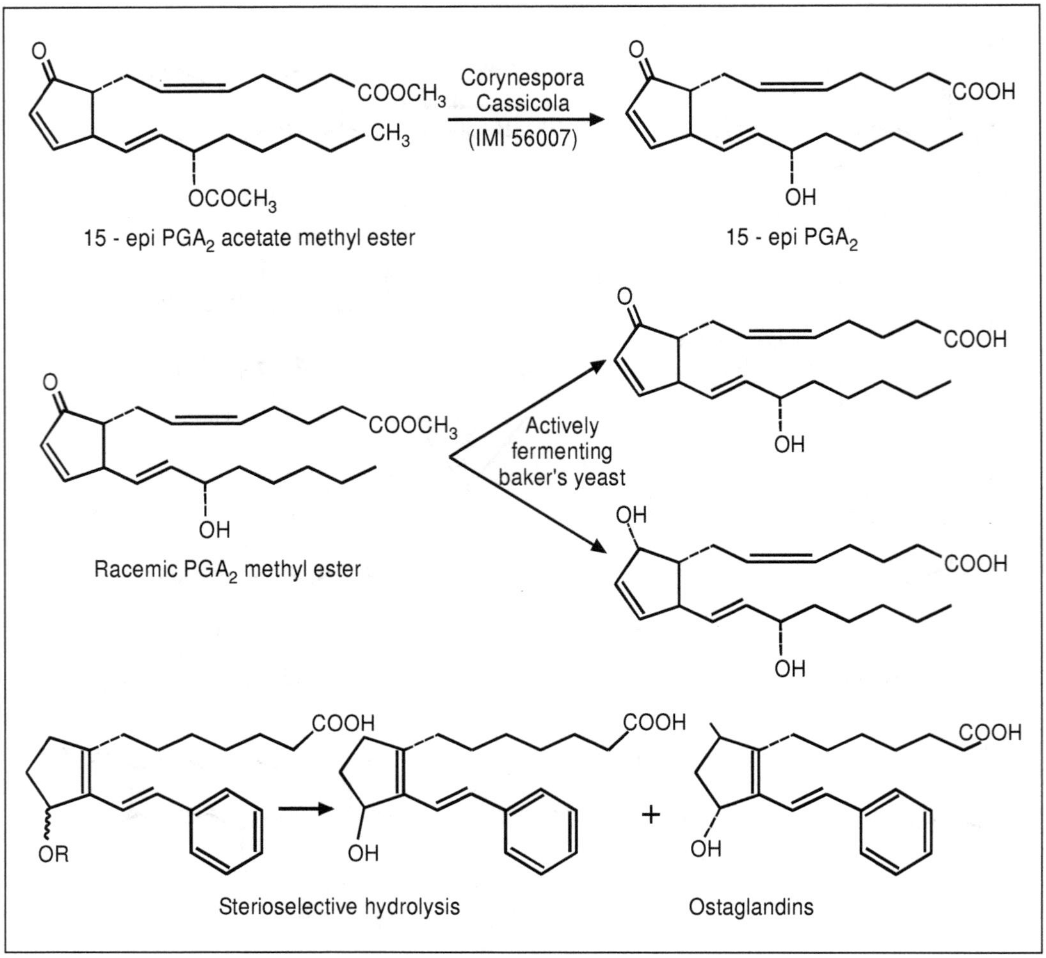

15 - epi PGA₂ acetate methyl ester → (Corynespora Cassicola IMI 56007) → 15 - epi PGA₂

Racemic PGA₂ methyl ester → Actively fermenting baker's yeast

Sterioselective hydrolysis

Ostaglandins

(E) Cyclization :

While designing a completely synthetic approach, the workers at Upjohn laboratories were inspired by the biosynthetic pathway of prostaglandins. They tried to synthesize prostaglandins from suitable polyunsaturated fatty acids with the aid of micro-organisms. Micro-organisms from five classes of fungi were employed namely Phycomyces, Ascomyces, Deuteromyces. Schizomyces and Basidomyces.

5.13 LIMITATIONS OF MICROBIAL BIOTRANSFORMATIONS OF PROSTAGLANDINS

(1) Prostaglandins exist as oily compounds which are sensitive to air oxygen (oxidation) and to even mild acidic or basic conditions. For example, PGE under acidic or basic conditions undergoes dehydration and get converted into PGA. The later isomerises to PGB under basic conditions. Hence, handling of prostaglandins and pH monitoring of the microbial medium needs special attention.

(5.18)

(2) Organic compounds present in the medium may influence the type and extent of the bioconversion.

(3) Depending upon the reaction involved, an inert atmosphere by the supply of nitrogen gas may be demanded.

(4) In order to inhibit an undesired degradation, the microbial oxidation has to be counter-attacked. This may be achieved by using divalent metal ions, chelating agents or the introduction of genetic mutations aimed at the enzyme responsible for initial attack.

5.14 SUMMARY

Although microbial bioconversion did not turn out to be as vital to prostaglandins as to steriod, their ease of handling and the mild physiological condition under which they operate, helped to increase the popularity as method to introduce chirality or chiral resolving agent.

Prostaglandins exhibit a broad range of biological activities, with a considerable depth of potency. Therefore, the possibility of their medicinal application led to the clinical trials which have shown encouraging result. For example, they could have a possible use in the termination of pregnancy and in controlling the various stages of the reproductive cycle. They also possess applications in the treatment of bronchial asthma (e.g., 10-halo derivative of PGA), nasal decongestion, hypotension and gastric hypersecretion. Thus in years to come prostaglandins may come to play an important therapeutic role in different medicinal fields. Associated with advantages and certain disadvantages of its own, microbial bioconversions have to play a role of valuable adjunct to the chemical methods for the synthesis of natural prostaglandins and their analogues.

Table 5.4: Clinically used Prostaglandins

Substance	Observed biological activity
PGD_2	Weak inhibitor of platelet aggregation.
PGE_1	Vasodilation. Inhibitor of platelet aggregation. Bronchodilatation. Stimulate contraction of Gl smooth muscle.
PGE_2	Stimulate hyperalgesic response. Renal vasodilation. Stimulate uterine smooth muscle contraction. Reduce secretion of stomach acid.
PGF_2	Stimulate uterine smooth muscle contraction. Stimulate breakdown of corpus luteum in animal.
PGI_2	Potent inhibitor of platelet aggregation. Potent vasodilator.

(B) MICROBIAL BIOCONVERSION IN ANTIBIOTICS

Biotransformation of antibiotics is far advantageous with respect to duration, safety, energy inputs, pollution and economics. Biochemical transformation of naturally produced antibiotics can potentially be used to alter their antimicrobial activity, spectrum of action, oral absorption, toxicity and allergic responses. Antibiotic biotransformation is achieved with the help of cell-free enzymes (biocatalysts) or microbes secreting such biocatalysts.

Characteristics of strain :

(i) It should be high yielding strain.

(ii) It should have stable biochemical characteristics.

(iii) It should not give undesirable product until the final product is obtained.

(iv) It should be easily cultivated on large scale.

Microbial Bioconversions in Antibiotics :

(i)

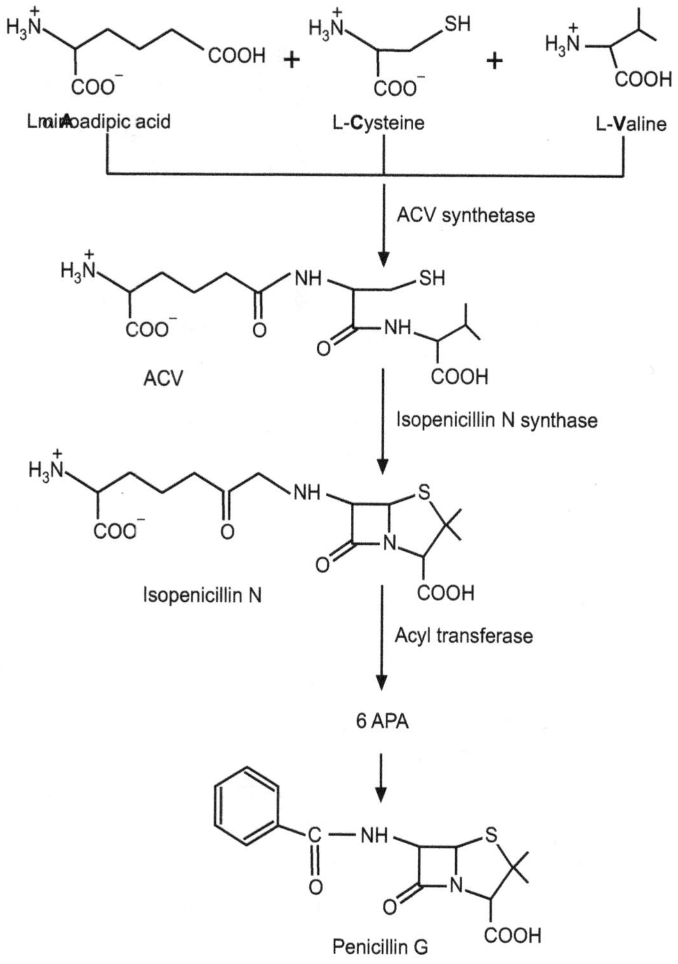

(ii)

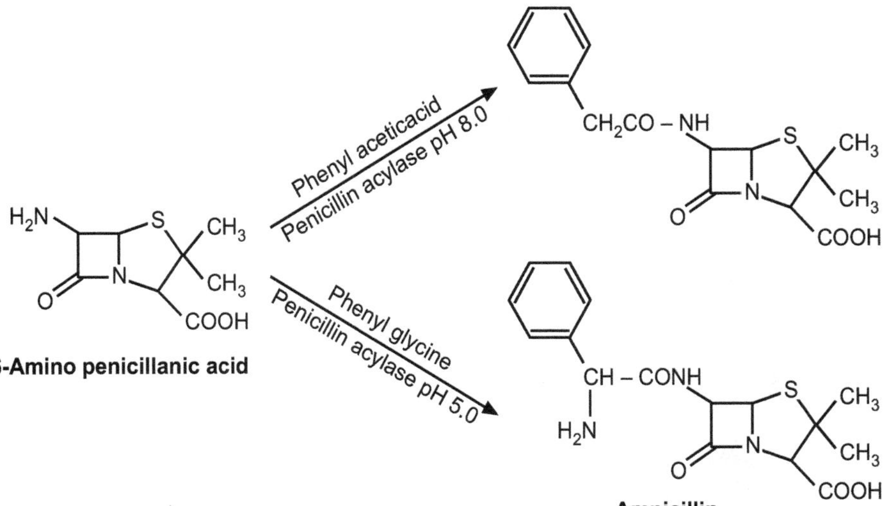

6-Amino penicillanic acid

Ampicillin

Biotransformation of β-lactum Antibiotic Acylation :

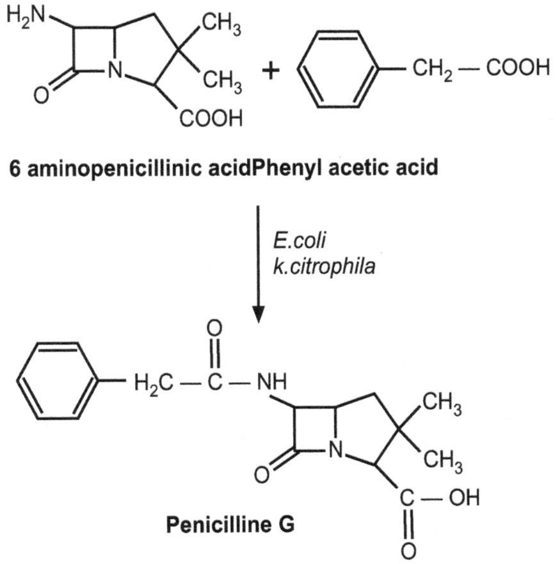

6 aminopenicillinic acidPhenyl acetic acid

E.coli
k.citrophila

Penicilline G

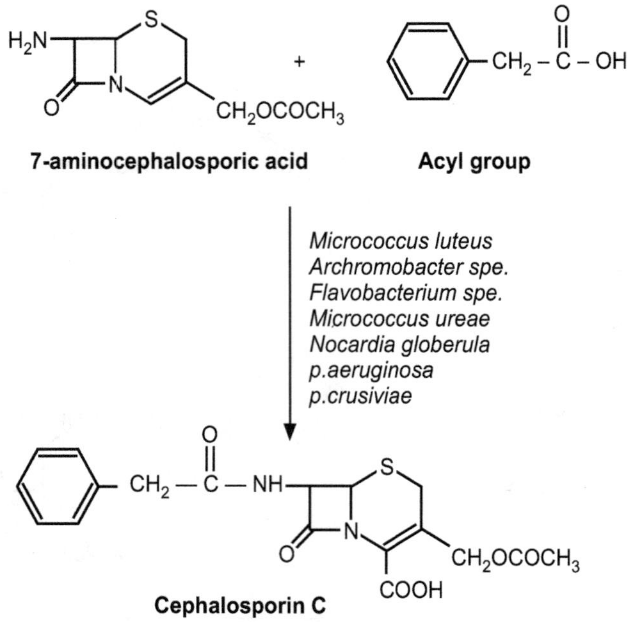

7-aminocephalosporic acid

Acyl group

Micrococcus luteus
Archromobacter spe.
Flavobacterium spe.
Micrococcus ureae
Nocardia globerula
p.aeruginosa
p.crusiviae

Cephalosporin C

Deacylation :

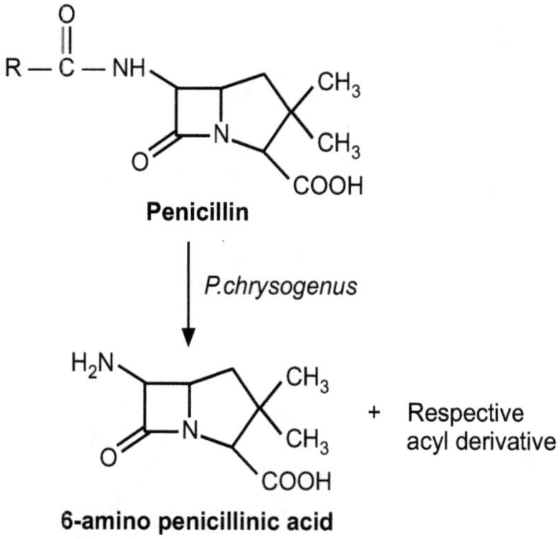

Penicillin

P.chrysogenus

+ Respective acyl derivative

6-amino penicillinic acid

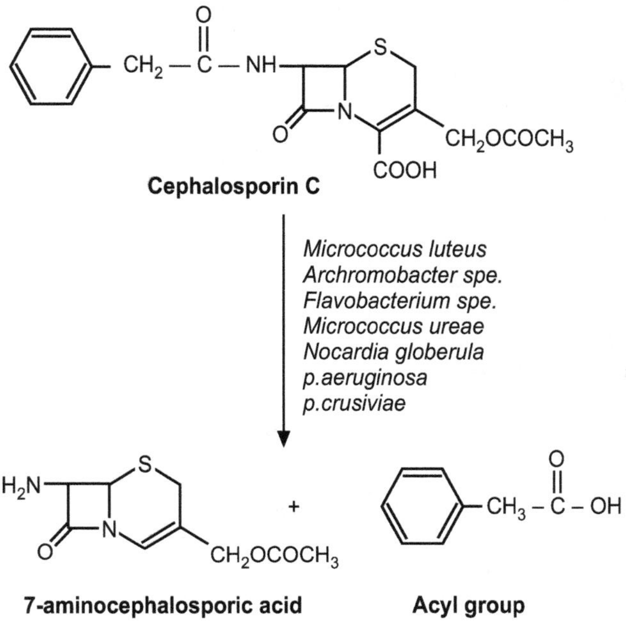

Cephalosporin C

Micrococcus luteus
Archromobacter spe.
Flavobacterium spe.
Micrococcus ureae
Nocardia globerula
p.aeruginosa
p.crusiviae

7-aminocephalosporic acid   **Acyl group**

Acetylation (position 3) :

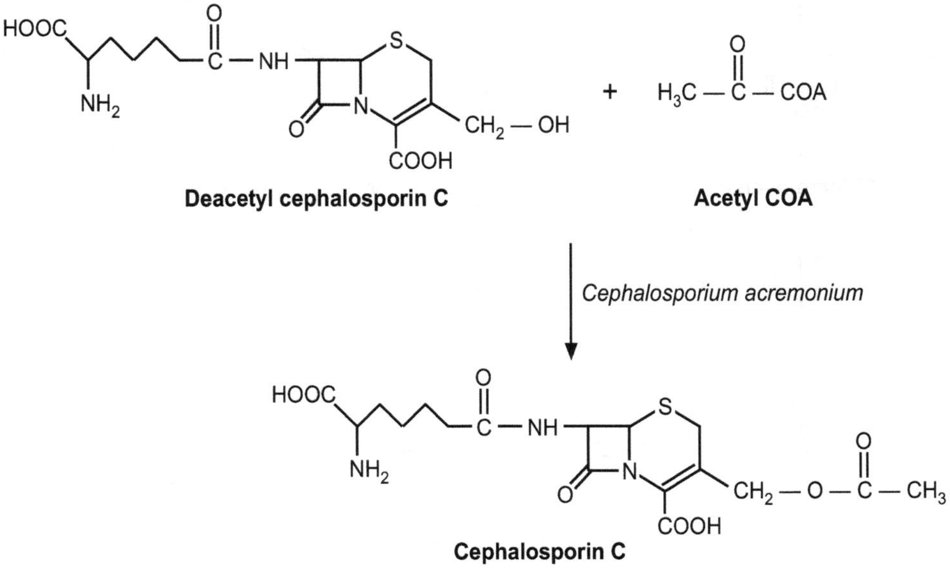

Deacetyl cephalosporin C   **Acetyl COA**

Cephalosporium acremonium

Cephalosporin C

Deacetylation :

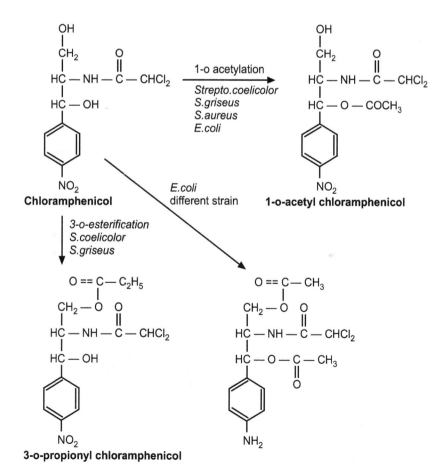

Biotransformation of Chloramphenicol :

Hydrolysis and reduction of chloramphenicol :

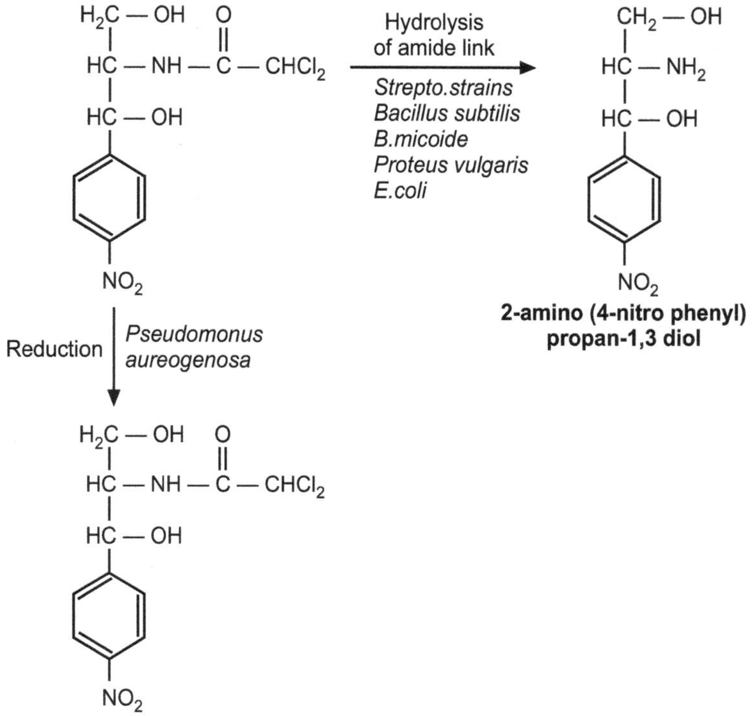

2-amino (4-nitro phenyl) propan-1,3 diol

Biotransformation of macrolide antibiotics :

Acylation :

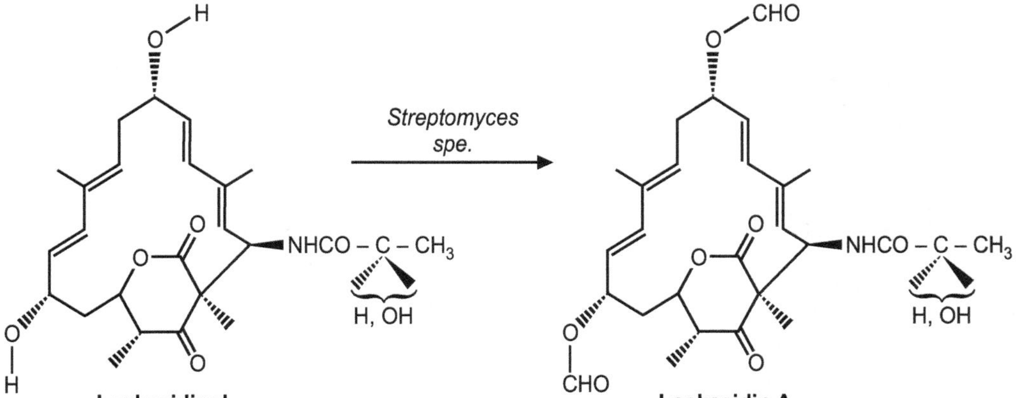

Lankacidinol acetate

Lankacidin A

Methylation :

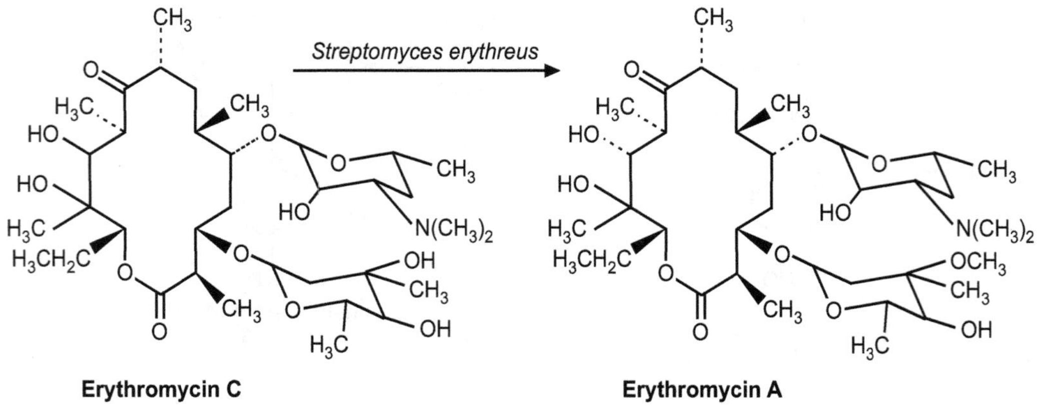

Erythromycin C   *Streptomyces erythreus*   Erythromycin A

Biotransformation of Antracycline Antibiotics :

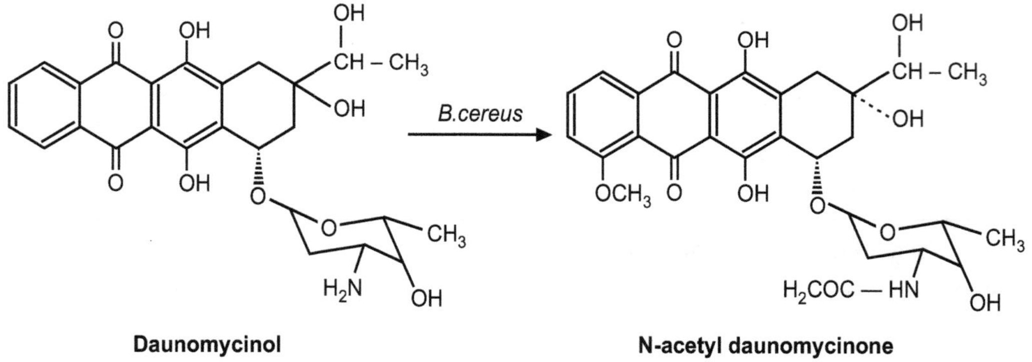

Daunomycinol   *B.cereus*   N-acetyl daunomycinone

Ketonic carbonyl reduction :

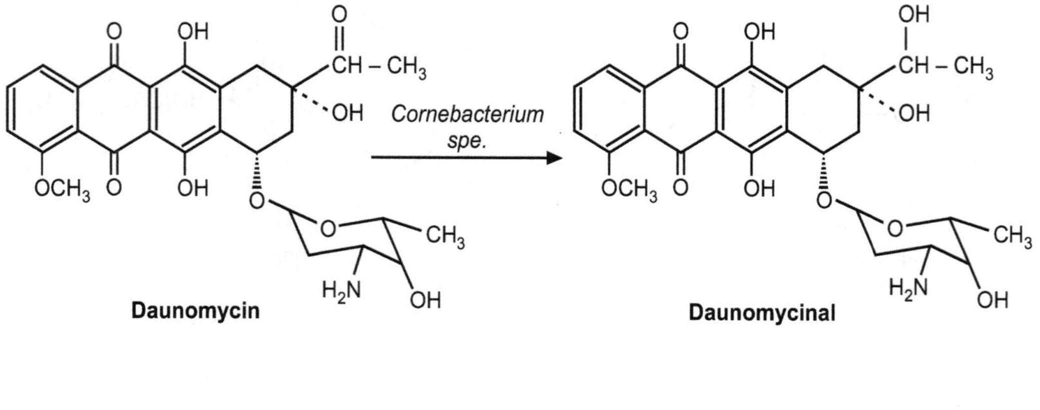

Daunomycin   *Cornebacterium spe.*   Daunomycinal

Biotransformation of Lincomycin :

Sulfoxidation :

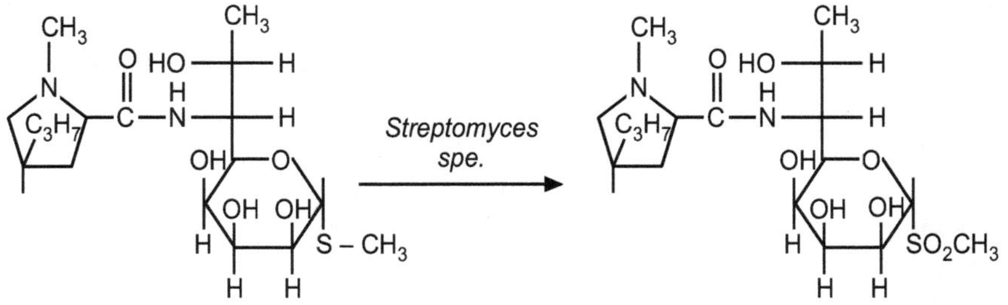

Lincomycin —*Streptomyces spe.*→ Lincomycin SULFOXIDE

Phosphorylation :

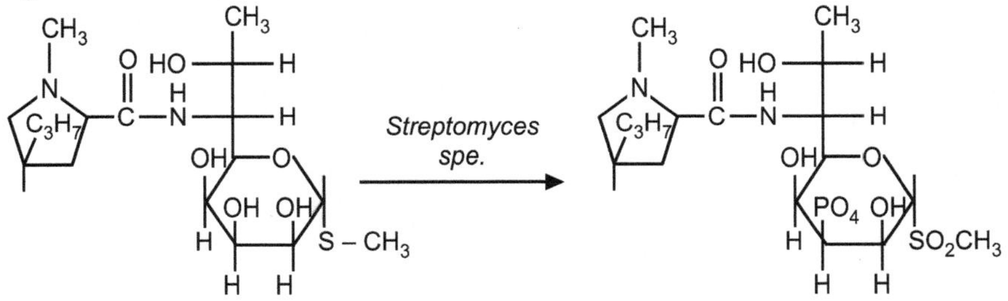

Lincomycin —*Streptomyces spe.*→ Lincomycin 3-phosphate

Demethylation :

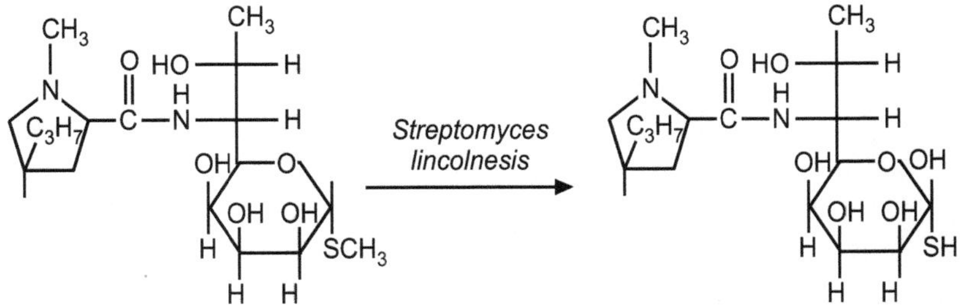

Lincomycin —*Streptomyces lincolnesis*→ Demethylthio 1-hydroxy lincomycin

Biotransformation of Griseofulvin :

Demethylation :

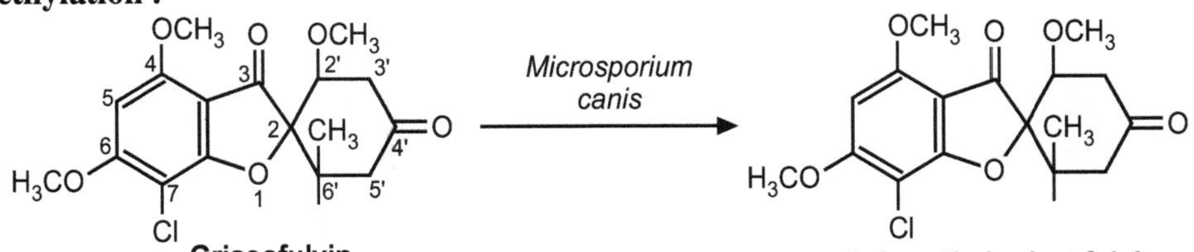

Griseofulvin —*Microsporium canis*→ 4-demethyl griseofulvin

6

NEUROTRANSMITTER

6.1 INTRODUCTION

All the important functions of the body are governed by two distinct and different systems, the endocrine and the nervous system. The endocrine system regulates principally the metabolic functions of the body through the secretion of hormones, which are carried by the blood stream to their target organs. The nature of the control mediated by this system is essentially long term and is exerted on growth, the initiation and maintenance of sexuality the rate of metabolism and the level of blood glucose. In contrast, the nervous system is known to mediate very rapid actions and responses such as muscular contractions, rapidly changing visceral events and even the rates of secretion of some endocrine glands.

By means of electrical and chemical transmission via a distinct of specialised cells, the nervous system produces reflex response to threats and emergencies, controls heart rate and blood pressure, lung function, digestion and recognizes even minute fluctuations in the external environment. It receives millions of bits of information from the different sensory organs and integrates all these information to finalize the response to be made by the body.

The human brain is believed to contain 10^{11} neurons. Except under rare conditions, in the synapse the signal passes only in the forward direction. This allows the signals to be conducted in the required directions for performing necessary nervous functions.

6.2 CENTRAL NERVOUS SYSTEM

The Central Nervous System (CNS) comprises the brain and spinal cord and is the thought and control center of the body. Most activities of the CNS are initiated by sensory information which enters the CNS through the spinal nerves and is conducted to multiple "primary" sensory areas in,

(a) the spinal cord at all levels,
(b) the reticular substance of the medulla, pons and mesencephalon,
(c) the cerebellum,
(d) the thalamus,
(e) the somesthetic area of the cerebral cortex.

While the motor functions of the nervous system are mediated through

(a) contraction of skeletal muscles,
(b) contraction of smooth muscles, and
(c) secretion of both exocrine and endocrine glands.

After the important sensory information has been selected, it is then channeled into proper motor regions of the brain to cause the desired responses. This channeling of information is called the integrative function of the nervous system. It is possible to locate the CNS regions concerned with sensory functions, motor activity, regulation of autonomic functions, control of respiration and memory. On this basis, the CNS can be divided into three major parts which include,

(a) the spinal cord level,
(b) the lower brain level,
(c) the cortical or higher brain level.

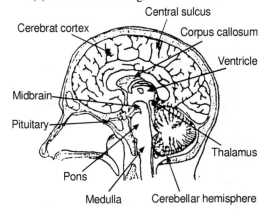

Fig. 6.1 : Major Regions of the Brain

The spinal cord level covers the region from the caudal end of the medulla oblongata to the lower lumbar vertebrae. It is mainly concerned with (i) walking movements, (ii) reflexes that withdraw portions of the body from objects, (iii) reflexes that support the legs to stand against gravity and (iv) reflexes that control local blood vessel and GI-movements.

The lower brain level includes medulla, pons, mesencephalon, hypothalamus, thalamus, cerebellum and basal ganglia. It controls the subconscious activities of the body like respiration, feeding reflexes and emotional responses.

The cortical level (i.e., cerebral cortex) functions as a memory store house of the body. Although the cerebral cortex is essential for most of our thought processes, it is the lower brain level that causes awakefulness and alertness in the cerebral cortex, thus helps to open its bank of memories to the thinking machinery of the brain. Similarly, with the help of memory store-house of cortex the raw and imprecise functions of the lower brain level are exercised in a very derminative and precise way.

(a) Limbic system :

It is sometimes called as visceral brain. It consists of cortical areas (e.g., olfactory and pyriform lobes, hippocampal gyrus) and subcortical structures (e.g., amygdala and septum). The hypothalamus, anterior thalamic nuclei, the epithalamus and ports of the basal ganglia are also included in the limbic system by some authors. The limbic structures through their connections with the extrapyramidal areas (basal ganglia) and the hypothalamus integrate emotional states with motor and visceral activites. The basal ganglia or neostriatum (the caudate nucleus, putamen, globus pallidus and lantiform nucleus) form an essential segment of the extra pyramidal motor system. While the hippocampus has been considered to be of importance in the formation of recent memory.

(b) Reticular activating system :

The brain stem consisting of the medulla, pons, midbrain and a portion of diencephalon accomodates a very important functional system, the Reticular Activating System (RAS). The RAS which consists of the reticular formation and non-specific thalamocortical projections to the cerebral cortex, is involved with central integration for co-ordination of essential reflexive acts (such as vomitting) and of cardiovascular and respiratory functions. However, RAS is primarily responsible for regulation of sleep and wakefulness. It is a major site for action of CNS stimulants as well as CNS depressant drugs.

6.3 NEUROTRANSMITTER

Along with acetylcholine and norepinephrine, other neuro-transmitters which function in the CNS include dopamine, epinephrine, serotonin, glycine, gamma amino butyric acid, aspartic acid, taurine, histamine, substance P, enkephalins and ATP.

It is usually difficult to establish an identity of any other substance as a candidate to function as neurotransmitter in CNS. Many drugs affect CNS functioning by influencing the release, action or metabolism of the neurotransmitter. In such cases, it can not be judged easily whether the altered CNS pattern is due to involvement of new neuro-transmitter or due to modulating effect of drug given. It can be decided by developing such specific agents that will block the specific form of the nervous activity in CNS that was supposed to be operated by the drug which was claimed to be a new neurotransmitter.

Acetylcholine has been searched out in the brain cortex, limbic system, extrapyramidal nuclei and reticular formation. It regulates the sensory function, short term memory, the classical phase of sleep and elimination of hormones, especially vasopressin.

Norepinephrine acts as a neuro-transmitter in limbic system, reticular formation, locus coeruleus, hypothalamus and medulla oblongata. It is involved in thermoregulation, memory, motor activity and vegetative functions.

Dopamine is present at higher concentration in the extrapyramidal nuclei and limbic structures. It regulates motor activity, emotional tonus, memory and release of hormones.

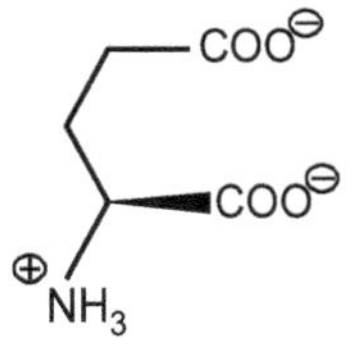

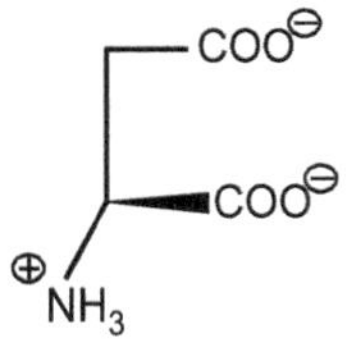

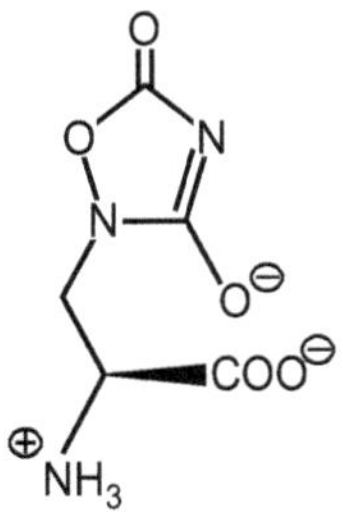

Table 6.1 : Excitatory Amino Acid Agonists and Antagonists

Endogenous agonists

L-Glutamate

L-Aspartate

Selective agonists

Quisqualate

Kainate

N-Methyl-D-aspartate (NMDA)

Ibotenate

Domoate

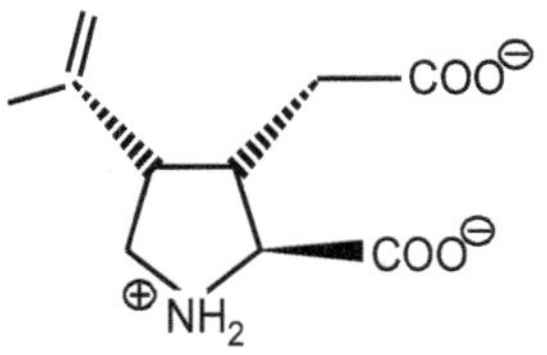

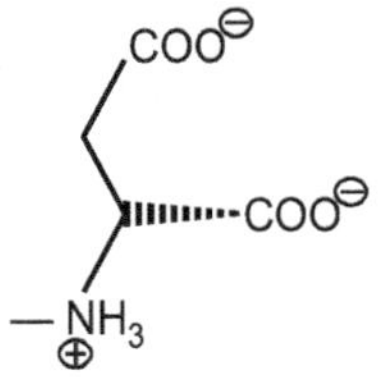

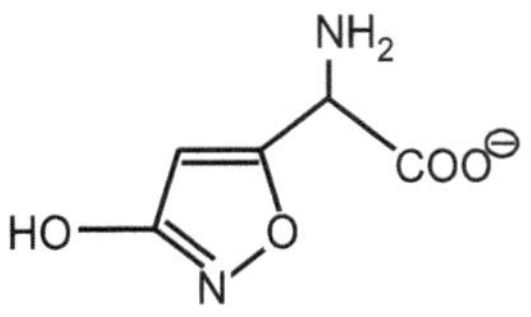

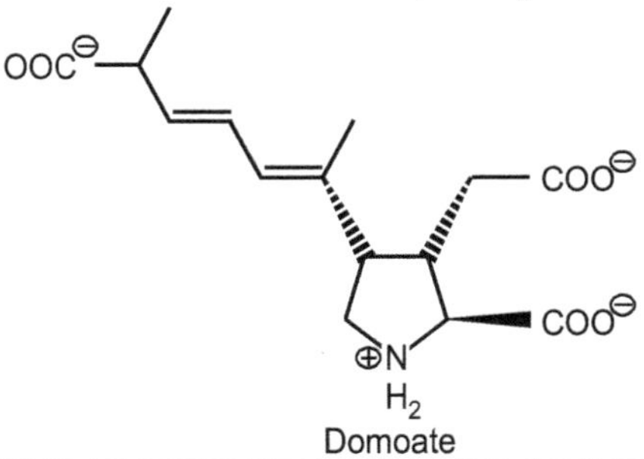

Antagonists

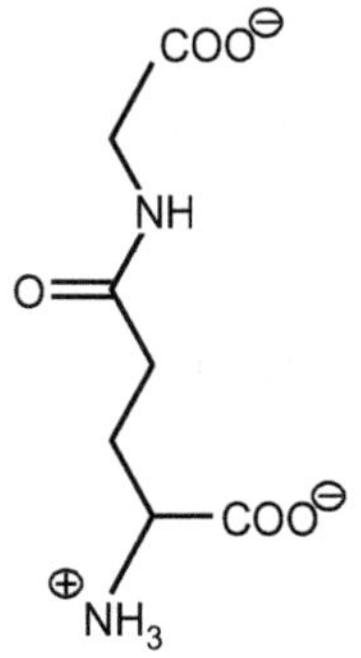

λ-D-Glutamylglycine (DGG)

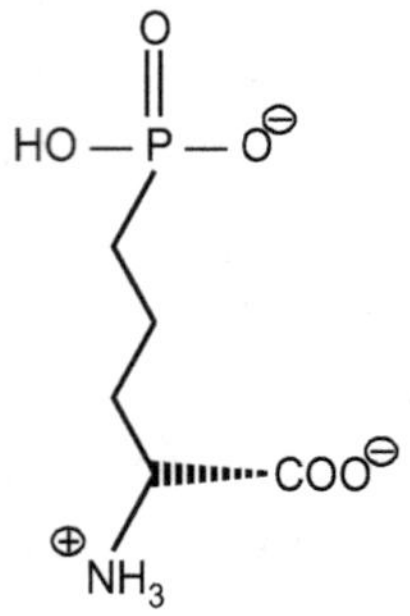

D-2-Amino-5-phosphonovalerate

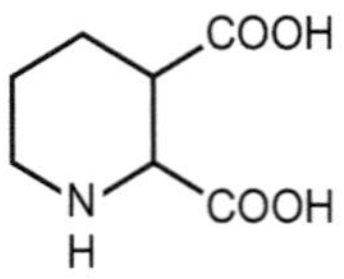

cis-2, 3-Piperidine dicarboxylic acid

Serotonin is a mediator which influences thermoregulation, learning, classical phase of sleep, analgesia and sensory functions. It is present in limbic system, hypothalamus, spinal cord and raphe nuclei. Lysergic Acid diethylamide (LSD) interferes in and reduces serotonin turnover in the brain. This explains the basis of hallucinogenic action of LSD. The depression of serotonin activity results in the inhibition of visual and other sensory inputs.

Substance P is an extremely active excitatory peptide neurotransmitter. It is involved in mediating pain responses peripherally as well as centrally. In the CNS, the effect of substance P is inhibitory, analgesic and is stimulated by the endogenous enkephalins. The second messenger involved is phosphatidylinositol which mobilizes Ca^{++}.

Glutamate and aspartate are the excitatory neurotransmitters found to be located in certain areas in the spinal cord, interneurons of the reflex arc and a pathway from the cortex to the striatum. They have been implicated in the mechanisms of information processing, learning and memory.

Similarly adenosine may act as modulator in both central and peripheral nervous system. Adenosine can affect a variety of physiological functions. The receptor mediated actions require the presence of guanyl nucleotide (G) binding subunit. Adenosine through its interaction with adenosine receptors linked to adenylate cyclase, can bring about vasodilation, hypotensive, anti-arrhythmic, sedative, anticonvulsant, analgesic and antipyretic effects.

Table 6.2 : Classification of Neuronal Receptors

Subtype	Selective agonist	Selective antagonist
(A) Adrenergic receptors		
α_1	Phenylephrine	Prazosin
α_2	Clonidine, guanfacine	Idazoxan
β_1	Dobutamine	Metoprolol
β_2	Terbutaline	Butoxamine
(B) Dopaminergic receptors :		
D_1	Dihydroxidine, SKF 38390	SCH 23390
D_2	Quinpirol PHN 0434	Domperidone, Sulpiride
(C) Serotonergic receptors		
$5\,HT_{1A}$	Buspirone	Spiperone
$5\,HT_{1B}$	Ru 24969	------
$5\,HT_{1C}$	LSD, methylsergide	------
$5\,HT_{1D}$	5 – methoxytryptamine	Metergoline
$5\,HT_2$	------	Spiperone
$5\,HT_3$	------	Zocopride
(D) Cholinergic receptors :		
M_1	McN-A-343, Oxotremorine	Pirenzepine
M_2	------	AF-DX-116
M_3	------	Hexahydrosiladifenidol
N (neuronal)	Dimethylphenyl, piperazinium	Trimethaphan
N (muscular)	Phenyltrimetyl ammonium	Tubocurarine
(E) GABA-nergic receptors :		
$GABA_A$	Muscimol	Bicuculline
$GABA_B$	Baclofen	Phaclofen
(F) Histaminergic receptors :		
H_1	Histamine	Pyrilamine
H_2	Histamine	Ranitidine
H_3	Histamine	Thioperamide
(G) Opiate receptors :		
μ	Morphine	Cyclic somatostatin
κ	Dynorphin	Norbinaltorphimine
σ	Haloperidol, N-allylnormetazocine	------
δ	Enkephalins	KI-176

6.4 ADRENALINE AND ADRENERGIC RECEPTORS

In the mammalian CNS, adrenaline is present relatively in low concentration, approximately 5-15 % of the noradrenaline concentration. It is synthesized from the amino acid precursor, tyrosine which is taken up from the bloostream by an active transport mechanism and concentrated within the brain.

Both tyrosine and phenylalanine are the normal constituents of mammalian brain, present in a concentration of about 5×10^{-5} M.

Certain drugs affect the biosynthesis of adrenaline by blocking the enzymes that catalyze the intermediate steps. They may be used to lower norepinephrine formation in patients with pheochromocytoma and malignant hypertension.

Table 6.3 : Enzyme Inhibitors Affecting Biosynthesis of Adrenaline

Enzyme	Enzyme Inhibitors
L-tyrosine hydroxylase	α-methyl-p-tyrosine, 3-iodotyrosine, α-methyl-3-iodotyrosine α-methyl-5-hydroxytryptophan
Dopamine – β-hydroxylase	D-cysteine, L-cyseine, glutathione, mercaptoethanol and copper chelating agents like disulfiram.

6.5 DOPAMINE AND DOPAMINERGIC RECEPTORS

Besides its role as intermediate in the biosynthesis of norepinephrine and epinephrine, dopamine is also accepted as a full fledged neurotransmitter. Drugs affecting dopaminergic neuronal functions are showing promising results in the treatment of schizophrenia and Parkinson's disease. The D_1 receptor is a glycoprotein having molecular weight of about 110-190 KD. The D_1 receptors are suspected to regulate the force of vascular smooth muscles.

(a) Dopamine synthesis inhibitors :

Carbidopa and benserazide are the DOPA decarboxylase inhibitors used to protect the DOPA from peripheral decarboxylation. They are administered in the treatment of Parkinson's disease. Because of their ionic character, both drugs, can not cross the blood - brain barrier which explains their exclusive peripheral mode of action.

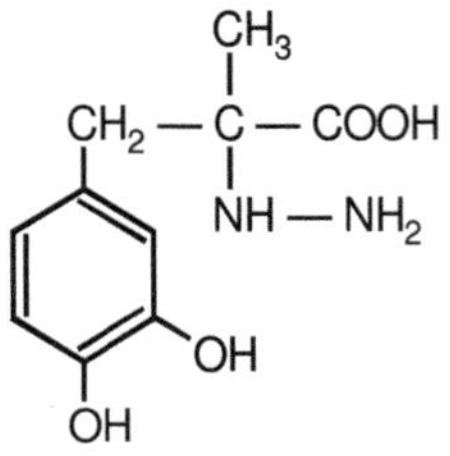

Carbidopa

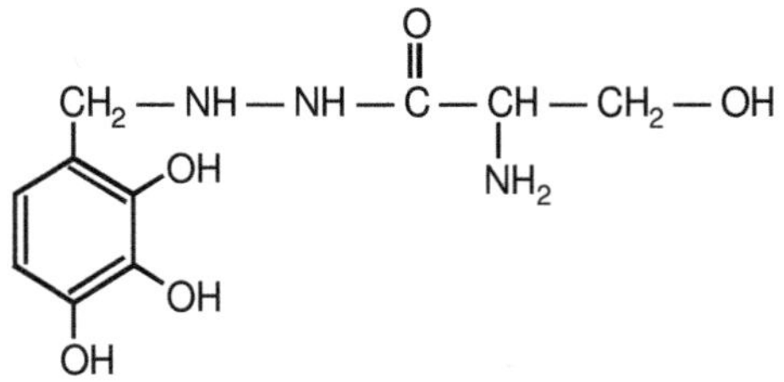

Benserazide

(b) Dopamine storage modulators :

High doses of amphetamine and amantadine (an antiviral drug) may become beneficial in parkinsonism, by promoting the release of dopamine while γ-hydroxy butyrate or its precursor, butyrolactone inhibits dopamine release.

(c) Dopamine reuptake inhibitors :

Following are the examples of specific DA uptake inhibitors. Except benztropine (an anticholinergic drug), rest of inhibitors may be used as potent antidepressants.

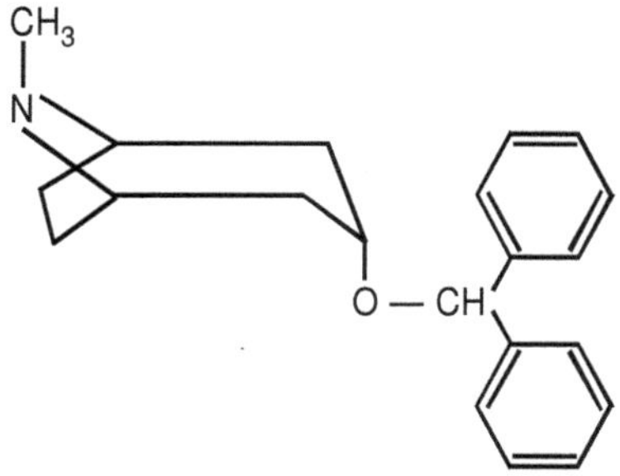

Benztropine

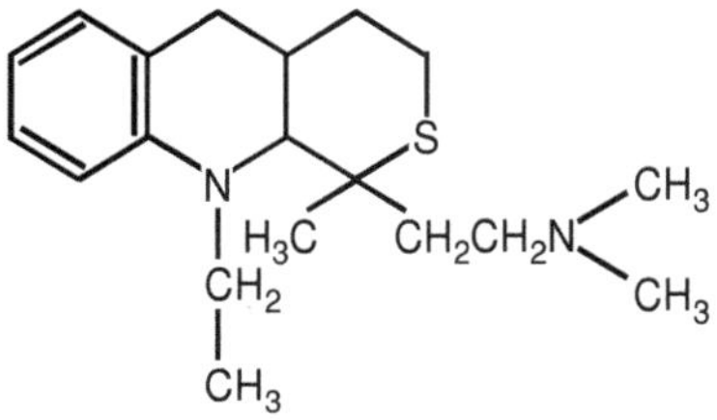

Tandamine

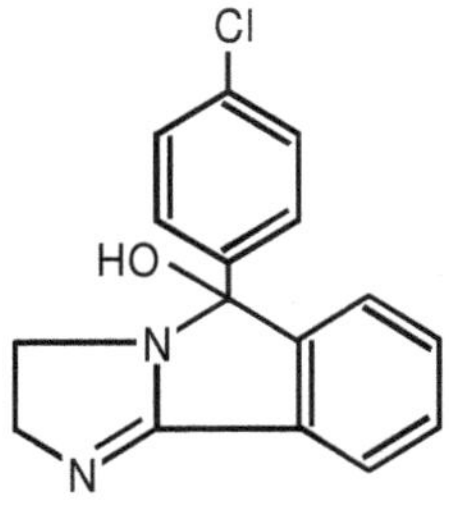

Mazindol

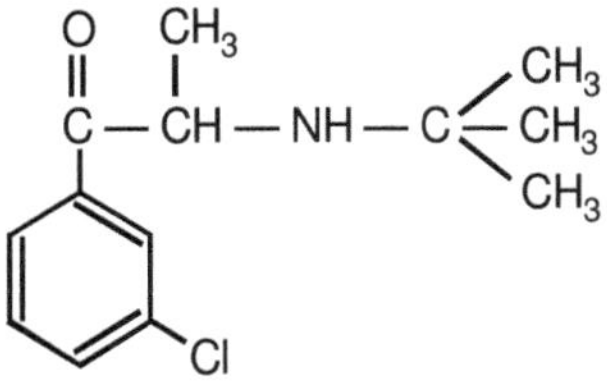

Bupropion

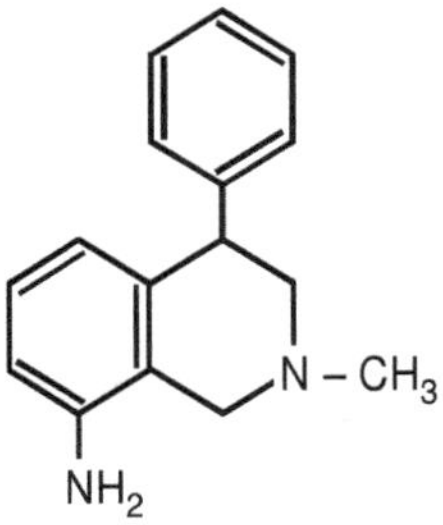

Nomifensine

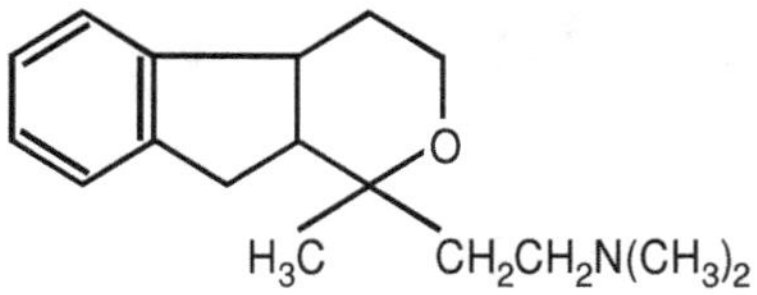

Pirandamine

(d) Dopamine agonists :

Presynaptic dopaminergic agonists like ADTN and 3-PPP act as potent antipsychotics by controlling DA release. Nomifensine is structurally related with ADTN but is used as an antidepressant drug. SKF 38390 is a ring homologue of nomifensine which acts as a selective D_1 - agonist and dilates the renal vascular bed without having any cardiac effects. While the related SCH 23390 is a selective D_1 - antagonist.

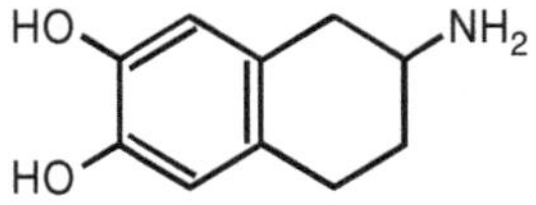

ADTN

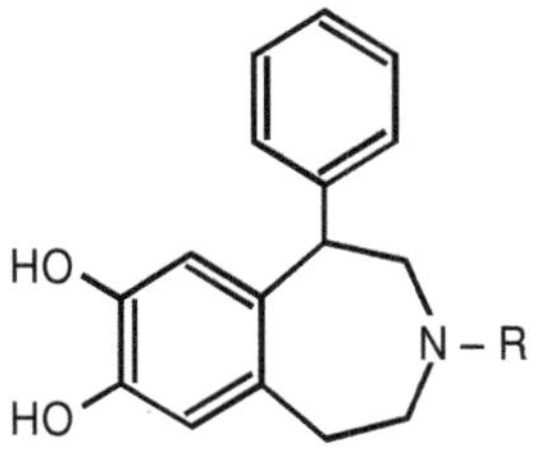

SKF 38393 (X = OH, R = H)

SCH 23390 (X = Cl, R = CH₃)

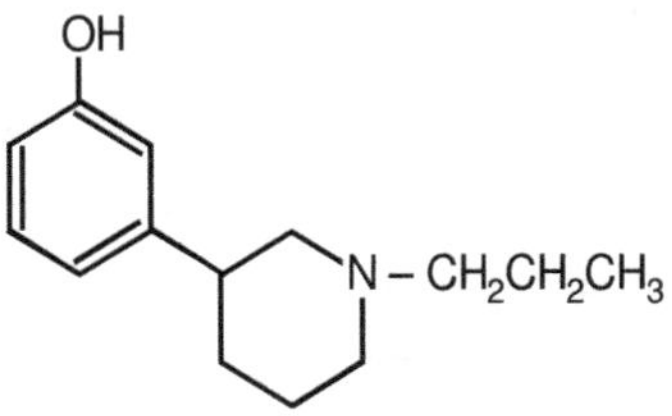

3-(3-Hydroxyphenyl)-
N-(n-propyl) piperidine (3-PPP)

6.6 SEROTONIN AND SEROTONERGIC RECEPTORS

Serotonin (5-hydroxytryptamine) is a central neurotransmitter which is also found peripherally in the intestinal mucosa and in blood platelets. In the CNS, the serotonergic neuronal system is found to be localized in the raphe region of the pons and brain stem, projecting to the medulla and spinal cord. Serotonin is an inhibitory neurotransmitter and operates through adenylate cyclaze. It is involved in the etiology of migraine headaches.

Serotonergic receptors are subdivided into three families - $5HT_1$, $5HT_2$ and $5HT_3$. Cyclic-AMP serves as a second messenger for $5\text{-}HT_1$ receptors while $5HT_2$ receptor uses phosphatidylinositol as second messenger. Both $5HT_1$ and $5HT_2$ receptors belong to the G-protein coupled receptor family. Whereas $5HT_3$ receptors are thought to be ion channels and are probably the members of the nicotine/GABA/glycine channel family. $5HT_1$ receptors have been associated in the periphery both with vasoconstriction and vasorelaxation, inhibition of transmitter release and centrally with behavioural effects, inhibition of transmitter release and reduction of blood pressure.

$5\text{-}HT_2$ receptors are well characterized in the periphery where they mediate vascular and non-vascular smooth muscle constriction and platelet aggregation, whereas centrally, behavioural effets have been reported.

$5\text{-}HT_3$ receptors have been extensively characterized in the periphery. Their localisation is neuronal and they modulate transmitter release. No second messenger system has, as yet, been described for $5\text{-}HT_3$ receptors. The activation of $5\text{-}HT_3$ receptors is suspected to be involved in pain mediation and drug induced vomitting phenomenon where increase, serotonergic function potentiates opiate analgesia.

(a) Serotonin synthesis inhibitors :

Tryptophan hydroxylase catalyzes the rate determining step in the biosynthesis of serotonin. p-Chlorophenylalanine blocks this enzyme and can be used as inhibitor of serotonin synthesis.

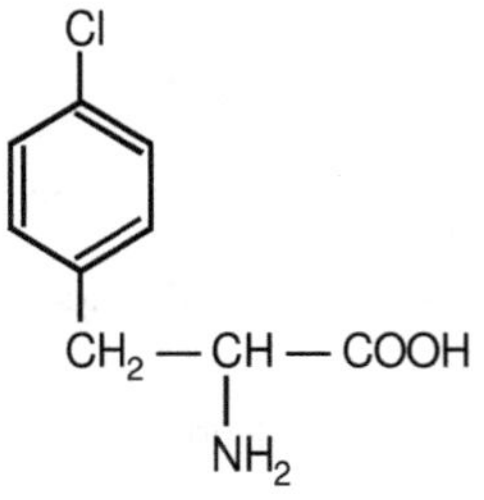

p-chlorophenylalanine

(b) Serotonin reuptake inhibitors :

Important members from this category include;

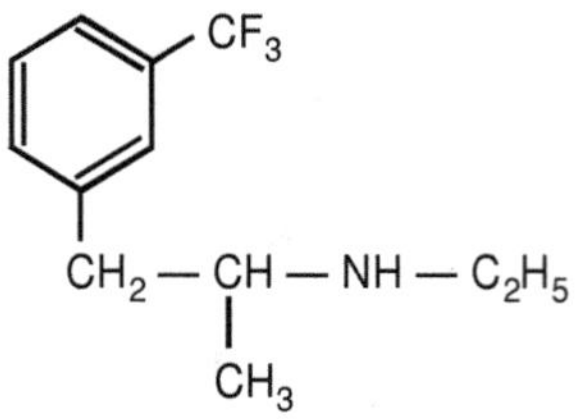

Fenfluramine

Table 6.4 : Serotonergic Receptor Sub-types

Type	Location	Function	Agonist	Antagonist
5HT$_1$	CNS, CVS skin, ileum	Vascular contraction, neuronal inhibition	8-hydroxy-2-(N-dipropyl) aminotetralin-5-carbamoyl tryptamine	Methysergide
5HT$_2$	CNS, CVS, platelets, respiratory system, urogenital system	Muscle contraction and platelet aggregation	α-Methyl serotonin	Ketanserin
5 HT$_3$	Neuronal	Pain, vomiting	2-Methyl 5-HT	ICS-205

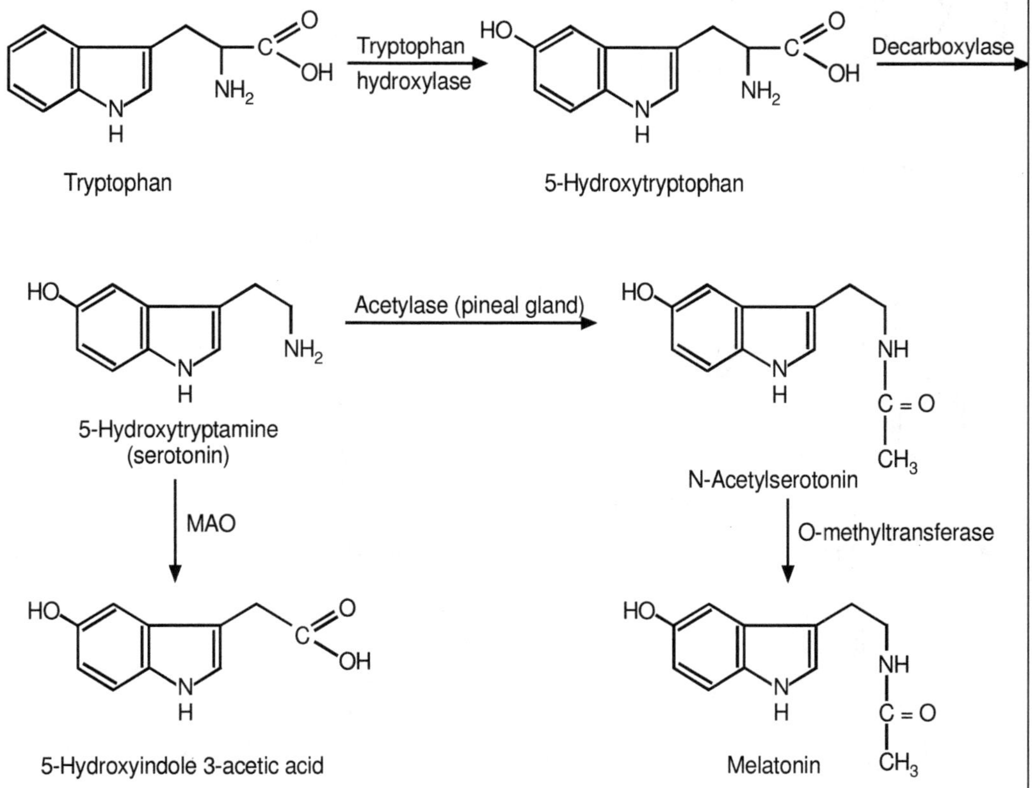

Fig. 6.2 : Biosynthesis and Degradation of Serotonin

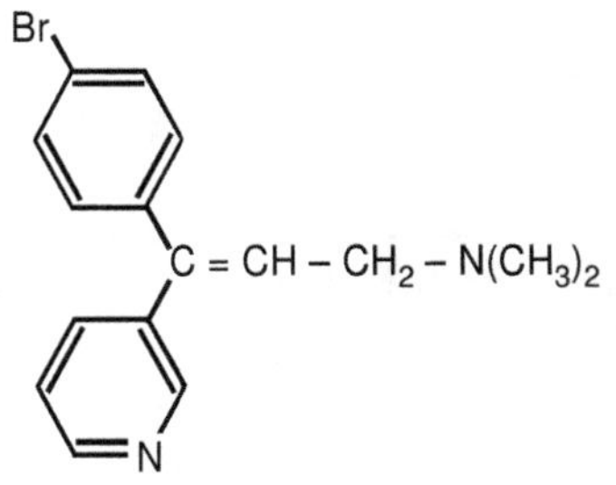

Zimelidine

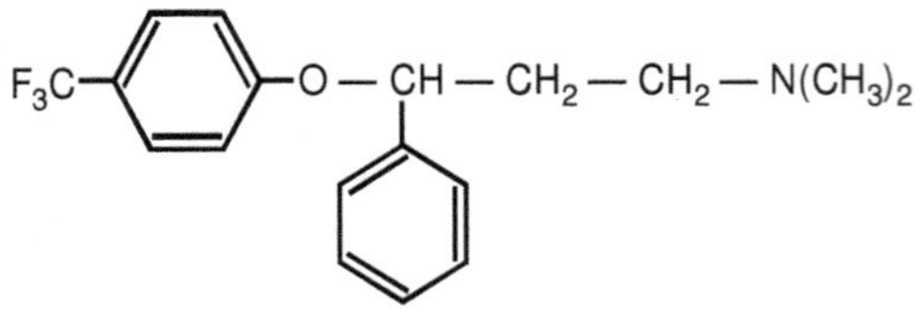

Fluoxetine (anorectic agent)

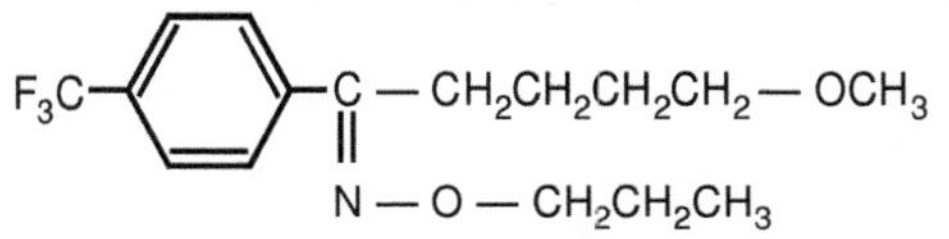

Fluvoxamine

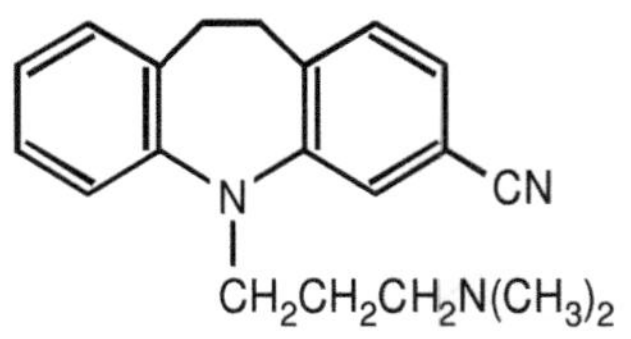

Cyanoimipramine

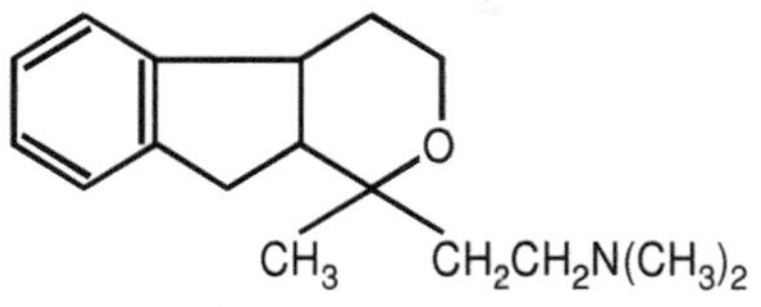

Pirandamine

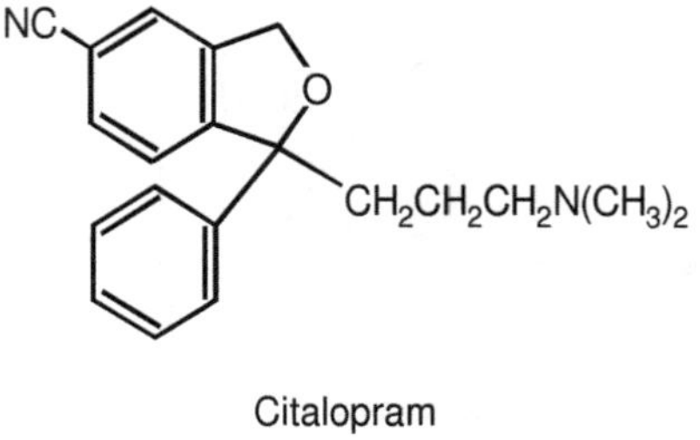

Citalopram

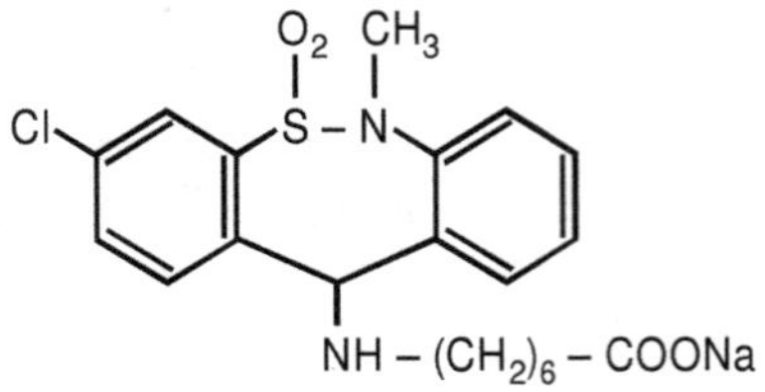

Tianeptine-Na

All these agents are potent antidepressants. This in turn suggests the role of serotonin in endogeneous depression.

(c) Serotonergic agonists :

The important serotonergic agonists include,

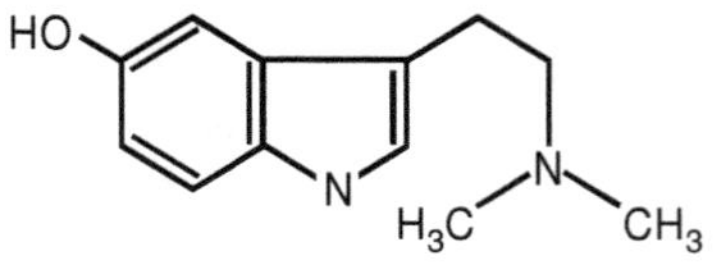

Bufotenin

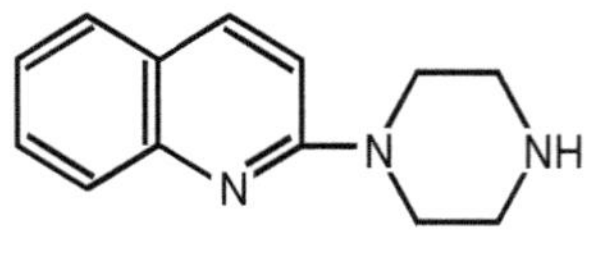

Quipazine

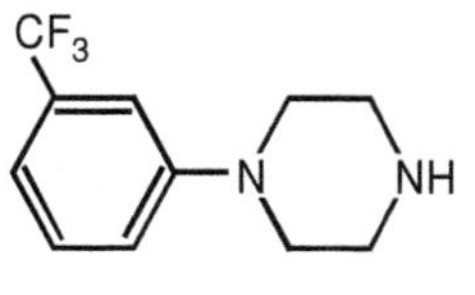

N-(3-trifluoro methylphenyl) piperazine

(d) Serotonin antagonists :

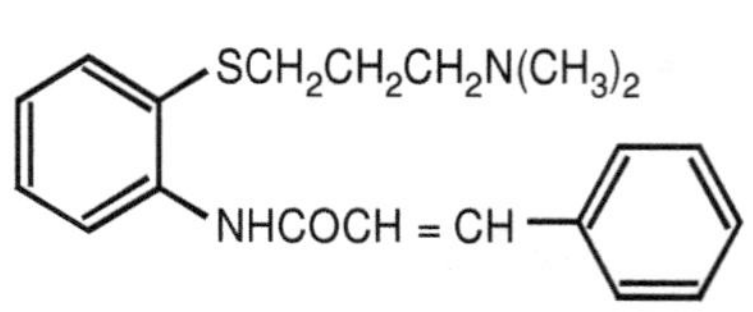

Cinanserin (analgesic and immunosuppressant)

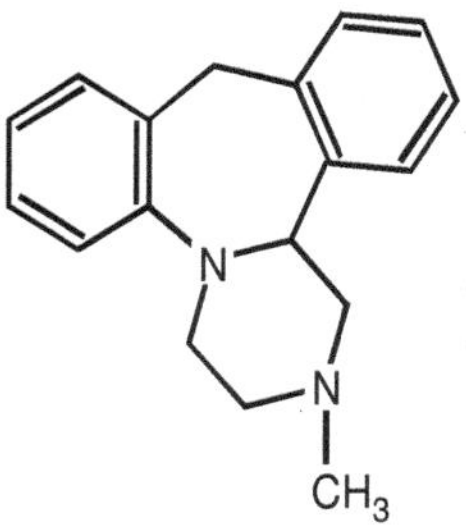

Mianserin (antidepressant)

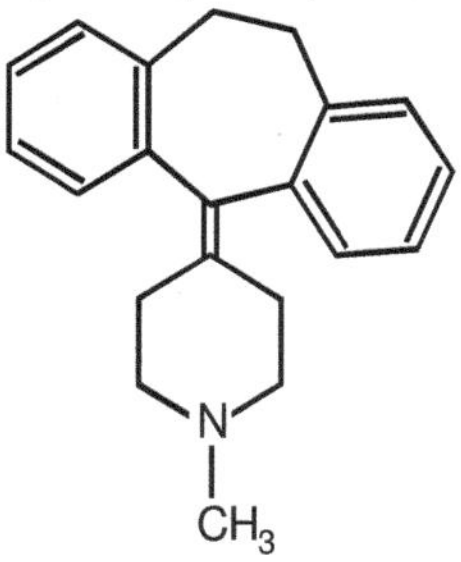

Cyproheptadine (antihistamine)

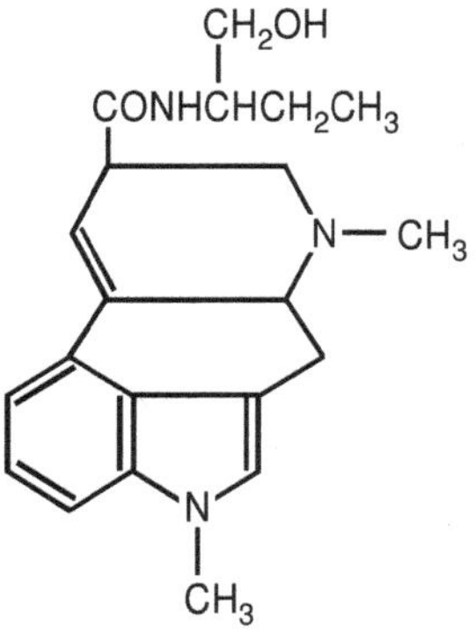

Methylsergide

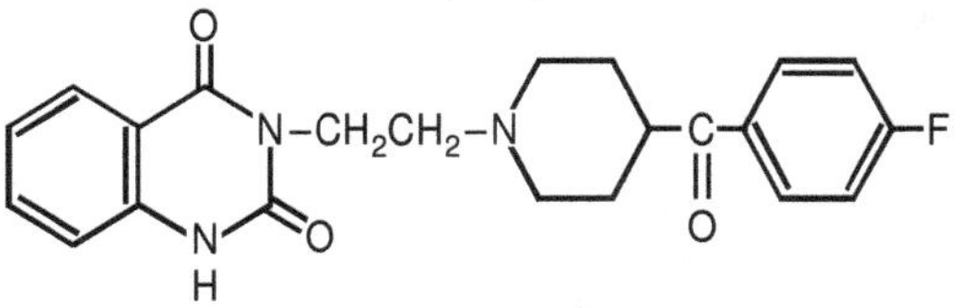

Ketanserin

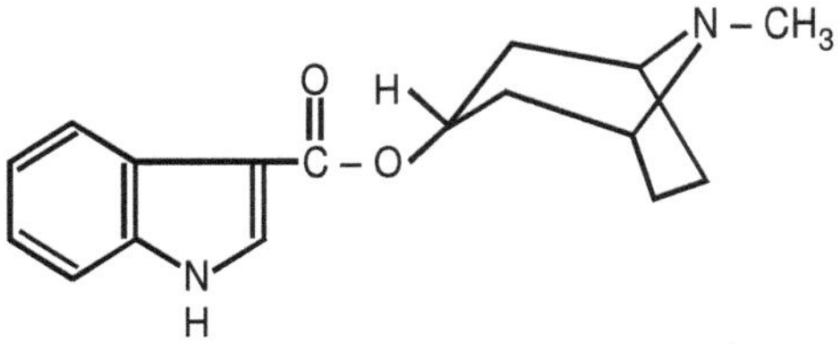

ICS 205-930

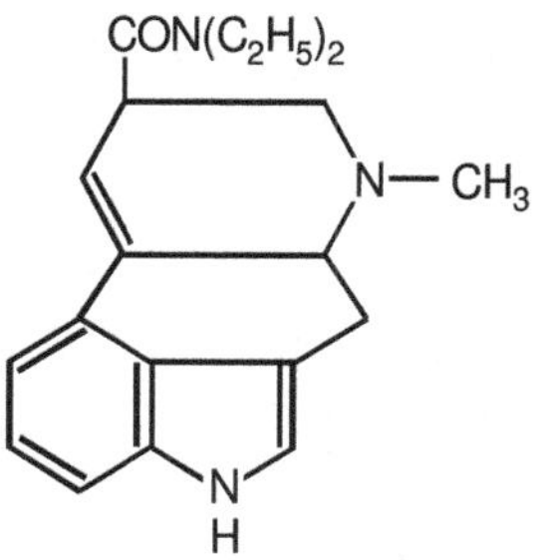

LSD

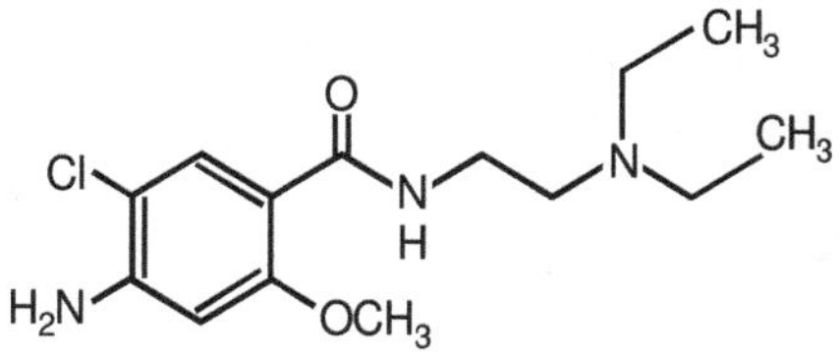

Metoclopramide

6.7 HISTAMINE AND HISTAMINERGIC RECEPTORS

Histamine is both a local hormone and a neurotransmitter. It is implicated in a variety of vegetative functions and behaviours ranging from cardiovascular and temperature control to roles in arousal and the regulation of neuroendocrine mechanisms. Histamine also stimulates the secretion of acid by stomach, relaxes uterus and imparts positive inotropic effect on the heart.

Chemical constitution of histamine :

Chemically, it is β-imidazolyl ethylamine. The structural features of histamine permit it to exist in ionic, tautomeric and conformeric forms which constantly get interconverted to each other. These forms differ mainly in the electronic charge distribution and in the position of hydrogen atoms.

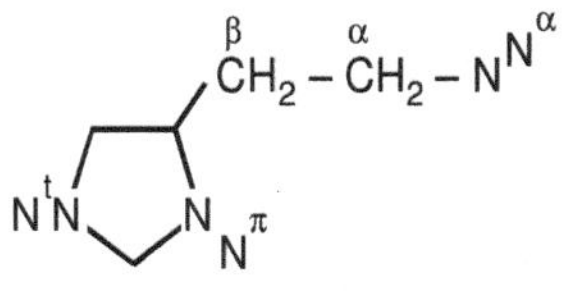

Histamine is comprised of an imidazole ring connected to an amino group through ethylene bridge. Both, imidazole ring and amino group are basic and get protonated under acidic condition. The imidazole ring is an aromatic system and exists in the rigid and planar form. It contains two types of nitogen atoms which are tautomeric and exist in neutral solution in two different forms in which only one of the imidazole nitrogen atoms carries a proton. The single bond in the side chain permits free rotation giving rise to different conformations of the molecule. All the nitrogen atoms in the histamine structure, are negatively charged. Since, there is a little net charge on the carbon atoms, the positive charge is distributed widely over all the hydrogen atoms in the molecule, tending to be concentrated on the N-H hydrogens.

Due to above properties, histamine exists in a solution as a mixture of many species undergoing rapid interconversion, viz. ionic forms, tautomers and conformers. These species differ in electronic charge, position of hydrogen atoms and overall shape. The overall shape of the molecule is determined by the orientation of the rigid planar imidazole ring (indicated by the angle ϕ_1) and by the conformation of the single bonds containing side-chain (indicated by the angle ϕ_2). Here ϕ_1 measures the rotation of imidazole ring while ϕ_2 measures rotation within side-chain. The change in these angles results in change in conformation and shape of the molecule.

For example,

(a)

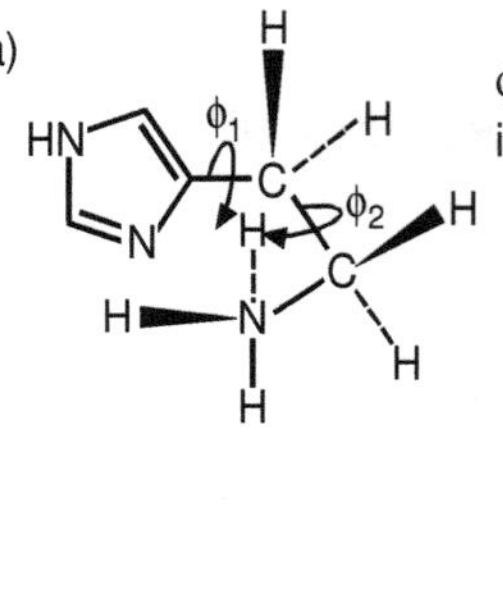

$\phi_1 = 180^\circ$ and $\phi_2 = 0^\circ$. It is eclipsed conformation.

(b)

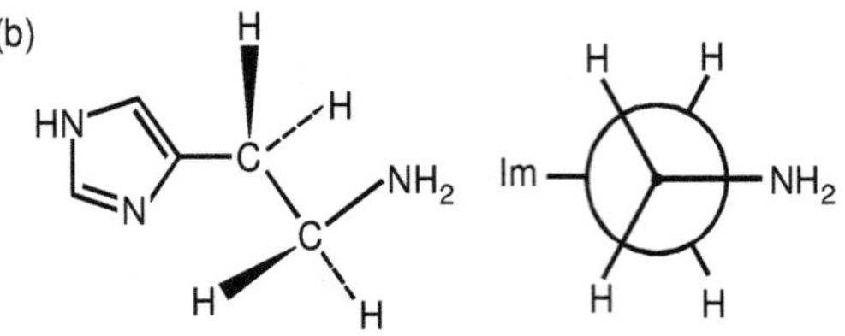

It is a trans (extended) conformation where $\phi_2 = 180^\circ$.

(c)

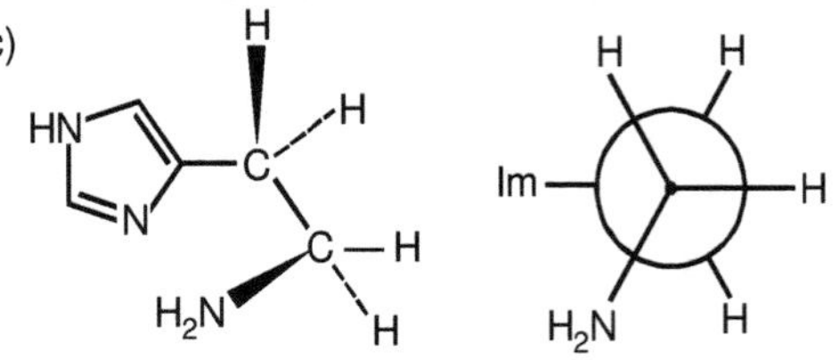

It is gauche (folded) conformation where $\phi_2 = 60^\circ$ or 300°.

Since the most stable conformers are those in which the H-atoms in the side-chain have a staggered arrangement (e.g. trans and gauche), in an aqueous solution, a mixture of approximately equal amounts of trans and gauche conformers is present.

Histamine is a very polar molecule. The partition coefficient of histamine was found to be 0.2 at pH 11.8 in n-octanol/water system. Because of such high hydrophilicity, over 80% of histamine remains in the aqueous solution. Histamine exists in various ionic forms whose population is a function of pH of the solution.

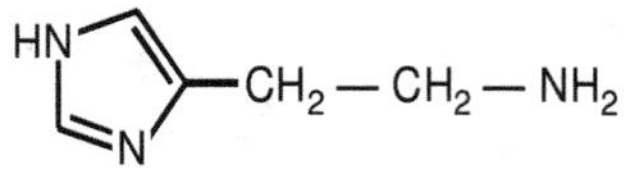

Uncharged free base

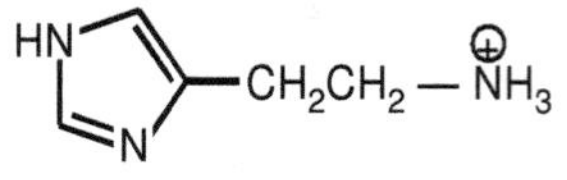

Monocation

Since, the population of monocation was found to be maximum at physiological pH, it suggests that the monocation is the physiologically important species. Thus, proton shift in imidazole ring leads to tautomers, free rotation in the side-chain allows formation of conformers and protonation of basic nitrogen results into formation of monocation. The sites for generation of tautomeric, conformers and ionic forms of histamine are shown in the Fig. 6.3.

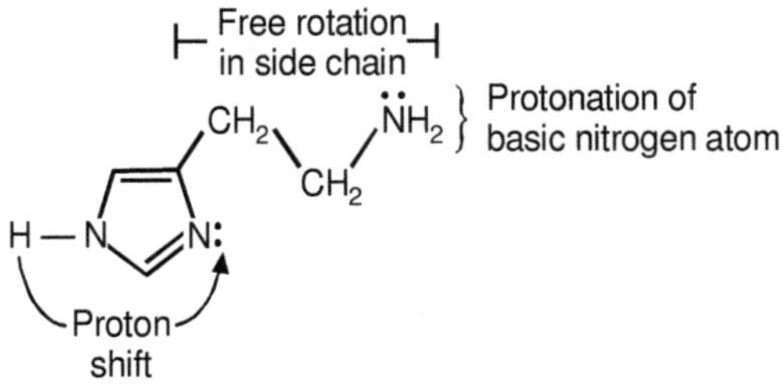

Fig. 6.3 : Sites of Generation of Tautomers, Conformers and Ionic Forms of Histamine

The tertiary amine N^α, N^α-dimethyl histamine is active at H_1 and H_2 receptors but the quaternary ammonium derivative, N^α, N^α N^α-trimethyl histamine is extremely weak. This suggests that atleast one hydrogen atom should be present on nitrogen (N^α) of the side-chain. If the main function of the proton was considered as H-bonding then activity would appear to reside exclusively with the monocation.

Kier (1968) proposed that the ability of histamine to interact with H_1 and H_2-receptors is due to ability of its monocationic form to adopt two distinct and preferred conformations. He assigned H_1-receptor activity to the trans monocation and H_2-activity to the gauche monocation. In trans rotamer, the carbon and nitrogen atoms are coplanar with the ring and there is a

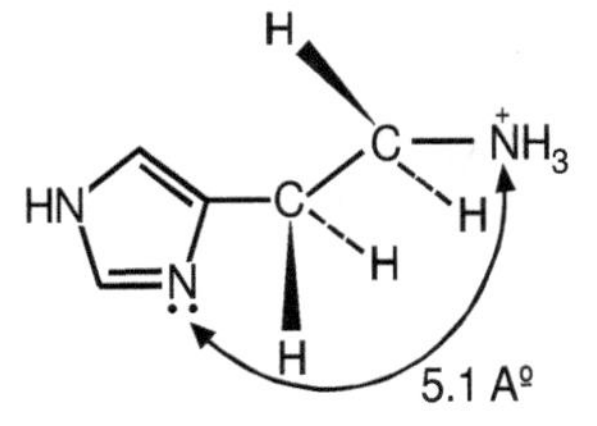

maximum separation (5.1 A°) between the charged ammonium group and the ring N^π-nitrogen atom. The H_1-essential conformation is not a minimum energy species, but has an energy of about 3 kcal/mol above the minimum. Thus at the H_1-receptor, imidazole tautomerism is not a functional requirement. However, the ring should achieve coplanarity with the side-chain.

Structural requirements of histamine as an H_2-agonist are considered to be the protonated side-chain nitrogen atom and the ability of the imidazole amidine system to undergo a tautomeric shift. It is suggested that the histamine monocation binds to the H_2– receptor via the formation of three H–bonds. Here the cationic ammonium group and the –NH– group of imidazole system are hydrogen donors, whereas, the $= N-$ atom of the imidazole ring acts as a hydrogen acceptor. The proton-shift at the receptor surface in addition to the tautomerism of the imidazole ring is believed to trigger the H_2-receptor stimulation.

Thus, the monocation of the side chain forms a H– bond with a basic moiety (X) present at the receptor where it may give up its

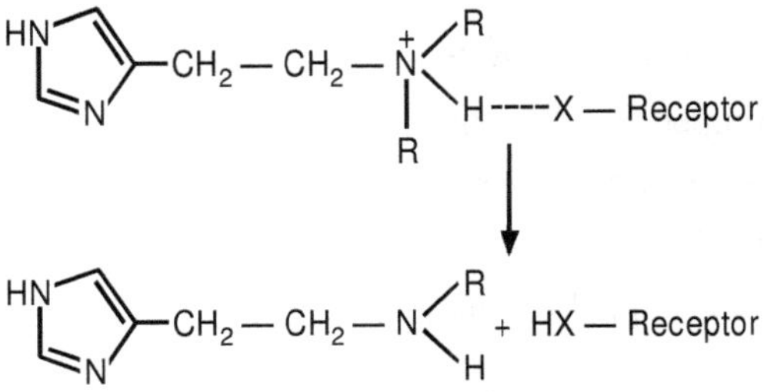

proton to the basic moiety of the receptor resulting into generation of uncharged histamine molecule. The uncharged forms may be required for an access or be involved in assisting imidazole - mediated proton - transfer at the receptor site.

Thus, at H₁-receptors, histamine shows agonistic activity because of following structural features :

(a) side-chain cation and N^t - H tautomer,

(b) heterocyclic ring with basic nitrogen with lone pair of electrons at ortho position, and

(c) the trans rotamer.

While to exhibit H₂-receptor agonist activity, histamine possesses following structural features :

(a) side-chain cation,

(b) ring which can undergo 1, 3-protropic tautomerism. Probably imidazole N^t – H tautomer may be involved in the bifunctional H–bonding.

Bifunctional H-bonding

(c) the gauche rotamer.

Thus at the H₂-receptor, the tautomeric property of the imidazole ring of histamine appears to be of importance and histamine might act as a proton-transfer agent in bifunctional H-bonding.

6.8 OPIOID AND OPIATE RECEPTORS

The original concept of opioid receptor was first postulated from the stereo - selective studies by Beckett and Casy (1954). They proposed that an opioid receptor is composed of three prominent parts.

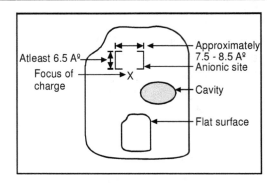

Fig. 6.4 : Opioid Receptor

(1) A flattened part which holds the aromatic portion of an analgesic molecule through Vander Waals forces.

(2) A cavity or hallow portion which entraps the ethylene bridge.

(3) An anionic site which holds the tertiary nitrogen which is assumed to be ionised at physiological pH.

GTP, GDP and the non-hydrolyzable analogue Gpp (NH) 1 reduce agonist affinity while divalent ions such as magnesium increase agonist activity. Sodium ions and Gpp (NH) P were found to decrease the binding of agonists to μ sites more effectively than to δ sites while binding to k site remains least affected.

The activity of morphine resides in D(–) morphine. In this structure, the piperidine ring and alicyclic ring remain in the horizontal plane while rest of the rings of the phenanthrene nucleus exist perpendicular to this. This arrangement helps the molecule to acquire 'T' shape. Because of this shape of morphine molecule, the receptor is considered to have a pouch shape in which the molecule has a perfect fit.

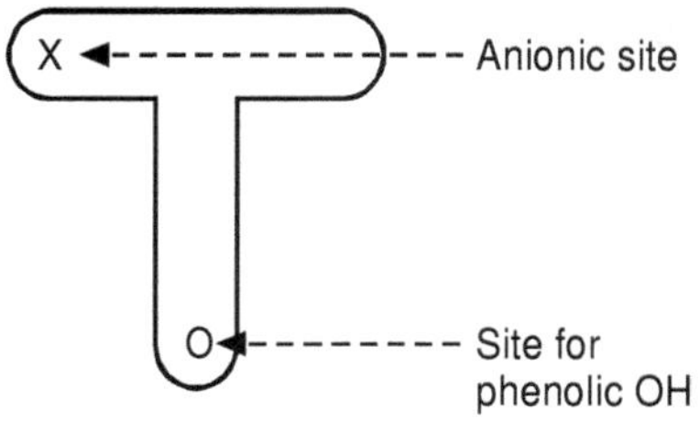

Endogenous opioids :

Enkephalins were the first endogenous ligands to be isolated from pig brain by Huges and Koesterlitz in the mid 1970s. The opioid peptides are formed in the brain, the pituitary gland and in the adrenal medulla by the proteolytic cleavage of three protein precursors. These are preproopiomelanocortin (ACTH- β-LPH precursor), preproenkephalin A (preproenkephalin) and prepro-enkephalin B (preprodynorphin). Over 1000 analogues of enkephalins have been synthesized. Greater stability towards metabolizing enzymes can be attained by conversion of the terminal carboxyl to $-CONH_2$ or by inserting a D-amino acid at position. The tyrosyl group which provides a link between the enkephalins and thebaine derivatives is an essential feature. A $10.0 \pm 1.1A°$ distance between the aromatic rings of Tyr 1 and Phe 4 may be important in the design of enkephalins with other aromatic moieties.

The enkephalins, both methionine and leucine type have the phenyl group of the phenylalanine moiety oriented in relationship to the tyrosine residue to correspond almost exactly to the relationship of the side chain phenyl group (7) to the phenolic aromatic ring of the oripavine nucleus.

Enkephalinase inhibitors might be of use as analgesic drugs. Schering-Plough are reported to have developed an orally active enkephalinase inhibitor, Sch-34862, which is currently under clinical trials.

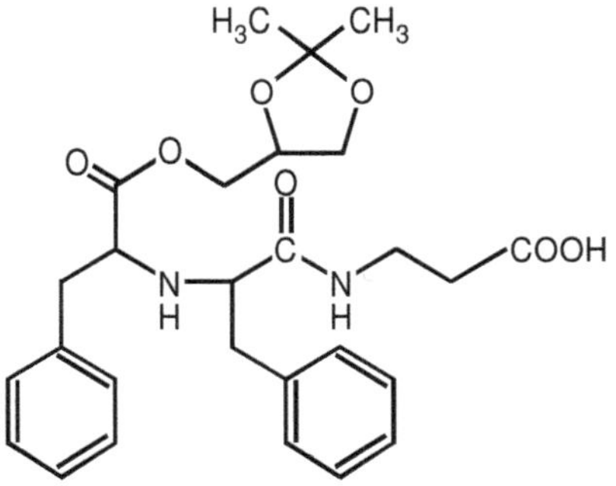

Sch - 34862

The δ-selective peptide (Tyr-D-Ala-Gly-Phe-D-Leu) has been found to produce effective analgesia after intrathecal administration in cancer patients who had become tolerant to the analgesic effects of morphine.

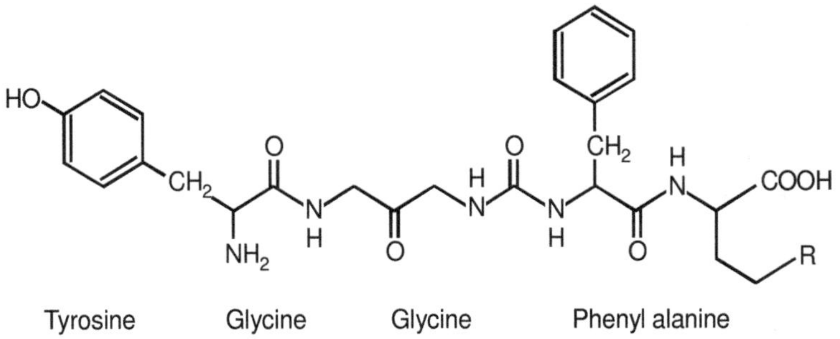

When   R = S – CH₃ → Methionine enkephalin

R = i – Propyl → Leucine enkephalin

Dissimilar Modes of Binding :

A variety of structures possessing narcotic analgesic activity has been shown to be antagonised by nalorphine. Since, the effects of certain highly potent analgesics do not appear to be completely antagonized by

(a)

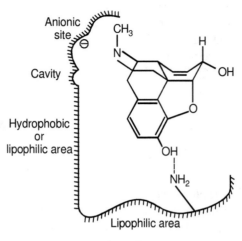

Fig. 6.5

nalorphine, it seems likely that there may be several different species of narcotic analgesic receptors. The latter have a degree of flexibility that allows interaction with a large variety of analgesic molecules than would rigid receptors. For example, the conformationally restricted compound (a) is as potent as morphine even though the aromatic ring is fixed in the equatorial position instead of the axial conformation as in morphine.

Unlike nalorphine, the N-allylnormeperidine is not an antagonist and possesses activity comparable to meperidine. This suggests that nalorphine and N-allylnormeperidine, are interacting with the analgesic receptors by dissimilar modes. There are some compounds which have the same pharmacological effects as that of morphine but they are not structurally similar to morphine. For example, morphine and methadone, both are narcotic analgesics.

Both of them have the same receptors but they do not show parallalism in SAR studies. The morphine molecule fits in receptor structure as shown in Fig 6.5.

Now, we have to consider methadone molecule. The structure is,

This molecule of methadone consists of an aliphatic chain but it is considered that there exist the bonds (weak) as shown by the dotted line and then a pseudo piperidine is formed.

Now, the nitrogen can have the interaction with the anionic site and C = O group can have the weak bond with NH_2 or a weak bond between lipophilic membrane and the benzene ring is also possible but the configuration of the molecule is such that if hydrogen bond is formed then the benzene rings go away from the lipophilic area and if the lipophilic area and benzene rings come together –OH goes away from NH_2 and thus only a anionic site remains complete bound, hence morphine has more intrinsic activity than methadone because it acts at all the sites on receptors. If different congeners of the morphine molecule are formed then the activity is changed but the same change in the activity with the similar modification in the structure of methadone, are not observed because though it has affinity for receptor, it shows less intrinsic activity and thus parallalism is not observed.

If the modes of interactions are quite dissimilar, then identical N-substituents attached to two different analgesiophores would experience different phsico-chemical environments on the receptors. Such a situation would give to non-proportional differences in ΔS and ΔH which would manifested by a non-parallel relationship.

The influence of phenolic hydroxyl group on the analgesic activity can be explained in similar way. The meta phenolic hydroxyl group enhances the analgesic activity by the interaction of the meta OH with a dipolar site on an analgesic receptor which aids in binding of the molecule. An ortho or para hydroxyl group or a non-phenolic aromatic ring may be responsible for incorrect aligning of the molecule which could result in loss of activity due to loss of affinity for the receptors. Thus, the mode of binding of phenolic and non-phenolic compounds may sometimes be quite dissimilar.

It is possible that an analogous situation exists for analgesic receptors, in that different sites on the same receptors have the potential for binding some common features of structurally dissimilar analgesiophores. An identical absolute stereochemistry of the more active analgesic enantiomers does not necessarily indicate that these structures are interacting with analgesic receptors by similar modes unless variation of the N-substituent produces at least a roughly qualitative parallel change in the activity.

The dissimilar modes of interaction may be used to account agonistic and/or antagonistic activity of opioids. It has been proposed that the observed agonist/ antagonist properties could be caused by the receptor binding interactions. An overlap of the basic nitrogen with that of morphine leads to agonism while an overlap of the m-hydroxyphenyl moieties without the overlapping of respective nitrogen leads to antagonism which remains independent of the nature of the substituent present on the nitrogen. This explains how a single compound could produce both agonist and antagonist activity by binding in this bimodal fashion.

Effect of N-substitution on SAR of Narcotic Analgetics :

(i) Morphine analogues :

The first narcotic antagonist, N-allylnorcodeine (IA), was discovered in 1915. Snyder has suggested that the steric effects of the C-14 hydroxy group of naloxone makes the N-allyl substituent equatorial and this stabilizes the receptor in an antagonist rather than in an agonist conformation.

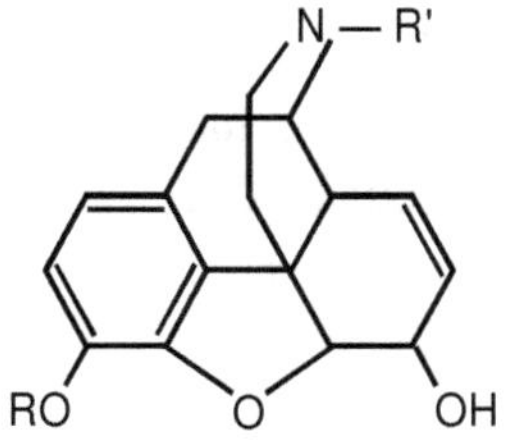

(A) R = $-CH_3$; R' = $-CH_2CH = CH_2$

(B) R = $-H$, R' = $-CH_2CH = CH_2$

(C) R = $-CH_3$, R' = $-CH_2-\triangleleft$

(D) R = $-CH_3$, R' = $-CH_2-\Diamond$

(E) R = $-H$, R' = $-CH_2-\triangleleft$

The key to antagonistic activity appears to reside in the alkylation of the piperidine nitrogen. In the homologous N-alkyl series of normorphine compounds containing a three-carbon side-chain with or without branching, such as propyl, allyl, isopropyl or 2-methylallyl have antagonistic activity. As the chain length increases to amyl and hexyl, agonistic activity is restored and these compounds are nearly as potent analgetics as morphine.

Within the five-ring structure of morphine, there appears to be a good correlation between the agonist potency of the N-methyl derivative and antagonistic potency of their respective N-allyl congeners. That is, the more potent the analgetic activity of the N-methyl compound, the more potent the antagonistic potency of its N-allyl derivative. Such a relationship breaks down in the six ring oripavine series.

The oxymorphone series is of great interest, since the N-allyl compound naloxone is known to being a pure antagonist of any of the compounds reported to date.

(ii) Benzomorphan analogues :

The triannular benzomorphan structure has been the most extensively explored in regard to analgetic-antagonistic activity.

The N-cyclopropylmethyl derivative (cyclazocine) is a potent antagonist and in addition it has a high degree of internuncial blocking and tranquilizing activity. Cyclazocine is a potent analgesic in man but produces too high a level of psychotomimetic activity to be clinically useful.

(iii) Meperidine series :

Replacement of the N-methyl group by an allyl radical did not lead to an antagonist. Indeed the compound behaved like a typical narcotic analgetic. A similar situation exists with N-cyclopropylmethyl derivative. This might be related to the lack of a phenyl-ethylamine fragment in the structure.

(iv) Oripavine derivatives :

In the most potent analgetic series where R = isoamyl, N-allyl and N-cyclo-propylmethyl, derivatives are not antagonists. They have a typical morphine like analgetic activity i.e., although they do not antagonize the anti-nociceptive activity of morphine, they do not add to it. When a shorter side chain (R = CH$_3$), is employed potent nalorphine like antagonists can be generated.

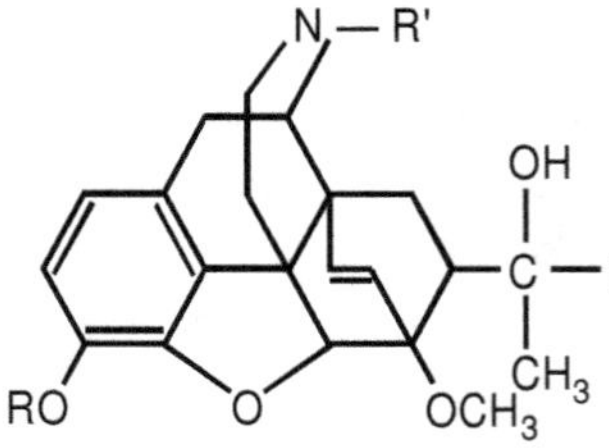

An N-allyl or an N-cyclopropylmethyl group frequently confers antagonist activity. However, there are numerous exceptions to this. For example, tonazocine (a) is an antagonist

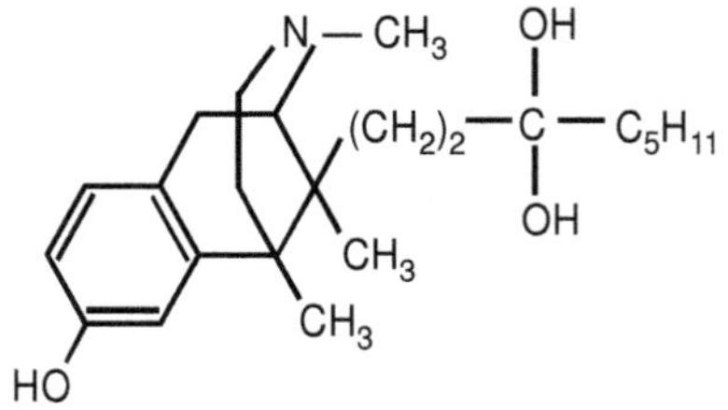

Tonazocine

(a)

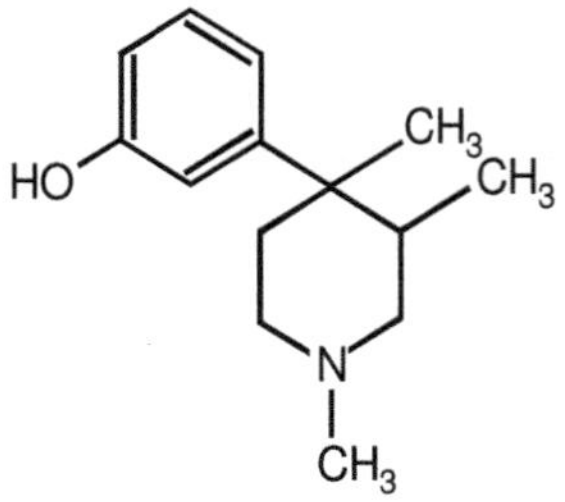

(b)

and the 4-phenylpiperidine derivative (b) has greater antagonist potency with an N-methyl than an N-allyl or N-cyclopropylmethyl substituent.

6.9 GABA AND GABA-NERGIC RECEPTORS

Epilepsy is one of such diseases where selectively acting drugs are still lacking. The prevalence of epilepsy is between 3 to 6 per 1000 population. Since, GABA hypofunction is thought to be one of the major etiological factors in epilepsy, during the last two decades most of the attention has been focused on the development of GABA-nergic anticonvulsants.

There seems to be numerous GABA-nergic pathways in the CNS. GABA is found in the highest concentration in the substantia nigra. It is also found in hypothalamus and occurs in low concentration in practically all brain structures as well as in the spinal cord. GABA-levels in brain are important to prevent the spread of the seizures.

GABA-receptor was thoroughly investigated in the early 1980s. The $GABA_A$ receptor is a high affinity binding site with fairly constant density. The $GABA_B$ receptor has a low binding affinity and shows great variation in receptor density in various brain areas. GABA receptor is regulated by a thermostable protein called GABA modulin, having a molecular weight of 150,000. This protein is an inhibitor of the Ca^{++} dependent and both C-AMP dependent and C-AMP-independent protein kinases. Its removal increases protein phosphorylation in the synapses by 20 fold which helps to increase the transmitter recognition ability of the receptor sites. The receptor assembly seems to be composed of GABA-receptor, GABAmodulin, protein phosphorylation site and the ionophore mediated chloride ion channel. The GABA-modulin binding site is apparently the same as benzodiazepine binding site.

The existence of peripheral GABA-receptors has been shown, since they are located at outer mitochondrial membrane. They may be involved in the modulation of intermediary metabolism.

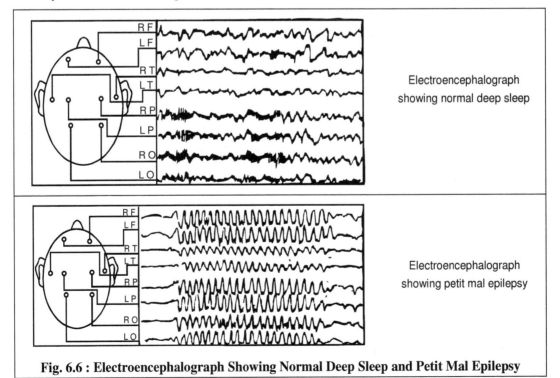

Fig. 6.6 : Electroencephalograph Showing Normal Deep Sleep and Petit Mal Epilepsy

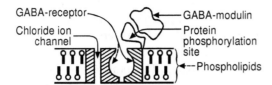

Fig. 6.7 : GABA-nergic Receptor

GABA is involved in feeding, sleep, hormonal secretion, CVS functions and in analgesia that is not mediated by opiate-sensitive neurons. The GABA-mimetic THIP (tetrahydroisoxazole-pyridinol), a non-addictive pain-relieving agent, is reported to be equivalent to morphine. The correlation may be enkephalinergic neurons involved in pain regulatory pathways, seems to be regulated in part by GABA-nergic neurons.

(a) Drugs affecting biosynthesis of GABA :

The concentration of GABA is regulated by two pyridoxal-5'-phosphate dependent enzymes, namely L-glutamic acid decarboxylase (GAD) which converts glutamate to GABA and GABA-amino transferase (GABA-AT) which degrades GABA to succinic semialdehyde.

The agents that decrease the concentration of GABA by trapping vitamin B_6, an essential cofactor for GAD include,

3-Hydrazinopropionic acid

Allylcine

(b) Drugs affecting GABA release :

The release of GABA is found to be inhibited by high doses of chlorpromazine, haloperidol and imipramine. While baclofen (orally active muscle relaxant) enhances the rate of release of GABA.

Baclofen

(c) Drugs that inhibit GABA reuptake :

Several GABA reuptake inhibitors have been reported in the literature. Important amongst them include nipecotic acid and its derivatives.

Nipecotic acid

(d) Drugs that inhibit metabolism of GABA :

The GABA metabolism inhibitors increase its duration of action by increasing life span of GABA molecules. Gabaculine and vigabatrin are the clinically used examples of GABA - AT inhibitors.

Gabaculine   Vigabatrin

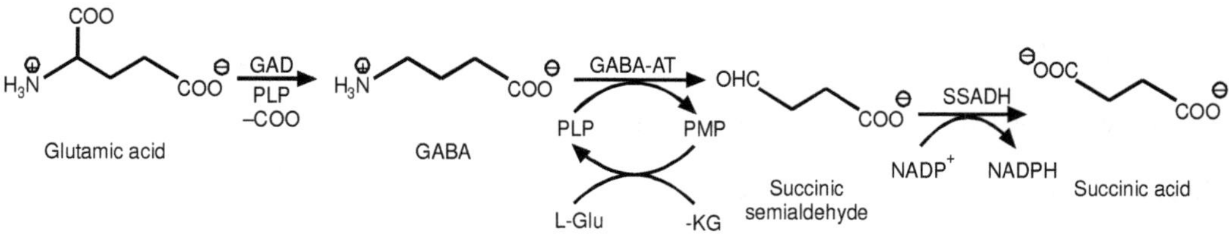

Fig. 6.8 : Biosynthesis and Metabolism of GABA

Because of the vinyl substituent in vigabatrin,

(a) Lipopilicity increases.

(b) Vinyl being an electron withdrawing substituent, has an effect of lowering the pKa of the amino group. This would increase the concentration of non-zwitter ion form which is more lipophilic than zwitter ion.

Similarly, valproic acid exerts anti-epileptic action by inhibiting succinic semialdehyde dehydrogenase, the enzyme oxidising the semialdehyde metabolite. As this metabolite accumulates, GABA-AT activity is decreased by end-product inhibition and the GABA concentration increases. The important derivatives of valproic acid include,

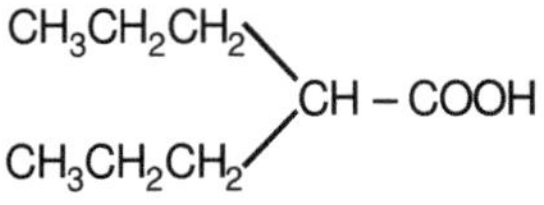

Valproic acid

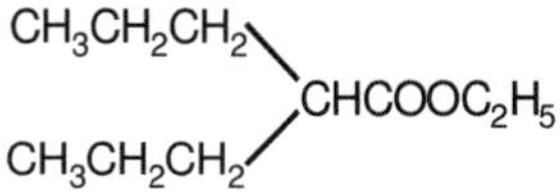

Valdice

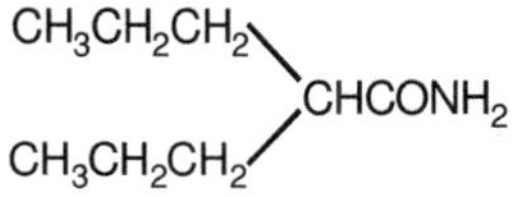

Valpromide

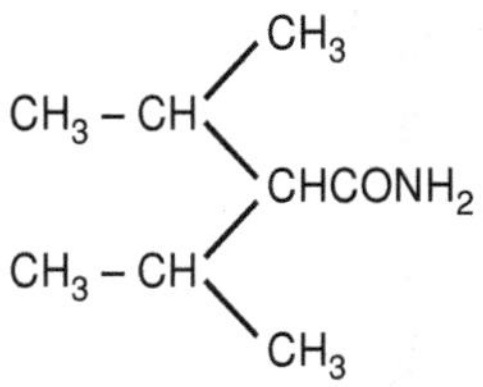

Di-isopropylacetamide

Valdice behaves as a prodrug as like valpromide. In di-isopropylacetamide, the amide linkage is protected from hydrolysis by two methyl groups present at β-position. The methyl groups prevent the attack of amidases through steric hinderance and make the compound more stable.

(e) Drugs that act as agonist at postsynaptic GABA-nergic receptors :

Muscimol is a naturally occuring isoxazole, isolated from the mushroom Amanita muscaria. It has hallucinogenic activity.

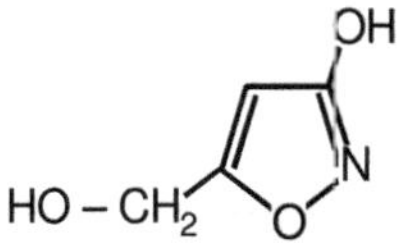

ISO-THAZ

Muscimol

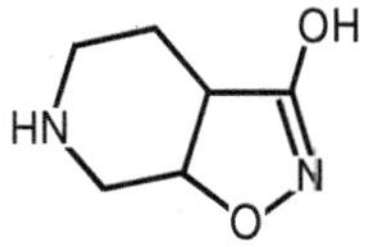

4, 5, 6, 7-Tetrahydro-isoxazolo pyridin-3-ol (THIP)

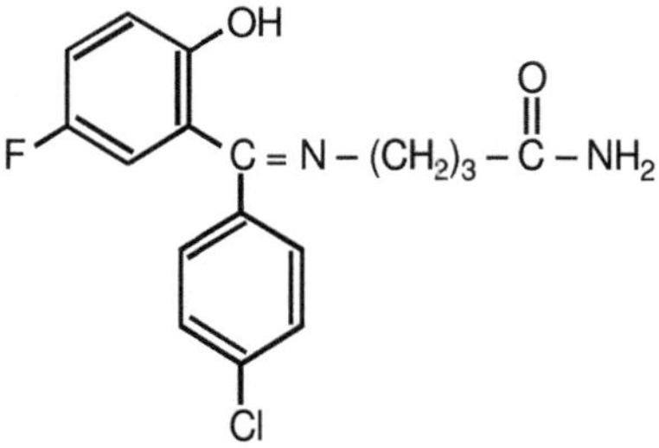

Progabide

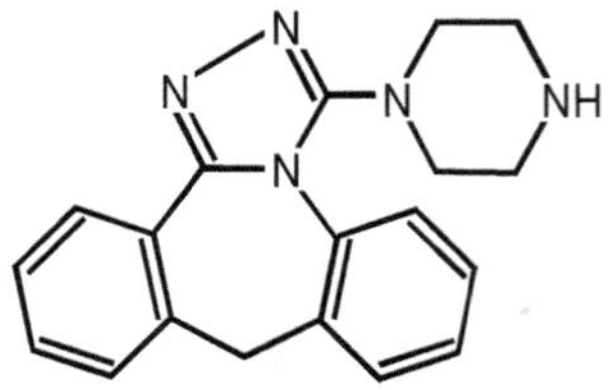

Pitrazepine

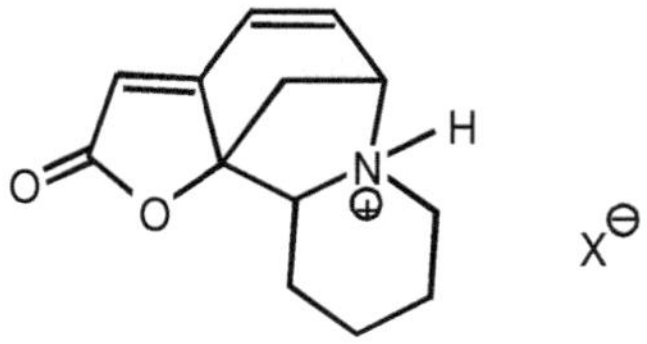

Securinine

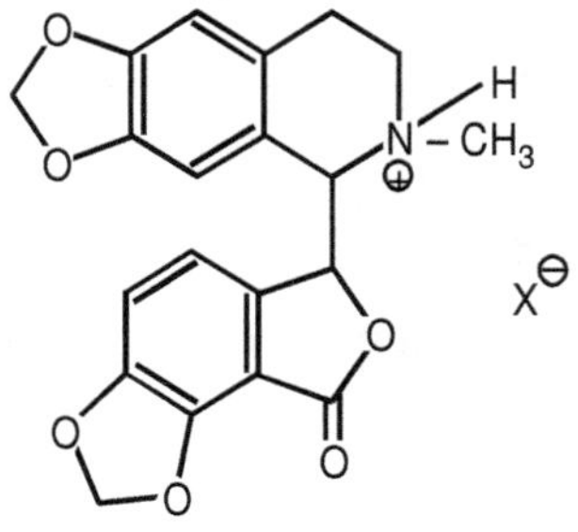

Bicuculline

(f) Drugs that act as antagonists at GABA-nergic receptor sites :

These drugs include pitrazepine, (+)-bicuculline, securinine, R-5135 and tubocurarine.

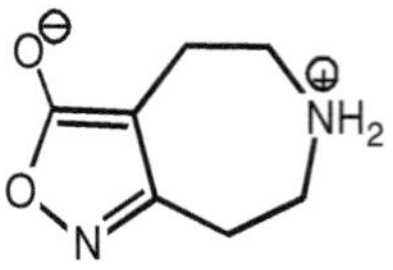

Table 6.5 : Some Animal Models for Evaluation of Anticonvulsant Activity

Model	Animals
1. Electroshock models :	
(a) Maximal electroshock	Rats and mice
(b) Minimal electroshock	Rats and mice
(c) Psychomotor electroshock	Mice
2. Chemical models :	
A. Mainly enhance excitatory systems :	
(a) Pentylenetetrazol	Rats and mice
(b) Convulsant barbiturates (CHEB, DMBB)	Mice
B. Block inhibitory systems :	
(i) **Block effect of GABA at receptors**	
Picrotoxin	Rats and crayfish
Penicillin	Cat and rat
Bicuculline	Rats
(ii) **Block GABA synthesis or release :**	
Isoniazid	Rats
(iii) **Block effect of glycine at receptor :**	
Strychnine	Rats
C. Block energy metabolism :	
Methionine, sulfoximine	Mice and rats
D. Ion transport inhibitors :	
(a) Cations - Ouabain	Rats
(b) Anions - SCN, ClO$_4$,	Rats

7

DRUGS ACTING ON CARDIO-VASCULAR SYSTEM

7.1 RENIN-ANGIOTENSIN-ALDOSTERONE SYSTEM

The renin-angiotensin-aldosterone system is an important physiological mechanism that regulates the blood volume, blood pressure and water-electrolyte balance in the body fluids. Human renin is an aspartyl protease which is synthesized, stored and secreted into the renal arterial circulation by the granular juxtaglomerular cells. The active form of renin is a glycoprotein having 340 amino acids. Renin and prorenin are both stored in the juxtaglomerular cells and circulate in the blood. The half-life of circulating renin is about 15 minutes.

The enzyme renin acts on a plasma protein substrate, an α_2-globulin known as angiotensinogen. As a result, a pressor material, angiotensin I (decapeptide) is generated. This decapeptide is cleaved by Angiotensin Converting Enzyme (ACE) to yield the active angiotensin II (octapeptide). This, in turn, undergoes hydrolysis by an aminopeptidase to yield the heptapeptide angiotensin III which is also active. Further cleavage yields peptides with little activity.

The renin-angiotensin system is involved in the regulation of aldosterone secretion. Angiotensin-II stimulates the synthesis and secretion of aldosterone by the adrenal cortex to raise blood pressure via direct constriction of the smooth muscles of the arterioles. Thus, the renin-angiotensin system plays an important role in the regulation of fluid and electrolyte balance, blood pressure and blood volume, as shown below :

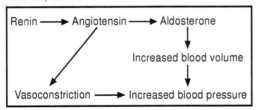

Fig. 7.1 : Homeostatic Role of Renin-Angiotensin System

7.2 ANGIOTENSIN CONVERTING ENZYME (ACE)

The substrate for renin is angiotensinogen, an abundant α_2-globulin that circulates in the plasma. Angiotensinogen is continuously synthesized and secreted by the liver, and its synthesis is stimulated by a number of hormones, including glucocorticoids, thyroid hormone, and angiotensin II itself. Human ACE is a large protein, containing 1278 amino acid residues. Although slow conversion of angiotensin I to angiotensin II occurs in plasma, its rapid metabolism in vivo is brought about by tissue-bound ACE.

7.3 INHIBITORS OF RENIN-ANGIOTENSIN SYSTEM

The interference in the functioning of renin-angiotensin system can be brought about at two levels. First approach involves designing angiotensin-II antagonists which block receptors for angiotensin-II. Second approach involves designing inhibitors of angiotensin converting enzyme. The ACE-inhibitors slow the rate of formation of angiotensin-II.

(a) Antagonists of angiotensin-II :

Many analogs of angiotensin-II have been synthesized. The removal of phenylalanine from angiotensin abolishes agonist activity in peripheral tissues. Most antagonists of angiotensin-II are designed by replacement of phenylalanine at position 8 with some other amino acid. The substituent selected should be resistant to enzymatic cleavage in order to increase its life in the circulation.

The first compound from this category was introduced in 1971 by Pals and Co-workers. This compound was developed by combining alanine at position 8 with sarcosine (N-methylglycine) in position 1. Chemically, it is [Sar[1], Val[5], Ala[8]] angiotensin-(1-8) octapeptide.

It competes with angiotensin II for its receptors. Saralasin commonly causes a fall in systemic blood pressure in patients with renovascular hypertension. A series of carboxybenzyl chloroimidazole compounds have recently been developed that are competitive antagonists of angiotensin-II. All such antagonists of angiotensin-II are found to be effective in the treatment of renovascular hypertension.

(b) Inhibitors of angiotensin converting enzyme :

In 1965, Ferriera and Co-workers demonstrated the presence of potent inhibitors of the bradykinase (kinase II or angiotensin converting enzyme) in the venoms of pit vipers. The ACE inhibitors found in snakes were peptides of 5 to 13 amino acid residues. Based upon their amino acid sequence, teprotide (first synthetic non-peptide BPF 9α) was synthesized which was found to lower blood pressure when given parenterally. Further studies of inhibitory action of teprotide were used to develop the orally effective enzyme inhibitor, captopril in 1977 by Cushman et al. The unique pharmacological intervention affored by captopril prompted a search for newer agents. This led ultimately to the synthesis of a series of carboxy alkanoyl or mercapto alkanoyl derivatives that acted as potent competitive inhibitors of the enzyme.

Because captopril contains a sulfhydryl (mercapto) moiety, it was associated with side effects like abnormal taste sensation, rash etc. Enalapril is a second generation oral, non-sulfhydryl, ACE inhibitor. Chemically, it belongs to the group of substituted N-carboxymethyl dipeptide which can inhibit metallodipeptidyl carboxypeptidases, despite lack of Zn^{++} - sulfhydryl interaction.

7.4 MECHANISM OF ACTION

The ACE-inhibitors are highly specific drugs. Most of the haemodynamic actions of renin-angiotensin-aldosterone system are mediated through angiotensin-II, which is a very potent vasoconstrictor and stimulator for aldosterone release. This leads to an increase in salt and water retention and potassium wasting thus further raising blood pressure.

The ACE-inhibitors prevent the conversion of the relatively inactive angiotensin-I to the active angiotensin-II or the conversion of angiotensin-I to angiotensin-III. These conversions take place primarily in the lungs, although other organs are also involved. The ACE-inhibitors bind strongly to both circulating and tissue angiotensin converting enzyme and prevent the formation of angiotensin-II. This leads to reduction in angiotensin induced vasoconstriction and aldosterone mediated salt and water retention. This explains a fall in blood pressure.

7.5 PHARMACOLOGICAL ACTIONS OF ACE-INHIBITORS

The ACE-inhibitors produce no significant changes in cardiac function indices such as heart rate, cardiac output, ejection fraction, stroke volume, left ventricular ejection fraction, left ventricular end systolic wall stress or pre ejection period/left ventricular ejection time ratio. They reduce total peripheral vascular resistance in a dose dependent manner. They improve arterial compliance and tissue perfusion. The ACE-inhibitors increase renal blood glomerular filtration rate and decrease renal vascular resistance. They are also shown to lower total cholesterol level and to raise high density

Table 7.1 : Clinically used ACE-inhibitors

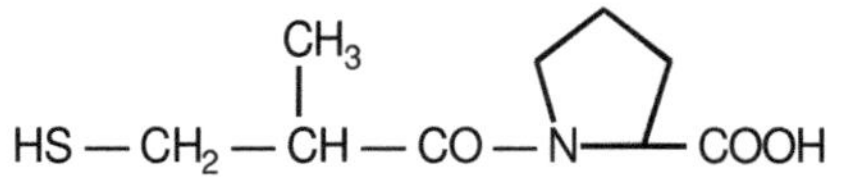

lipoprotein levels. Hence, they can be used in combination with thiazide diuretic to prevent diuretic induced hyperlipidemia.

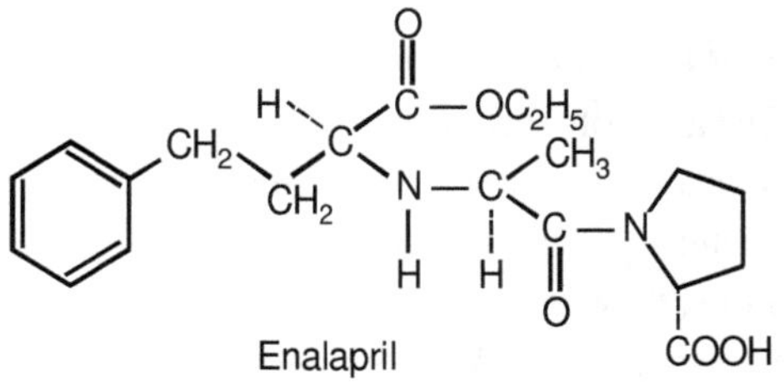

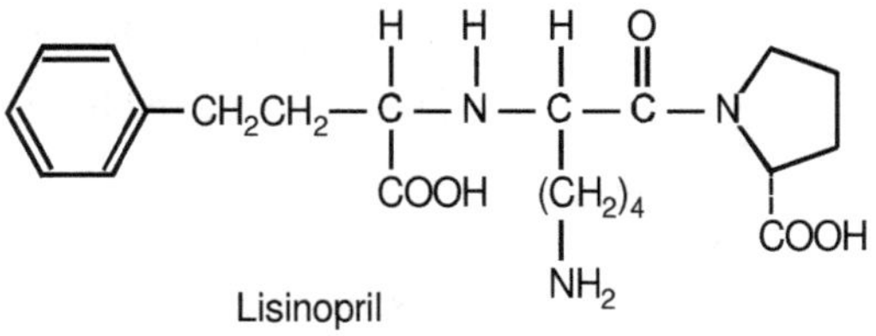

Enalapril is a prodrug that is not itself highly active. It must be hydrolyzed to the active parent dicarboxylic acid, enalaprilate. This conversion is accomplished by a serum esterase. While lisinopril is the lysine analogue of enalaprilate. Unlike enalapril, lisinopril itself is active.

Table 7.2 : Pharmacokinetic Parameters of ACE-inhibitors

Drugs	Oral % Absorption	Half-life (hr.)	Excretion in urine
Captopril	65	2-3	About 40% captopril + Metabolite
Enalapril	70	11	Metabolites
Lisinopril	30	12	No metabolism

Besides above clinically used ACE-inhibitors, the ACE-inhibitors under investigation include zofenopril, fosinopril, ramipril, alacepril and cilazapril.

Table 7.3 : Physiological Actions of Angiotensin-II

(A) Central Actions :
- Increase in sympathetic efferent nerve activity,
- Increase in water intake,
- Secretion of vasopressin,
- Secretion of adrenocorticotrophic hormone,
- Modulation of baroreflex activity,
- Reduction in vagal activity.

(B) Peripheral Actions :
- Inhibits reuptake of noradrenaline,
- Potentiates release of noradrenaline at sympathetic nerve,
- Facilitates transmission in sympathetic ganglia,
- Increases biosynthesis of noradrenaline,
- Release catecholamines from adrenal medulla,
- Potentiates post-junctional action of noradrenaline.

7.6 CLINICAL USES OF ACE-INHIBITORS

(a) Antihypertensive action :

Because of several advantages like oral effectiveness, favourable pharmacokinetics and high safety profile associated with the ACE-inhibitors, they are preferred in the treatment of hypertension. The ACE-inhibitor therapy in patients with mild to severe hypertension causes reduction in both systolic and diastolic blood pressure with no orthostatic hypotension or change in heart rate or cardiovascular reflexes. The antihypertensive effect is greater in patients who are sodium depleted due to any cause and/or have a high plasma renin activity. Diuretics and ACE-inhibitors act synergistically. The ACE-inhibitors blunt the hypokalemic responses of thiazide diuretics and therefore, concomitant use of potassium sparing diuretics is not recommended.

(b) Congestive heart failure :

Vasodilators are effective in the treatment of acute heart failure but their utility is questionable in the management of chronic congestive failure. Physiological compensatory mechanisms for the failing heart include increase in sympathetic activity and circulating catecholamines and activation of the renin-angiotensin-aldosterone system. Marked increase in afterload (vasoconstriction) adversely affects the changes that increase cardiac output and preload. The ACE-inhibitors are particularly useful as in adjuvant therapy in combination with diuretics and digitalis for the treatment of moderate and severe congestive heart failure. The ACE-inhibitors not only induce systemic arteriolar dilatation, and thereby reduce afterload, but they also cause venodilatation, lessen fluid retention, and thus reduce preload. The overall result is increased cardiac output, amelioration of signs and symptoms of congestion and prolongation of life in end-stage congestive heart failure. Thus, ACE-inhibitors prevent the onset of clinical heart failure and improve survival rates.

(c) Renal diseases :

Acute and chronic renal disease and unilateral and bilateral renal artery stenosis are usually associated with a high plasma level of renin, which in the presence of ACE activity leads to increased levels of angiotensin II with associated increase in sympathetic tone, sodium and water retention, peripheral vascular resistance and blood pressure.

ACE-inhibitors reverse these actions of angiotensin-II in patients with bilateral renal artery stenosis or sodium depletion. However, therapy also needs the use of renin inhibitors.

(d) Diabetes mellitus :

The ACE-inhibitors may be used to improve the glomerular filtration rate and to decrease albuminuria in diabetic patients with the renal disease.

7.7 ADVERSE EFFECTS OF ACE-INHIBITORS

The most common adverse effects associated with the ACE-inhibitors include dizziness, headache and fatigue. These are mild and transient in nature. Other less common side-effects of these agents include nausea, diarrhoea, rash, skin hypersensitivity, cough and hypotension. Hyperkalemia is reported to occur in patients receiving supplemental potassium or potassium sparing diuretics. These agents must be used with caution in patients with bilateral renal artery stenosis which may otherwise lead to deterioration of renal function.

7.8 CALCIUM ION

The main dietary sources of calcium include milk, cheese, green vegetables, eggs and some fish. Calcium can be absorbed from all parts of the small intestine by an active transport mechanism. Average daily intake for calcium in adults is about 800 - 1000 mg while the minimum requirement in an adult is about 400 mg per day. However, greater amounts of calcium are required in children and during pregnancy and lactation. About 99% of total body contents of calcium are found in the skeleton.

The normal range for total plasma calcium is 2.2 - 2.6 m mol/litre (i.e., 8.8 - 10.4 mg/ 100 ml). Just about half of this is bound to plasma proteins, a small fraction is complexed with citrate and phosphate and the balance amount circulates in blood as ionised calcium. It is this calcium which plays an important role in the functioning of nerves and muscles. If the ionised calcium concentration is low, tetanic spasms or convulsions may occur and if ionised calcium concentration is high, cardiac functions get disturbed. Calcium is mainly excreted in sweat, urine and faeces.

Calcium plays an important role in cellular regulation, where its major function is activation. It is because of its ability to carry positive charge, which allows calcium entry through highly regulated membrane channels to initiate and modify membrane depolarisation. The entry of positively charged calcium ions through calcium channels in the plasma membrane generates an inward (depolarizing) current that contributes to pacemaker activity, whereas calcium entry in the atrioventricular (AV) node provides the major depolarizing current during AV conduction. In addition, calcium serves as an intracellular messenger that binds to members of a family of intracellular calcium-binding proteins that include troponin and calmodulin. Calmodulin in case of smooth muscles and troponin in case of cardiac cells which results in contraction. In the heart, calcium binding to troponin initiates systole, and formation of the calcium-calmodulin complex in vascular smooth muscle initiates a series of reaction that leads to vaso constricition.

7.9 EFFECT OF CALCIUM ON THE ELECTRICAL ACTIVITY OF THE HEART

In resting cardiac and smooth muscle, the cell interior has a negative charge; systolic potassium concentration is high and sodium and calcium concentrations are low. In both the sinoatrial (SA) and atrioventricular (AV) nodes, calcium is the major ion responsible for depolarization. In the former, the control of the intrinsic pacemaker activity (i.e., the heart rate) is governed by the calcium. It also acts as a major determinant of AV conduction by conducting impulses from the atria to the ventricles. However in the rapidly conducting cells of the His-Pukinje system and in the working myocardial fibers of the atria and ventricles, the incoming impulse is carried over further by sodium ions.

A number of diverse cellular functions (contraction, secretion, etc.) are known to be regulated by fluctuations in the free calcium ion concentration in the cytosol. One important source of these divalent ions is the calcium reservoir in the extracellular fluid. Ca^{++} ions can be mobilised from this external pool by the operation of Ca^{++} - channel that are anchored in the plasma membrane. Since, Ca^{++} acts as a major regulator of smooth muscle contraction, Ca^{++} channel blocking agents may be used as antiarrhythmics. hypotensives and antianginal agents.

7.10 CALCIUM ION CHANNEL

A Ca^{++} channel residing in the membrane of a eukaryotic cell is viewed as being a macromolecular structure consisting essentially of one or more glycoproteins. Its configuration is presumed to be roughly cylindrical with an aqueous pore at its centre. The permeation of extracellular calcium ions through the pore into the cytosol is accomplished.

Within the aqueous pore of the calcium channel, the driving force acting to propel the cation inward will be countered by steric configurations and reactive groups or, in other terms, by energy barriers that act to impede the flow of ions through the channel. It appears that one of these barriers may be sufficiently high and uniquely structured to permit some types of cations to pass through, but halt any further forward movement of others. This barrier has been labelled as selectivity filter. In addition to establish the ion specificity of the channel, the selectivity filter as well as other energy barriers, serve to regulate the speed at which a permeant cation will move through the aqueous pore of channel.

The ions that have the capacity to traverse the selectivity filter and pass through the channel pore, can do so only when the channel is in an open conformation. Ca^{++} channels found in a number of different types of cells appear to have a gating mechanism that is similar to that of sodium channel, in that it operates to transform the channel into any one of three different conformations or states :

(a) activated state or open conformation

(b) the deactivated state and

(c) the inactivated state. The last two are closed conformations.

Based on the type of excitatory stimulus required to convert a channel to the activated state, Ca^{++} channels are divided into

(a) Voltage-dependent Ca^{++} channel : It will be activated when the membrane potential has been reduced to an appropriate level.

(b) Receptor operated Ca^{++} channels : Channels closely linked to membrane receptors and activated by agonist - receptor interactions. They received much less scrutiny than the Ca^{++} channels activated by membrane depolarisation.

(c) To some extent, extracellular Ca^{++} ions may also reach the cytosol via a small membrane leak and perhaps via a sodium - calcium exchange mechanism.

Functional studies have proved the existence of several distinct types of calcium channels. The two most prominent calcium channels of the heart are the T- and L-type channels. Most important is the L-type channel, which is the calcium channel whose functions were described above. Most of calcium channel blockers bind to and inhibit only the L-type channels.

In general, these channels are glycosylated membrane proteins made up of several peptides. They contain tetramers made up of 4 subunits that surround the water - filled pore through which the ions cross the phospholipid bilayer. The channel subunits are made up of six putative membrane - spanning helices. Two, S_5 and S_6, are hydrophobic and so are likely to interact with the hydrophobic core of the bilayer in which the channel is imbedded. The S_1 and S_3 membrane-spanning helices, which contain negatively charged amino acids, and the S_2 helix, which contains both positively and negatively charged amino acids, probably surround the water - filled pore. Most interesting is S_4 which contains a "ribbon" of positively charged arginine and

Table 7.4 : Peptide Components of Voltage -dependent Calcium Ion Channel

Subunit	Number	Approximate Mol. wt (Daltons)
α_1	1	212,000
α_1	1	175,000
α_2	1	140,000
β	1	54,000
γ	1	30,000
δ	1	27,000

lysine residues. It is believed to be the activation gate that opens the channel when the membrane is depolarized. Thus, the S_4-membrane spanning helix is known as the activation gate whose movement in the membrane opens the channel. While the cytoplasmic loop connecting the S_6-membrane spanning helix and S_1-membrane spanning helix acts as an inactivation gate, which is responsible for the refractoriness that follows the transition of the channel from the open to the closed state.

Two forms of this α_1-peptide are found in the muscle. A large, 212,000 dalton molecule is found in the cardiac conductance channels that carry the depolarizing calcium currents. It binds to the members of all three classes of calcium channel blockers : dihydropyridines, benzothiazepines and phenyalkyl-amines. The smaller α_1-peptide, which is similar to the 212,000 dalton peptide but lacks 320 amino acids at the C-terminal end and has a lower molecular weight of about 175,000 Da, is involved in the opening of the intracellular calcium release channels in the skeletal muscle when the muscle is depolarized.

Many of the smaller peptides associated with the calcium channel appear to play a role in channel regulation. Thus the β peptide, like the α_2 peptide, is a substrate for c-AMP-dependent protein kinase that, when phosphorylated, activates the channel.

The voltage - sensitive ion channels could exist in three functional states - open, closed (resting), and closed (inactivated). Starting front the closed state, calcium channels can flicker in two open states : brief opening and long - lasting opening. The ability of these ion -channels to exist in open states not only differ in their duration but in the amplitude of the current they allow to cross the membrane. These different conductance states may arise from graded interactions among the channel subunits. The effects of the calcium channel blockers are therefore to modify the probability that the channels shall be in one or another of these states, rather than simply to "plug" the channels. In the case of the calcium channels of the cardiovascular system, the ability of drugs to modify these transitions is of considerable importance in modifying the function of both the heart and vascular system.

7.11 CLINICAL UTILITY OF CALCIUM CHANNEL BLOCKERS

Calcium ions play an important part in the functioning of the cardiovascular system e.g. calcium ions determine the force of cardiac contraction, maintain coronary and peripheral arterial smooth muscle tone and influence pacemaker activity in the S.A node and conduction through AV node.

So by blocking calcium ion entry with a calcium channel antagonist, we can get a spectrum of effects, some of which can be used clinically. These effects include,

Table 7.5

Effect	Clinical use
(I) Interfers with excitation in muscle contraction coupling	
(A) Smooth muscle - vascular	
(i) Coronary vasodilation	Ischemic heart disease, coronary vasospasm, acute myocardial infraction
(ii) Peripheral vasodilation	Ischemic heart disease, hypertension, congestive heart failure, migraine headache, cerebrovascular spasm
(iii) Pulmonary vasodilation	Pulmonary hypertension
(B) Smooth muscle - non vascular	
(i) Pulmonary bronchodilation	Asthma
(ii) Uterine relaxation.	Dysmenorrhea premature labour
(iii) Oesophageal relaxation	Oesophageal motility disorders
(iv) Bladder relaxation	Bladder motility disorders
(C) Cardiac muscles	
(i) Negative inotropic effect.	Hypertrophic cardiomyopathy
(II) Inhibits the slow inward current of depolarisation	
(A) Cells of SA and AV node	Slow ventricular rate in atrial fibrillation and flutter
(B) Abnormal atrial and ventricular tissue	Arrhythmias associated with ischemia, glycoside toxicity
(III) Interferes with secondary processes	
A) Insulin secretion from β cells	Insulinoma (Excess of insulin in the blood).
(B) Oxytocin and vasopressin release from neurolypophysis	Asthma
(IV) Interferes with hemostasis and platelet aggregation	Ischemic heart disease
(V) Prevents injury induced calcium flux	Intraoperative protection of ischemic myocardium and acute myocardial infraction

7.12 CALCIUM CHANNEL BLOCKING DRUGS

In 1964, Fleckenstein reported that verapamil and prenylamine had the same inhibitory effect on cardiac muscle as did the withdrawal of extracellular calcium ions. These compounds were originally called as calcium antagonists because their inhibitory effects could be reversed by increasing the Ca^{++} ion concentration in the extracellular medium.

Since, other vasodilators do not exert any direct effect on the heart and verapamil does not possess any affinity for beta adrenergic receptors present on the heart muscles, it was suggested that verapamil inhibited the movement of calcium ions into cardiac cells. Hence, verapamil and similar drugs are termed as the calcium channel blocking agents. Calcium antagonists is not a recommended term, since it implies that calcium ions and the drug bind to the same site. Examples of the drugs from this category includes verapamil, diltiazem, nifedipine, felodipine, nitrendipine, bepridil, isradipine etc.

Ca^{++} channel blockers include :

(a) Drugs that induce or prevent changes in membrane potential.

(b) Drugs that alter the extracellular and /or intracellular concentration of calcium ions.

(c) Drugs that modify biochemical reactions involved in the operation of calcium channel (i.e., phosphorylation and dephosphorylation reactions etc.).

(d) Drugs that potentiate or prevent the activation of membrane receptors closely linked to calcium channels.

They are divided into different subgroups.

Group I consists of nifedipine and related 1, 4-dihydropyridines such as nitrendipine, nisoldipine, nimodipine.

Group II contains verapamil, D 600, diltiazem and diclofurime.

Group III contains diphenylalkylamine compounds like cinnarizine, fendiline, flunarizine and prenylamine.

Nitrendipine, a dihydropyridine calcium entry blocker, is a potent dilator of the peripheral vasculature. The primary action of nitrendipine is inhibition of calcium movement through the voltage-dependent 'slow' channels in the plasma membranes. The blockade of calcium-dependent contractile activity by nitrendipine results into relaxation of peripheral arterial vascular tone with a subsequent decrease in systemic vascular resistance. This leads to reduction in the blood pressure. High affinity binding sites are located in the region of the slow channels in the sarcolemma of cardiac tissues. Binding of nitrendipine to these sites regulates the influx of calcium through the 'slow' channel.

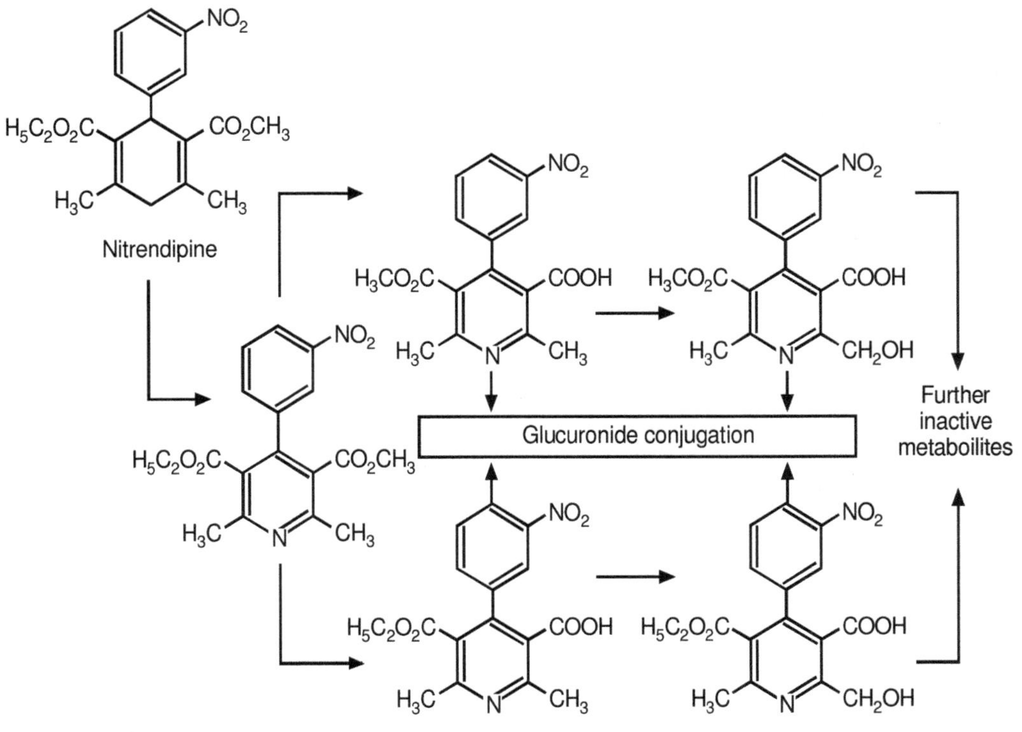

Major metabolic pathways for nitrendipine

Nitrendipine is very extensively metabolised. Major routes of metabolism are dehydrogenation to the pyridine analogue, cleavage of ester groups and hydroxylation of methyl groups with subsequent glucuronide conjugation in the bile.

All five known metabolites are 1000 times less potent than the parent drug. Hence, entire dihydropyridine ring is thought to be essential for activity.

7.13 CLASSIFICATION OF CALCIUM ANTAGONISTS

Calcium antagonists can be classified by three ways.

(1) According to the specificity of the drug :

(a) Potent specific agents : These agents have little or no secondary effects on sodium and magnesium channels e.g. Nifedipine, verapamil.

(b) Less specific agents e.g. perhexiline and prenylamine.

(2) According to the chemical nature :

(a) 1, 4 dihydropyridines e.g. nifedipine.

(b) Diphenylalkylamines e.g. verapamil, D600.

(c) Benzothiazepine derivatives : e.g. Diltiazem.

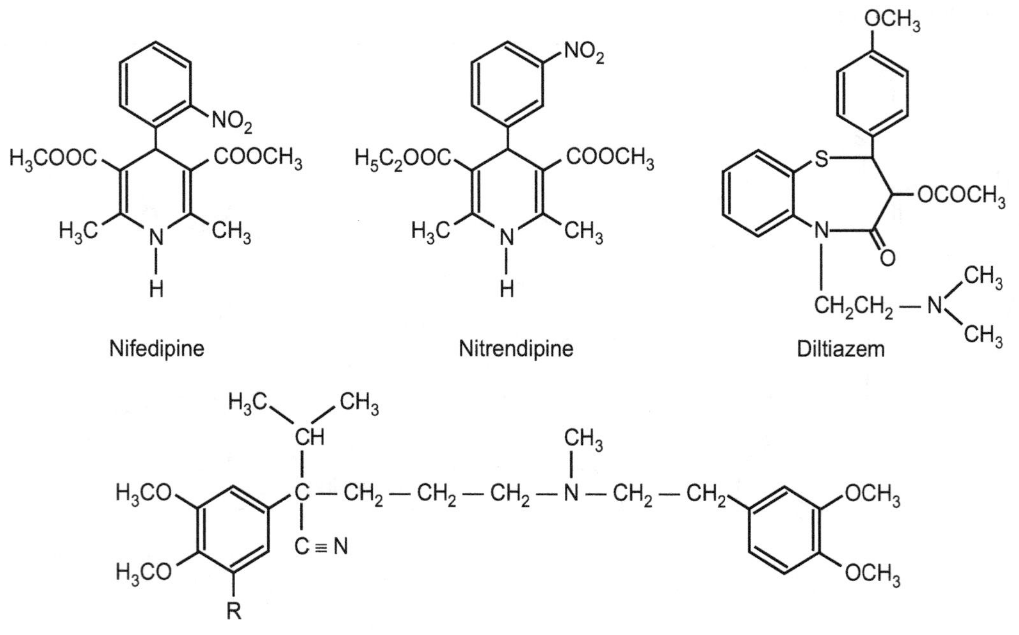

Verapamil (Gallopamil); R = H
Compound D-600; R =–CH–OCH$_3$

Fig. 7.2 : Structural Formulae of Nifedipine and Nitrendipine (Dihydropyridines), Diltiazem (Benzothiazepine) and Verapamil

(3) According to site of action, the calcium ion channel blocking agents can be categorized as follows :

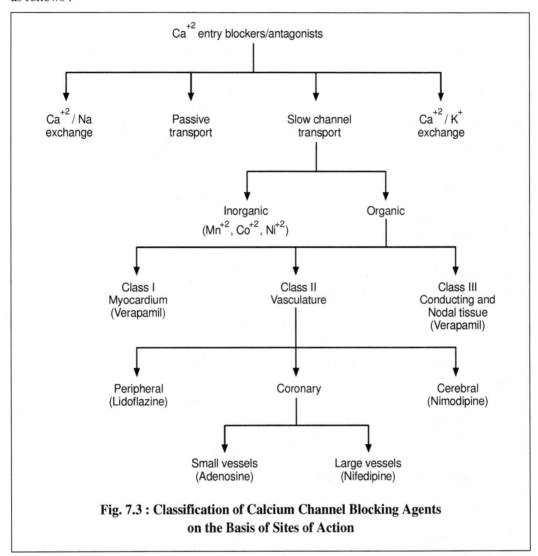

Fig. 7.3 : Classification of Calcium Channel Blocking Agents on the Basis of Sites of Action

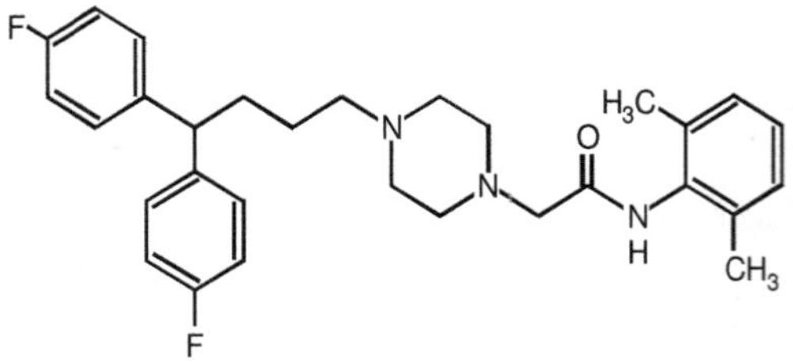

Lidoflazine

7.14 PHARMACOLOGY

(a) Excitation of β-adrenergic receptors in membranes increase, whereas excitation of muscarinic cholinergic receptors decrease the amplitude of Ca^{++} currents initiated by membrane depolarisation (i.e., powerful Ca^{++} channel stimulation).

The drug-receptor interaction induces an increase in C-AMP level in cytoplasm, resulting into activation of C-AMP dependent protein kinases. They cause phosphorylation of membrane proteins presumed to be part of or some manner, to potential Ca^{++} channels. The channels could assume the activated conformation. The net result was a larger inward Ca^{++} current.

(b) The reduction in Ca^{+-} current brought about by the interaction of cholinergic agonists and cholinergic receptors in cardiac cells may possibly involve cyclic GMP.

(c) Sometimes, a receptor induced breakdown of inositol phospholipids is responsible for the opening of calcium channel gates.

Calcium channel blockers primarily exert their activity by inhibiting calcium entry into the cells, thereby affecting calcium dependent functions. Calcium channel blockers mainly affect the slow calcium channels of SA and AV node, cardiac and vascular smooth muscle cells. As a result, they cause vasodilation of both the coronary and peripheral arteries. Inhibition of slow calcium channels in nodal and cardiac cells results in decreased chronotropic and inotropic effects, respectively.

Skeletal muscle cells, unlike cardiac and smooth muscle cells are not as dependent upon extracellular calcium to initiate contraction and are therefore less affected by calcium channel blockers.

All of the clinically used calcium channel blockers are primarily metabolised in the liver, and undergo appreciable first pass metabolism.

Table 7.6 : Pharmacokinetic Parameters of Calcium Channel Blockers

Drug	Absorption (%)	Protein binding (%)	Biological Half-life (hr.)	Active metabolites
Verapamil	90	90	3 – 7	Yes
Diltiazem	80 – 90	78	3 – 5	Yes
Nifedipine	90	96	2 – 5	No
Nitrendipine	80	98	12 – 20	Yes
Felodipine	100	99	10	No

7.15 MECHANISM OF ACTION

The primary action of calcium channel blockers is the inhibition of calcium movement through the voltage dependent 'slow' channels in plasma membranes. Binding of these drugs to high affinity binding sites in the region of slow calcium ion channel, occurs in a stereospecific, saturable and reversible manner. Thus, the blockade of calcium dependent contractile activity results into a relaxation of peripheral arterial vascular tone with a subsequent decrease in systemic vascular resistance. This leads to a decrease in the blood pressure.

So, it has been proposed that there are three binding sites on the calcium channel and they are allosterically connected. It means binding of one drug changes the conformation of the binding sites of other two. This has been proved by the fact that verapamil and D600 inhibit the binding of H^3 nitrendipine in a non-competitive manner in heart, brain, ileum, aorta, coronary artery.

(1) The Ca^{++} channel blockers probably enter or cross the cell - membrane in order to gain access to the appropriate site of action in or on the channel.

(2) There they complex with two specific groups of membrane sites; a low affinity-high capacity group and a high affinity-low capacity group.

(3) A prominent feature of the blockage produced by these agents is use dependence. In a cell stimulated repeatedly (i.e. one whose membrane is depolarised repeatedly for short periods), a drug exhibiting use dependence will induce an increasingly greater degree of inhibition with each successive stimulation until a steady - state level of inhibition is reached.

(4) Diltiazem interacts primarily with the inactivated Ca^{++} channels, whereas verapamil, D600 and nitrendipine interact with activated Ca^{++} channels.

7.16 ADVERSE EFFECTS

Most of the reported adverse effects for the calcium channel blockers relate to their vasodilating properties. Headache, flushing, dizziness and gastrointestinal side-effects are reported for all of the calcium channel blockers. Verapamil and diltiazem can also cause bradycardia, AV - block, worsening of congestive heart failure and constipation. The dihydropyridine derivatives (e.g., felodipine, nifedipine) with less negative inotropism but more vasodilatory properties are more likely to cause tachycardia and ankle oedema than the other calcium channel blockers.

7.17 THERAPEUTIC USES

The calcium channel blockers have been used for a variety of indications which include :

(a) Essential hypertension :

All of the calcium channel blockers have been used in the treatment of essential hypertension.

(b) Angina :

Exertional angina (angina pectoris) and chronic stable angina have been successfully treated with all of the calcium channel blockers.

Variant or vasospastic angina is associated with a decrease in coronary blood flow secondary to increased coronary arterial tone. Nifedipine, diltiazem and verapamil are all effective.

The calcium channel blockers act by both decreasing oxygen demand and by increasing coronary blood flow. Currently, the combination of a beta-blocker and a nitrate is considered as the treatment of choice for patients with unstable angina, although calcium channel blockers may be beneficial when added to the regimen.

(c) Myocardial infarction :

Calcium channel blockers are known to limit the area affected by infarction. They also help to minimize ischemia-reperfusion injury following myocardial infarction.

(d) Supraventricular tachyarrhythmias :

Both diltiazem and verapamil are categorized as class IV anti-arrhythmic agents. They are found to be effective in the long-term prophylaxis of supraventricular tachy arrhythmias. Intravenous verapamil is usually effective in controlling the ventricular response to atrial fibrillation. It also helps to change supraventricular tachyarrhythmias to sinus rhythm.

(e) Raynaud's syndrome :

It is characterized by intermittent restriction of blood supply to the fingers and toes (and sometimes the ears and nose), most often in response to cold. The signs include mumbness, tingling, pain and pallor of the affected extremities, occasionally with blueness. Warmth relieves the symptoms after some time as the dilation of the boold vessels occur with sometimes painful felling. Raynaud's syndrome may be a symptom of more serious underlying vascular, neurological or collagen disorder. Nifedipine is found to be effective in its treatment.

Nifdipine is selective for vascular smooth muscles and is therefore an excellent antihypertensive. Since, it causes tachycardia, it is usually prescribed with β-blockers. Verapamil and diltiazem are ideal antianginal agents because of lack of tachycardia.

Other recently introduced Ca^{++} - channel blockers include :

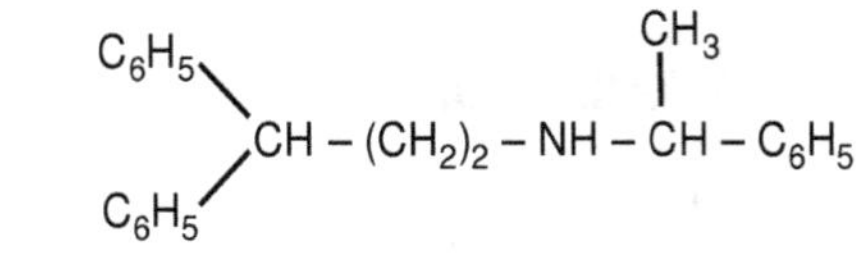

Fendiline

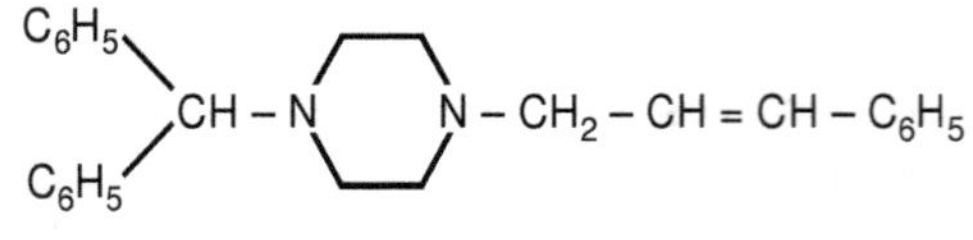

Cinnarizine

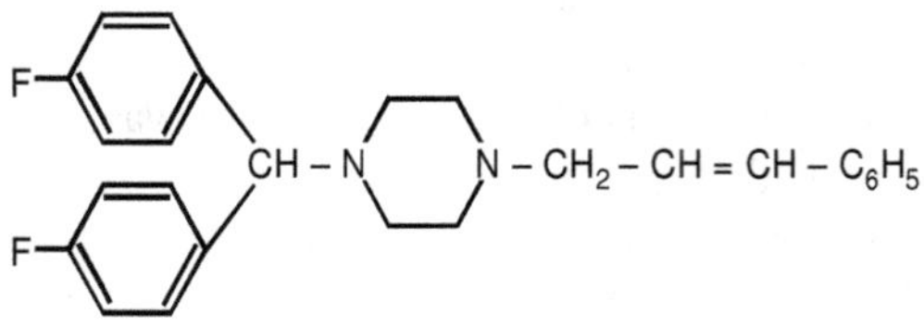

Flunarizine

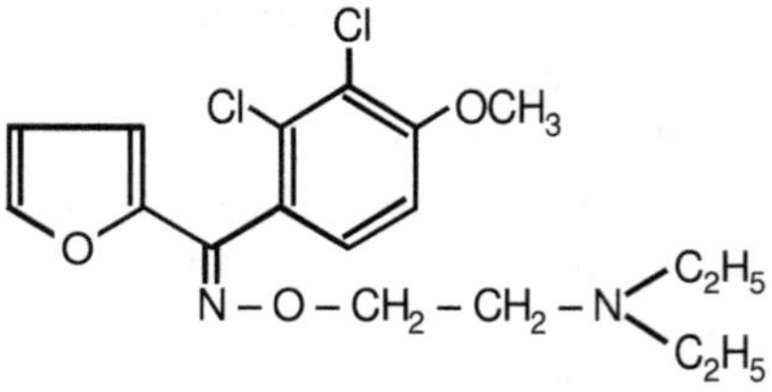

Diclofurime

Flunarizine is used in the migraine and dizziness prophylaxis. It also possesses H_1-histaminergic receptor blocking- activity.

7.18 CALCIUM ION CHANNEL AGONISTS

Ca^{++} channel agonists lead to vaso-constriction and exert a positive inotropic action. One of such agent (BAYK-8644) is a dihydropyridine derivative which shows promising results in the treatment of congestive heart failure.

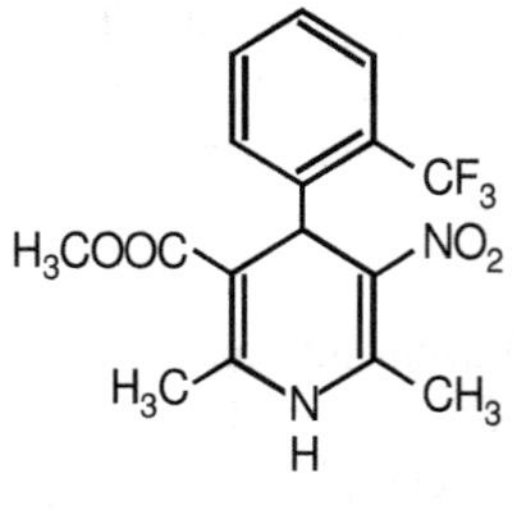

BAYK-8644

Table 7.7 : New Calcium ion Channel Blocking Agents

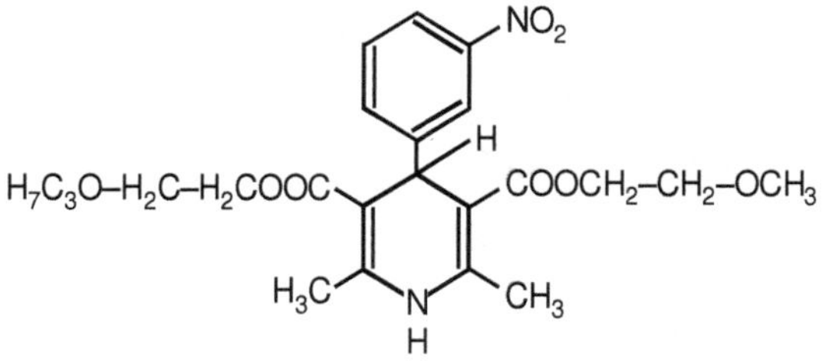

Niludipin

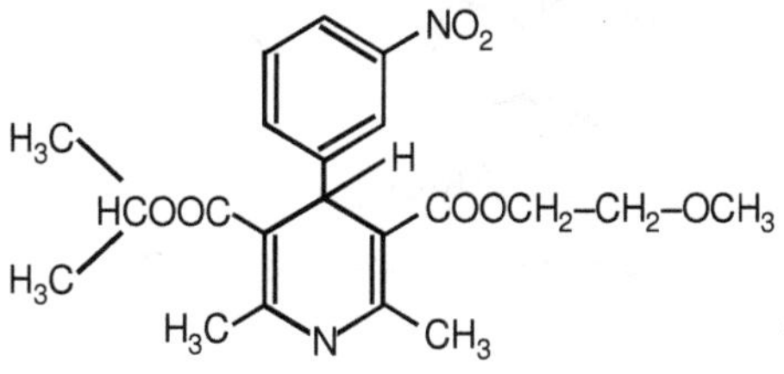

Nimodipine

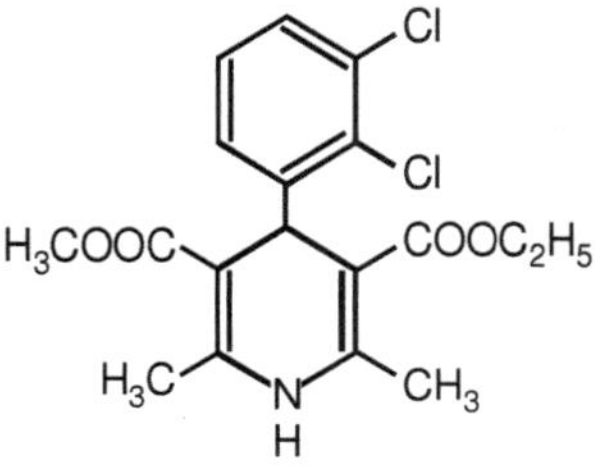

Felodipine

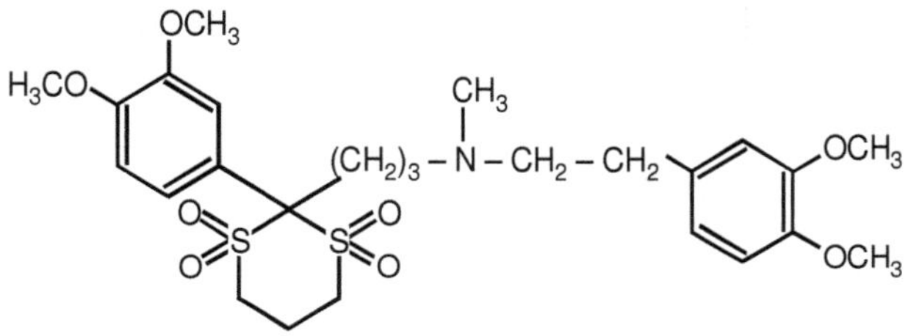

Tiopamil

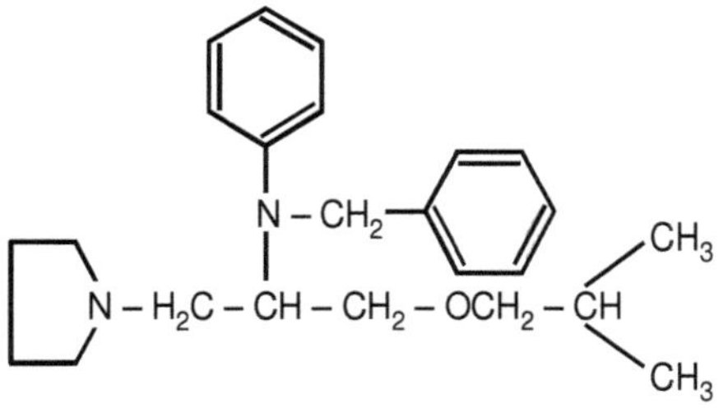

Bepridil

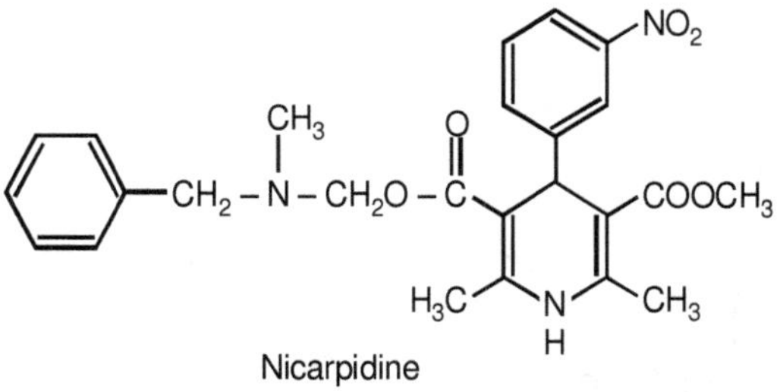

Nicarpidine

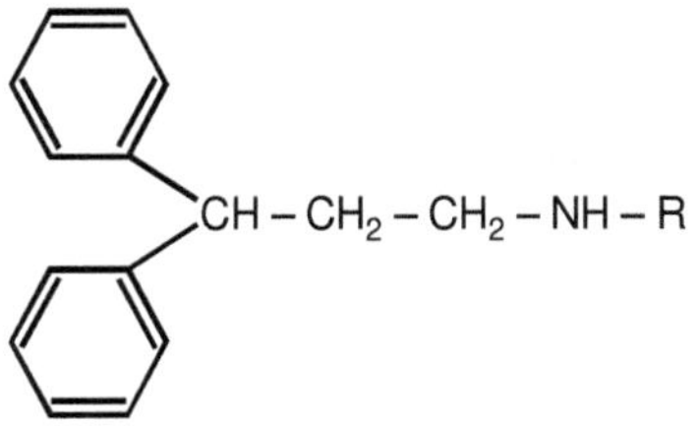

Prenylamine : R = – CH – CH₂

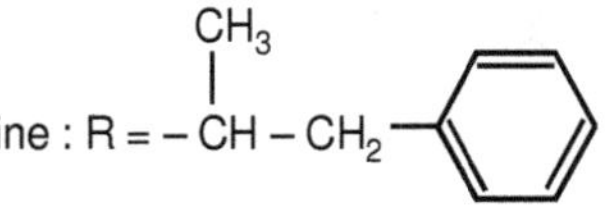

Fendiline : R = – CH

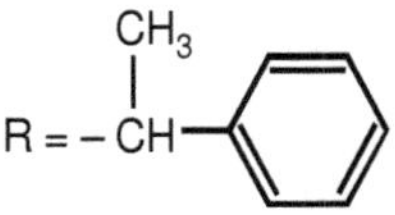

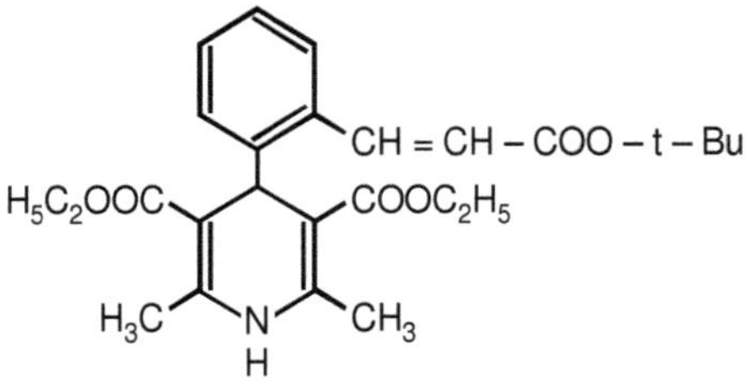

Lacipidine

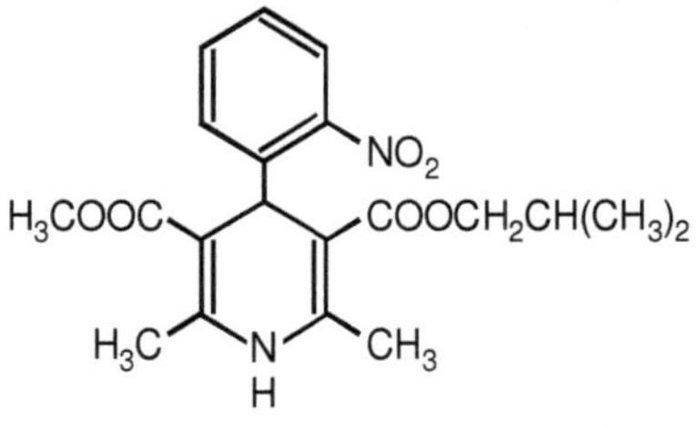

Nisoldipin

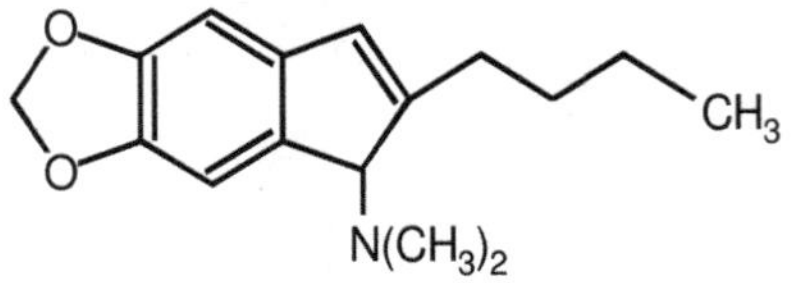

Drug Design   7.16   Drugs Acting on Cardio-Vascular System

2-n-butyl methylene-dioxyindene (MDI)

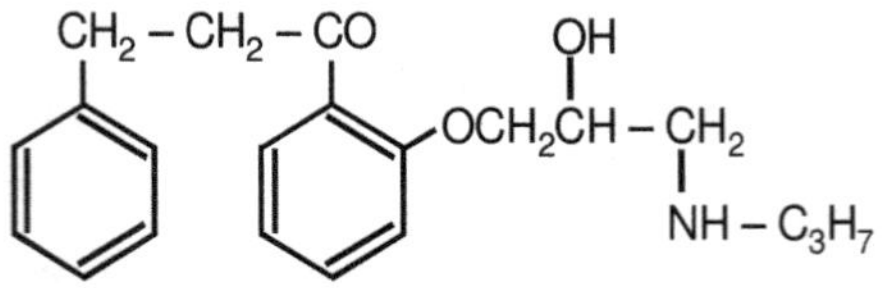

Propafenone

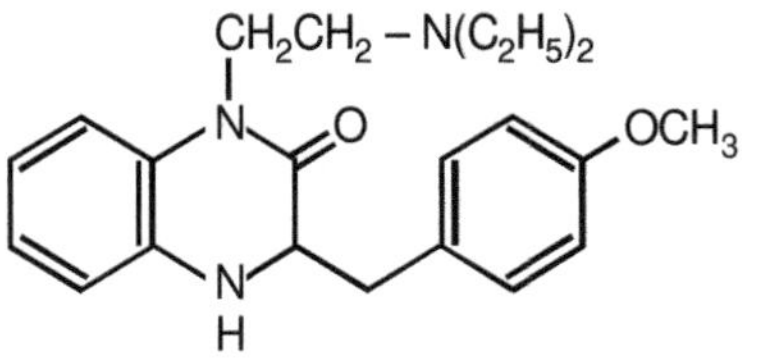

Caroverine

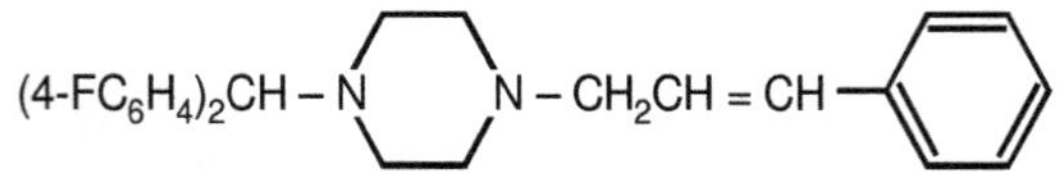

Flunorizine

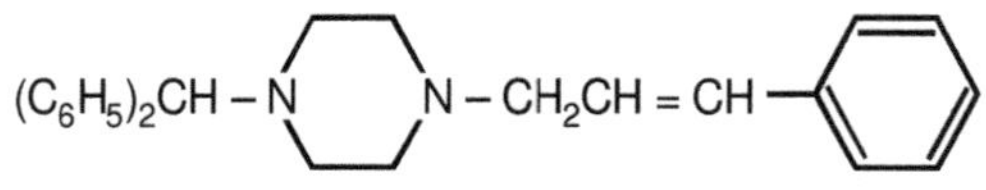

Cinnarizine

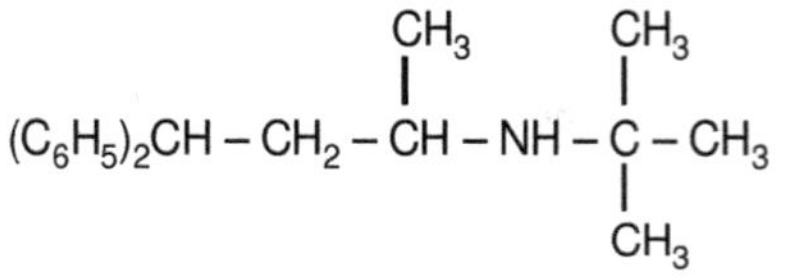

Terolidine

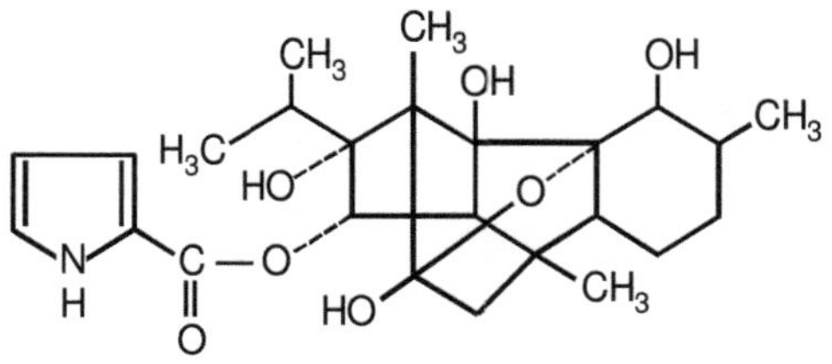

Ryanodine

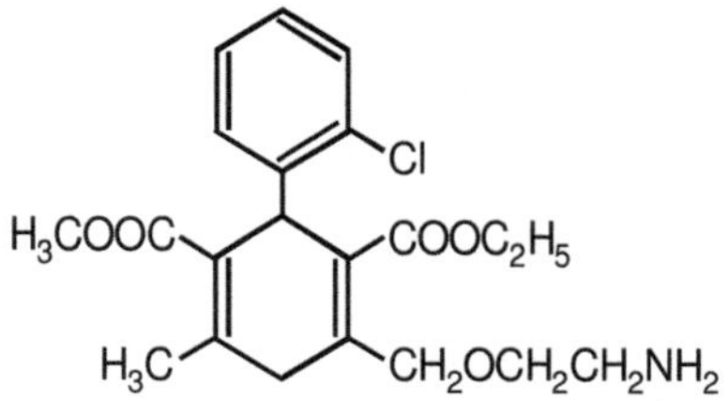

Amlodipine

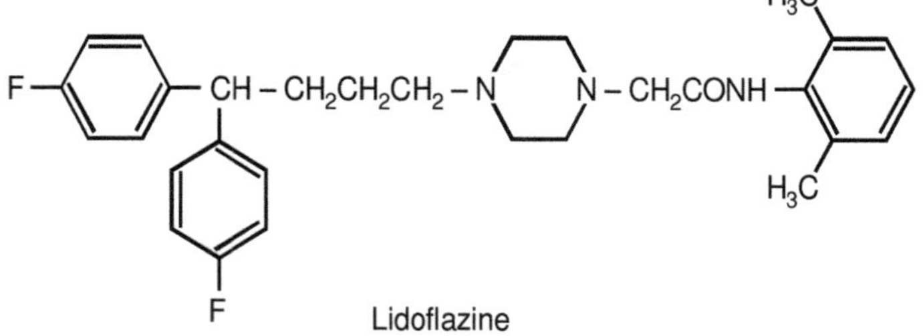

Lidoflazine

7.19 ANTI-HYPERTENSIVE AGENTS

Blood pressure is a bio-physical parameter which is closely related to the mechanisms that control perfusion or irrigation of blood to various tissues. A highly complex regulatory system operates for perfusion of blood into various tissues. The fluctuations in the vascular environment are nullified through the activation of baro- and chemo-receptors which maintain the blood pressure at a constant value. The elevated blood pressure may cause death through certain deleterious effects like stroke (i.e., damage to cerebral blood vessels), heart failure and kidney failure. In heart, the increased systemic pressure leads to an increase in the cardiac workload. The resulting cardiac overwork then becomes a prominent cause of left ventricular hypertrophy. While in kidneys, renal arteriosclerotic lesion of the afferent and efferent arterioles develop, resulting into renal failure.

Sustained hypertension may seriously affect the functioning of vital systems like cardiovascular system, central nervous system and renal system. It may disturb the functioning of CNS, resulting into vertigo, dizziness, occipital headaches, dimmed vision, vascular occlusion and hemorrhage.

7.20 GENERAL CONSIDERATIONS

Drugs affecting sympathetic tone produce their hypotensive action by affecting the biosynthesis. Storage, uptake, release, metabolism and adrenoceptor activation by sympathomimetic amines.

Agents acting at both, central sites (reserpine, guanethidine) and at peripheral sites (cardioselective β_1-antagonists) are included in this class. The adverse effects include increased renin secretion and development of tolerance. Other effects include sedation, dry mouth and depression.

The lowering of blood pressure by drugs like methyldopa and clonidine is brought about probably by stimulation of central presynaptic α_2-adrenoceptors, thereby reducing the release of efferent sympathetic traffic from CNS.

Guanethidine may be considered as a representative example of the drugs that depress the functioning at adrenergic neurons. Drugs in this class appear to act by more than one mechanisms. These agents mainly act by causing a gradual depletion of catecholamine stores from central and peripheral adrenergic nerve endings resulting into reduced sympathetic tone. Unlike clonidine, the therapy with reserpine and methyldopa is usually associated with extrapyramidal side-effects.

Alpha adrenoceptors are sub-classified as postsynaptic α_1-adrenoceptors and presynaptic α_2-adrenoceptor. The α_1-receptors are predominantly present in smooth muscle cells or arterial walls. While α_2-receptors are present on the presynaptic adrenergic neurons and exert inhibitory influence over the release of norepinephrine.

Activation of postsynaptic α_1-receptors leads to arterial vasoconstriction resulting into an increase in peripheral vascular resistance. Hence, α_1-adrenoceptor blocking agents can be clinically used as antihypertensive agents. Examples include, prazosin, trimazosin and indoramin. They appear to exert vasodilatory effect through the blockade of α_1-adrenoceptors. Prazosin is the first member of this class, reported in 1974 followed by trimazosin. Both are quinazoline derivatives. They mainly affect the venous vascular bed but become more balanced during long term treatment. They affect to varying degree, the functioning of renin-angiotensin system resulting into sodium and fluid retention. They tend to produce tolerance if used chronically. They are mainly used in the treatment of hypertension and heart failure.

β-adrenoceptors are mainly present in heart, pulmonary vessels, vessels supplying blood to skeletal muscles and are also involved in glycogenolysis and lipolysis. The β-adrenoceptor blocking agents act by the competitive inhibition of the effect of catecholamines on β-adrenoceptors. Previously, it was proposed that the antihypertensive effect of these drugs results due to a downward suppression of functioning of baroreceptors. But now the antihypertensive effect of β-adrenoceptor blocking agents is explained in the following lines.

(a) Decreased renin release occurs due to inhibition of β_1-receptors while renal plasma flow and rate of glomerular filtration are reduced by blockade of β_2-receptors.

(b) Decreased norepinephrine release occur from the postganglionic sympathetic nerves due to the blockade of presynaptic β-receptors.

(c) Central mechanism has been proposed for some lipophillic β-blockers, and

(d) The cardioselective β_1-blockers act by exerting a reduction in rate and force of heart contraction. However, such cardioselectivity is of relative nature and seen only at low doses.

Due to interference in glycogenesis, these drugs may cause hypoglycemia-like symptoms during chronic treatment.

Dichloroisoproterenol was the first β-blocker introduced in 1960s. All β-adrenoceptor blockers are analogues of adrenoreceptor agonist, isoproterenol.

The β-blockers compete with agonist molecules at three principle reactive sites. They are characterized by a substituted aromatic ring and a side-chain.

The nature of aromatic substituent affects receptor activation ability (i.e. intrinsic activity) while the side-chain appears to govern affinity of these antagonists for the β-adrenoceptors. Usually, affinity is proportional to chain-length. The configuration of asymmetric-carbon atom is crucial to define the pharmacological activity of the compound. The aromatic substituents also govern the lipophilicity of the compounds and thus their central effects.

Due to the presence of asymmetric-carbon atom in the side-chain, these compounds usually exist as pairs of enantiomers. The laevoisomers are much more potent (50 - 100 times) β-blockers than their dextroisomers. Except timolol (laevoisomer), all other β-blockers are available commercially in the form of their recemic mixture.

Dichloroisoproterenol, due to its weak antagonistic property was soon replaced by pronethalol. But it was also withdrawn from clinical testing because of reports that it caused thymic tumours in mice. However soon after, propranolol, a close structural relative of pronethalol, was developed. It is a non-selective β-blocker, having almost negligible Intrinsic Sympathomimetic Activity (ISA). It is considered now as a prototype of β-blocker series. It was then followed by atenolol, acebutolol, metoprolol, nadolol, practolol and tolamolol.

Practolol was found to induce mucocutaneous reactions while tolamolol was reported to initiate tumour development. For these reasons, both these drugs have been withdrawn from clinical use.

The relative lack of postural hypotension and sexual disfunctioning coupled with good therapeutic index are the added advantages of β-blockers over other antihypertensive agents. The membrane stabilizing or *'quinidine like'* effect associated with certain β-blockcrs (e.g., propranolol) do not play any significant role at the doses needed for their antihypertensive action.

The β_2-receptors are predominantly present in lung, particularly in bronchial muscles. The β_1 to β_2 receptor ratio in human lung is estimated to be nearly 30 : 70. Hence, β-blockers besides exerting their antihypertensive action, may antagonise lung β_2-receptors causing bronchial constriction, a case contraindicated in hypertensive patients suffering from bronchial asthma. The ratio of cardiac to lung activity has been evaluted for propranolol (2:1), practolol (15:1) and for atenolol (200:1). Atenolol and metoprolol are the examples of cardioselective β_1-antagonists that have much greater affinity for β_1-receptors in the heart than the β_1-receptors present in other tissues. While non-selective β-antagonists (e.g. propranolol) are mainly reserved for the treatment of migraine and tremor. The elevated peripheral resistance is the main cause behind most of the hypertensive cases. Vasodilators act by inducing vascular smooth muscle relaxation, thereby normalizing the elevated peripheral resistance which is the main hemodynamic abnormality in this condition.

The drawback of vasodilator therapy is the reflex activation of compensatory mechanisms such as sympathetic activation (resulting into an increase in the heart rate and cardiac output) and activation of renin-angiotensin-aldosterone system (resulting into increased extracellular fluid due to salt and water retention). The latter effect is much pronounced with hydralazine and diazoxide that cause mainly arterial dilation. This elevation induced by vasodilators can be minimized by concurrent administration of a diuretic along with β-adrenoceptor blocking agent.

Vasodilation can be brought about by using :

(a) Pure vasodilators e.g., hydralazine, minoxidil.

(b) Indirect vasodilator :
   (i) α_1-adrenoceptor blocking agents and
   (ii) Angiotensin converting enzyme inhibitors.

Renin is a proteolytic enzyme involved in the synthesis of a decapeptide, angiotensin-I. The latter is convened to an octapeptide, angiotensin-II by a peptidyldipeptide hydrolase (converting enzyme) in the vascular endothelial cells and epithelial cells of the proximal tubule and small intestine. The converting enzyme is a metalloenzyme (Zn^{++}) and requires the presence of chloride ions. Its activity is suppressed by hypoxia. Angiotensin II is a potent vasoconstrictor and initiates the release of aldosterone. It also independently controls Na^{++} transport by epithelial cells in the gut and kidney.

Thus, activation of renin-angiotensin-aldosterone system leads to vasoconstriction and hypertension. Hence, drugs that antagonise the effect of renin, angiotensin or aldosterone can be used in the treatment of systemic hypertension, congestive cardiac failure and pulmonary hypertension. The drugs from this class can be subcategorized as :

(a) Renin antagonists

(b) Aldosterone antagonists

(c) Angiotensin-II antagonists

(d) Converting enzyme inhibitors.

At present renin antagonists do not have therapeutic potential while aldosterone antagonists may principally be used as diuretic agents. Saralasin is an example of angiotensin-II competitive antagonist while captopril (1977) is an example of orally effective converting enzyme inhibitor.

Sodium retention and consequent fluid retention usually serve as an initiating factors in hypertension. Certain antihypertensive drugs (e.g. adrenergic neuron blocking agents, vasodilators) could not retain their efficacy due to reflex activation of plasma renin. In such cases diuretics can bring about impressive results by suppressing renal tubular reabsorption of sodium, thus reducing the blood volume and the cardiac output. They exert antihypertensive action by promoting the loss of salt and water through the kidneys. However they too, are not free from adverse effects and may induce reflex renin activation and metabolic changes like, hypokaemia, alkalosis, hyperglycemia and hyper uricaemia. Sexual dysfunction is also reported with the long term treatment of diuretics.

From the forgoing discussion, it becomes clear that none of the above categories qualifies the test for ideal anti-hypertensive agent. Their efficiency is largely paralyzed due to emergence of compensatory reflex mechanisms in the body. For example, vasodilators lead to reflex tachycardia and elevation of plasma renin activity while sympatholytics gradually lose their effectiveness due to fluid retention. The sympatholytics can abolish reflex tachycardia associated with vasodilator therapy while the fluid retention caused due to sympatholytics and vasodilators can be effectively neutralized by the use of diuretics. Such a combination of a sympatholylic, vasodilator and a diuretic agent presents most effective antihypertensive treatment where very low incidences of side-effects result due to comparatively low doses of each of the three components.

7.21 DRUGS AFFECTING SYMPATHETIC TONE

In the begining of 1960s, Helmut while working on decongestive imidazolines (e.g., tolazoline, phentolamine) observed that the imidazoline nucleus is connected with an aromatic ring by a methylene bridge. With previous experience, he predicted that replacement of $- CH_2 -$ by $- NH$ group may lead to increase in decongestive activity. The resulting compounds when tested by Dr. Wolf who administered a few drops of 0.3% solution to Mrs. Schwandf for common cold, decongestive activity was found far less than its potent antihypertensive activity. The compound (clonidine) then developed for this new indication and introduced in therapy in 1966. Clonidine is a potent agonist of presynaptic inhibitory α_2-adrenoceptors.

Clonidine   Lofexidine

Introduction of two chlorine atoms in the imidazolidine molecule proved important for the activity of clonidine, as (a) two substituents at ortho position forced the molecule into a non-planar conformation with the two rings approximately perpendicular to each other so as to meet the steric requirements to fit α-adrenoceptor. The presence of two chlorine atoms at ortho position helps to prevent free rotation of two rings. This contributes to better complimentary fit at α-receptor. (b) two chlorine atoms also make the molecule sufficiently lipophilic to cross blood-brain barrier.

Thus clonidine may be viewed as the norepinephrine analogue with a limited degree of conformational freedom. Other cyclic analogues of norepinephrine with limited degree of conformational freedom include,

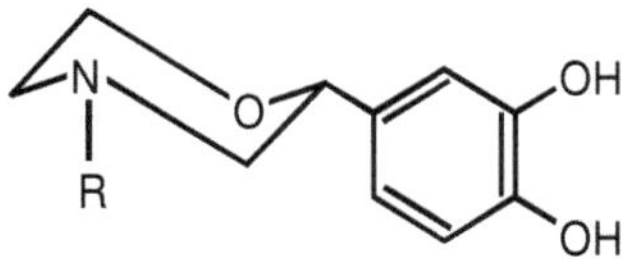

(a) 2-(3, 4-dihydroxyphenyl) morpholines

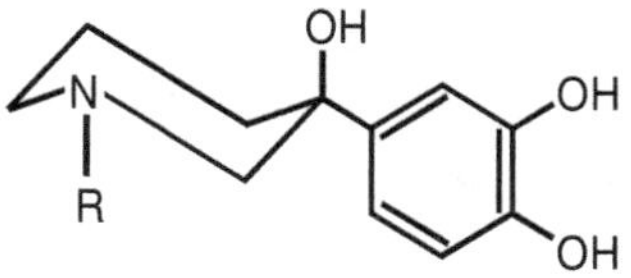

(b) 3-(3, 4-dihydroxyphenyl) -3- piperidinols

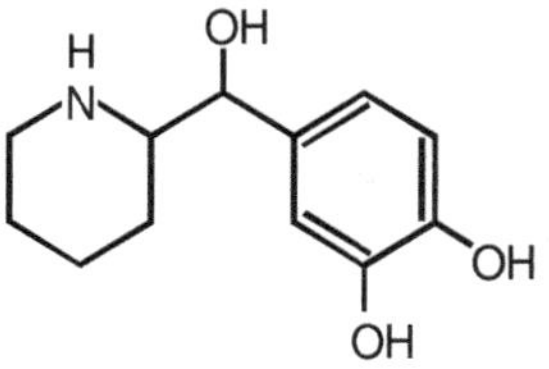

(c)

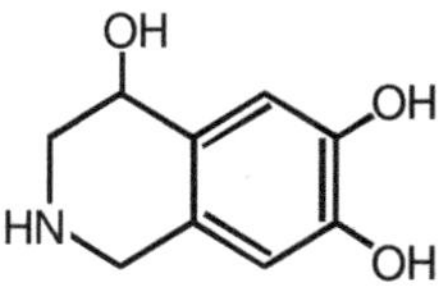

(d)

Adrenoceptor blocking agents :

While investigating toxicity of antimalarial compounds, Moe et al, in 1949 found that various quinolines produced appreciable anti-α-adrenergic effects. As a result, a series of 6, 7-dimethoxy quinolines was synthesized in Norwich laboratory. The potent hypotensive agents include,

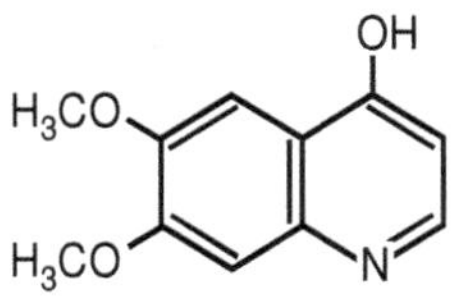

U-558

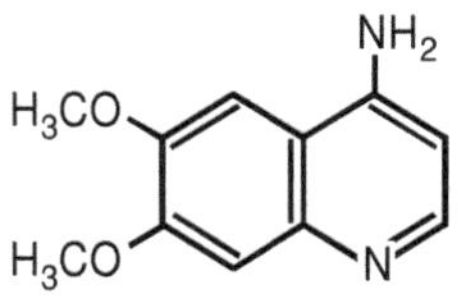

Amiquinsin

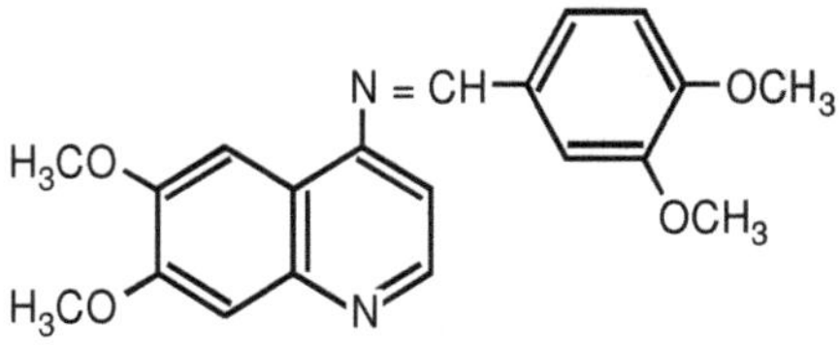

Leniquinsin

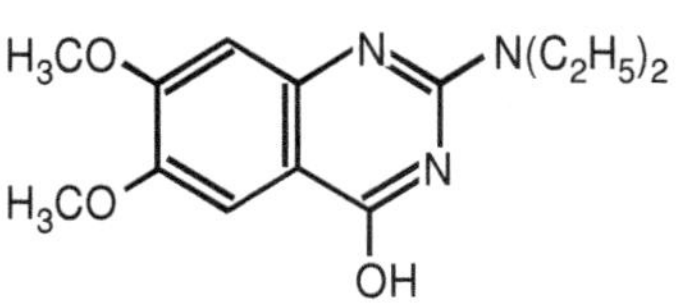

XV

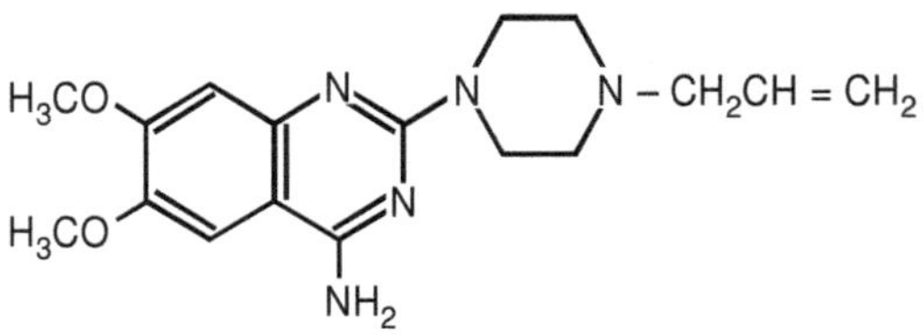

Quinazosin

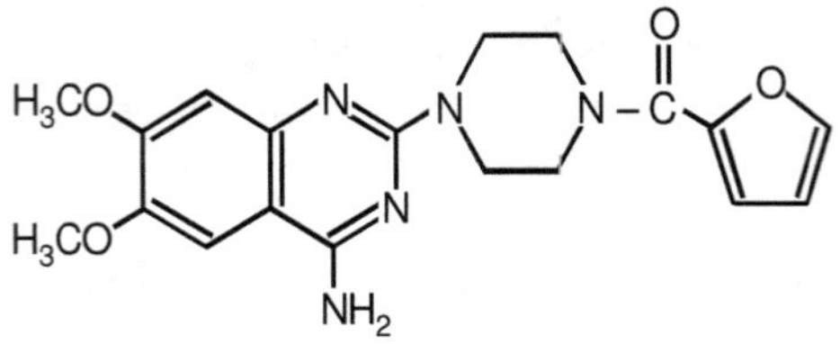

Structures (top box): Prazosin, 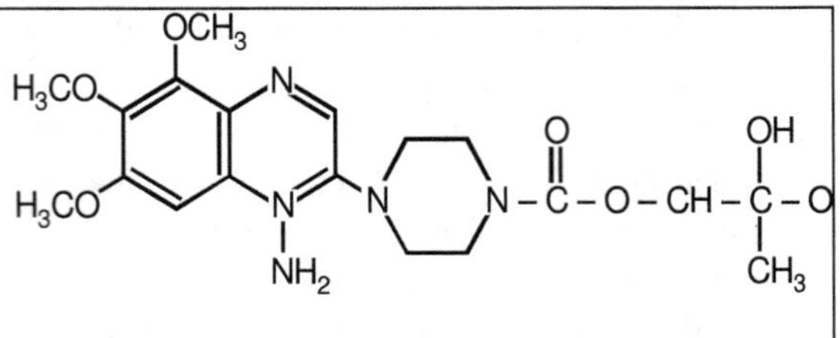 Trimazosin, 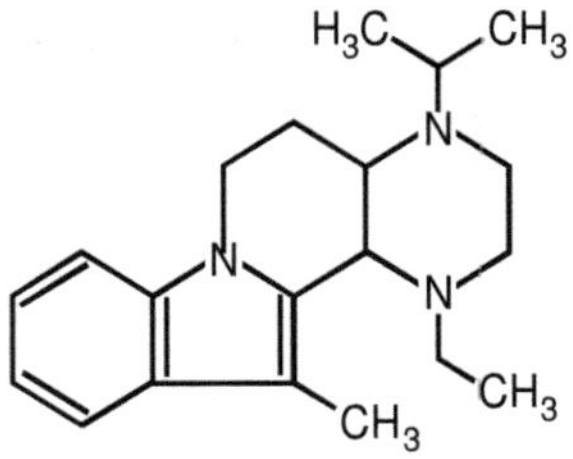 Aliprosin, 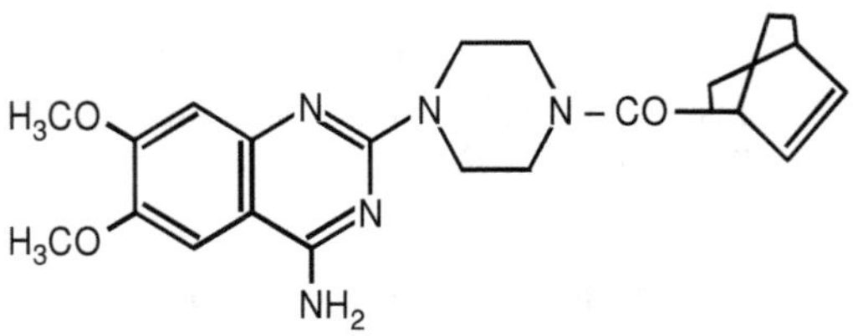 SM 2470

Prazosin (1974) exerts its antihypertensive action by blocking post-synaptic α_1-adrenoceptor resulting into vascdilation of the arterioles. The decreased arterial vascular resistance and reduction in arterial and venous tone are the effects mainly due to vasodilation caused by blockage of vascular α_1-receptors.

Indoramin is yet another example of vascular α_1-receptor blocking agent. Chemically, it is 1-[2-(3-indolyl ethyl] derivative of 4-benzarnido piperidine and resembles with the structure of procainamide.

7.22 β-ADRENOCEPTOR BLOCKING AGENTS

The concept of β-adrenergic blockade was pioneered in 1960's. All cardioselective β_1-adrenoceptor blocking agents are more hydrophilic than propranolol and their cardioselectivity can be attributed to the fact that β_1-receptors are hydrophilic while β_2-receptors are lipophilic.

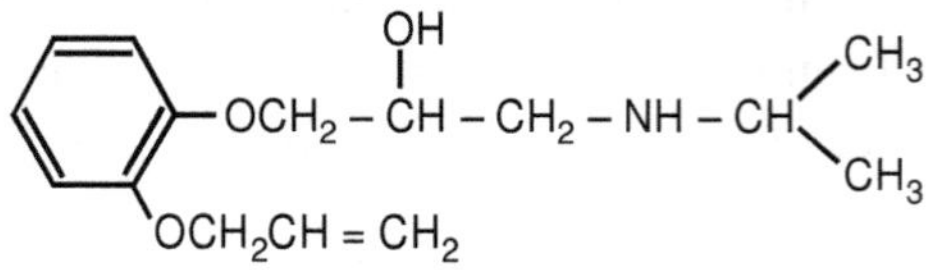

CIBA

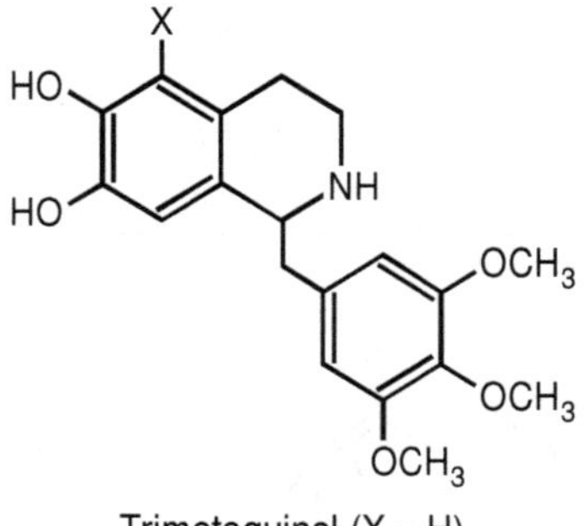

Trimetoquinol (X = H)

Trimetoquinol is a competitive inhibitor of human platelet aggregation. It also has a non-specific β-adrenergic agonistic activity. The changes in β-adrenoceptor activation were correlated to differences in phenolic pKa attributed to the electronic influence of X.

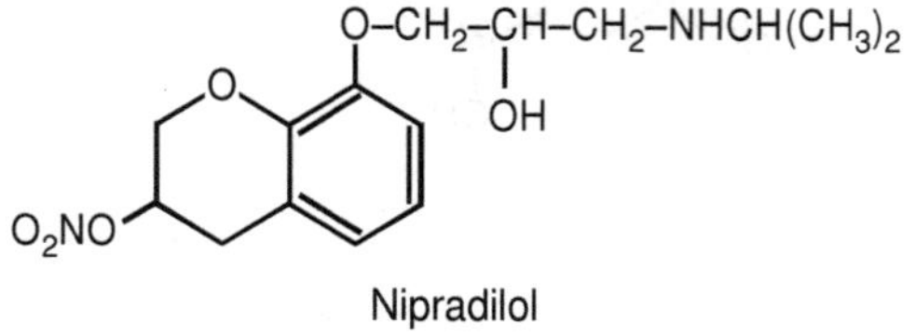

Nipradilol

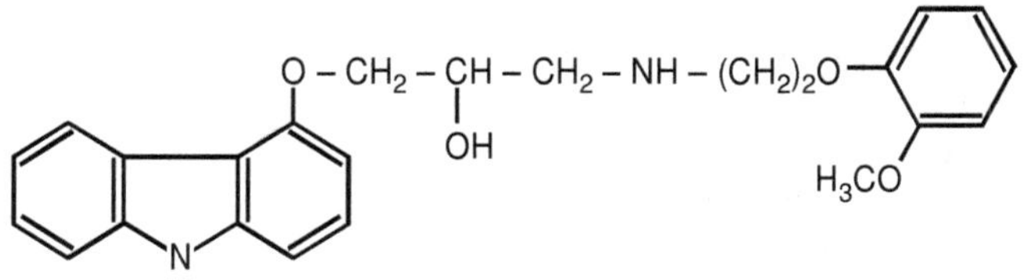

Carvedilol

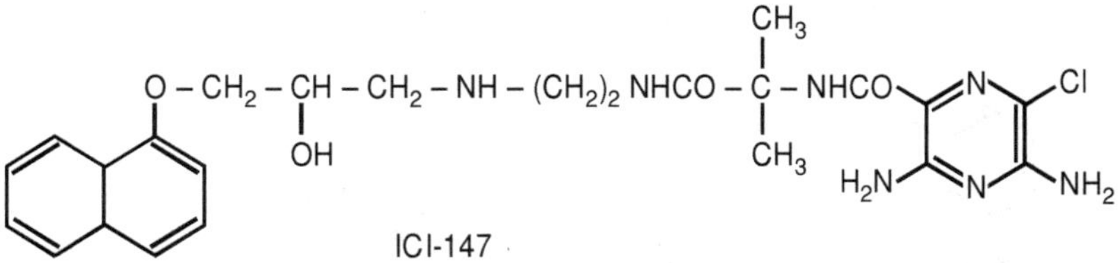

ICI-147

Since vasodilators reduce blood pressure by relaxing peripheral vascular smooth muscles, the reduction in blood pressure leads to a reflex increase in sympathetic tone, followed by increases in heart rate, cardiac output and plasma renin activity which partly nullify the anti-hypertensive effect. Hence, a combination of a vasodilator and a β-blocker is usually done to take care of these undesired effects of vasodilators. The vasodilators at the same time, control the possible increase in peripheral vascular resistance induced by β-blockers. Nipradiol and carvedilol are the examples of drugs having both vasodilation and β-adrenoceptor blocking activities. While ICI-147 has both diuretic and β-adrenoceptor blocking properties.

7.23 CALCIUM ION CHANNEL BLOCKERS

The elevated peripheral vascular resistance is the main cause behind most of the hypertensive conditions. The calcium channel blockers, unlike direct vasodilator cause dilation of coronary arteries and markedly affect the automaticity, conduction velocity and refractory period in myocardial cells.

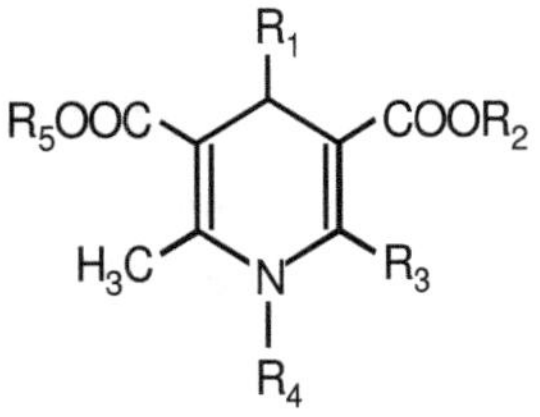

1, 4-Dihydropyridines

Name	R_1	R_2	R_3	R_4	R_5
1. Nimodipine	$3-NO_2C_6H_4$	$-CH(CH_3)_2$	CH_3	H	$OCH_2CH_2OCH_3$
2. Nisoldipine	$3-NO_2C_6H_4$	CH_3	CH_3	H	$OCH_2CH_2OCH_3$
3. Nicardipine	$3-NO_2C_6H_4$	$-(CH_2)_2NHCH_2C_6H_5$	CH_3	H	CH_3
4. Lacidipine	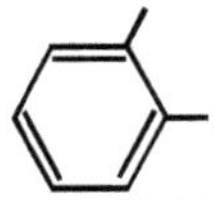 – CH = CH – COO.t-Bu	C_2H_5	CH_3	H	C_2H_5

Certain steric hindrance at ortho position is required to fix the dihydropyridine structure in favourable conformation in which the aromatic group is approximately perpendicular to dihydropyridine ring. Agents with slower onset and longer duration of action can be developed from dihydropyridine category by optimizing the ester and aryl substituents. For example,

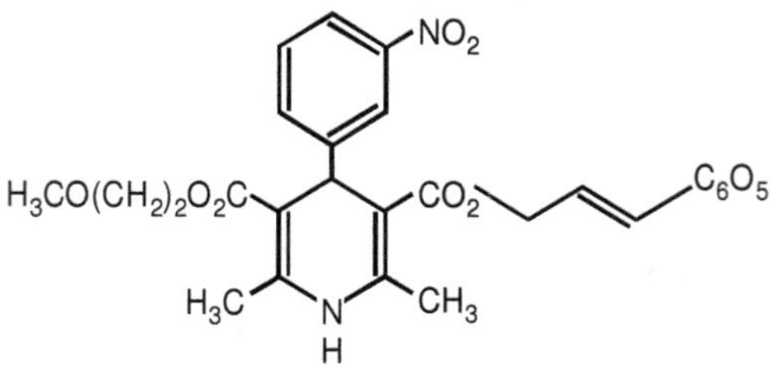

FRC – 8653

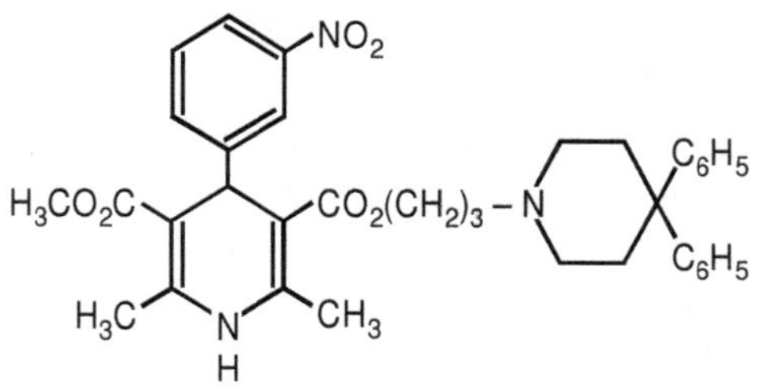

B – 844 – 39

Attempts were made further to develop a dual acting calcium channel blocker/ β-adrenoceptor antagonist which resulted into YM-16151 and (a).

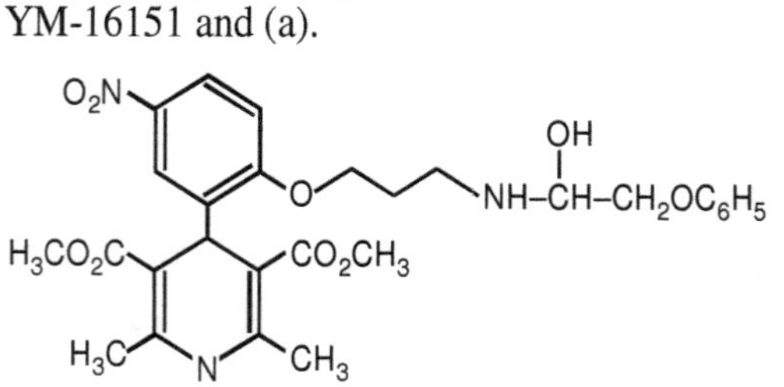

YM – 16151

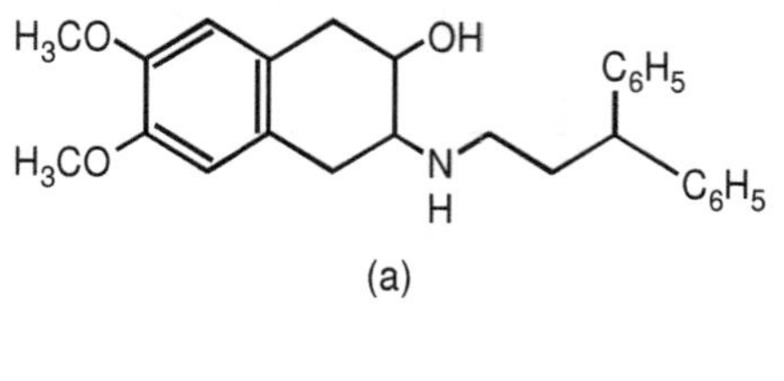

(a)

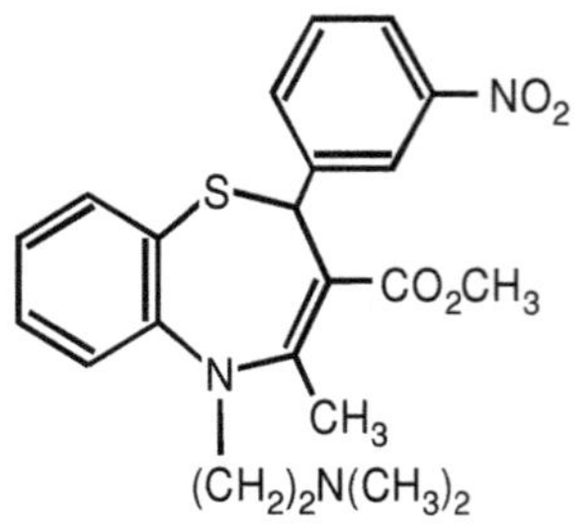

(b)

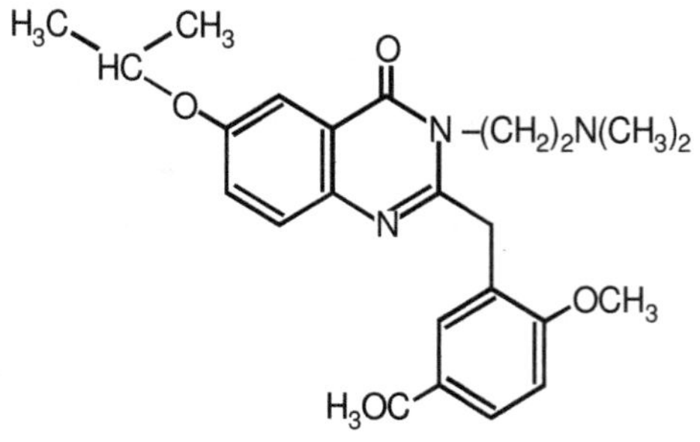

MCI - 176

Attempts were also made to develop a structuaral hybrid of nifedipine -diltiazem (b) and a non-dihydropyridine calciumn ion channel blocker, MC1- 176.

Organic nitrates (e.g., nitroglycerine, nicorandil) promote vasodilation by increasing c-GMP production in various vascular smooth muscles. Simultaneous use of calcium antagonist and nitrate compound clinically enhances the therapeutic anti-hypertensive effect with few side-effects. So the combination of nitro-like and calcium ion channel blocking action in a single molecule was also tried to get a potential vasodilating activity. Similar attempts ware also made to club nitro-like and β_1-adrenoceptor blocking activity in a single molecule. Example include nipradilol.

7.24 AGENTS ACTING ON RENIN-ANGIOTENSIN-ALDOSTERONE SYSTEM

The renin-angiotensin system is one of the important homeostatic mechanisms that regulate hemodynamics and water and electrolyte balance. Manipulation of the renin-angiotensin system and the blockade of renin, in particular, currently constitute the major areas of investigation for novel anti-hypertensive agents. The feasibility of long-term control of blood pressure by active immunization against human renin was searched.

Table 7.8 : Important Renin Inhibitors

R = CH_3; CGP - 38259
R = t-Bu; CGP - 38560

(Ciba Geigy; CGS - 38560)

(Hoechst)

CGS - 38651 (Ciba Geigy)

(Hoechst)

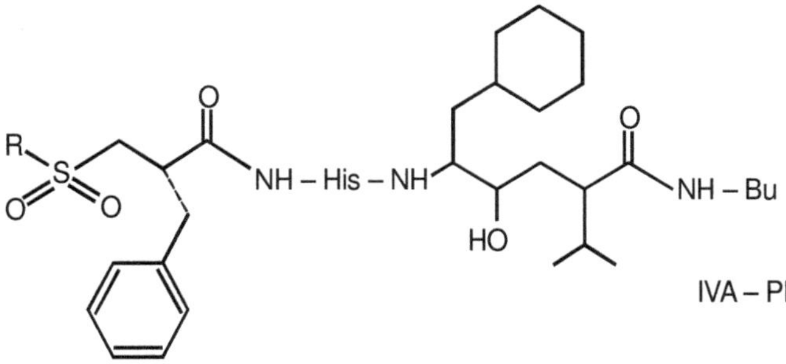

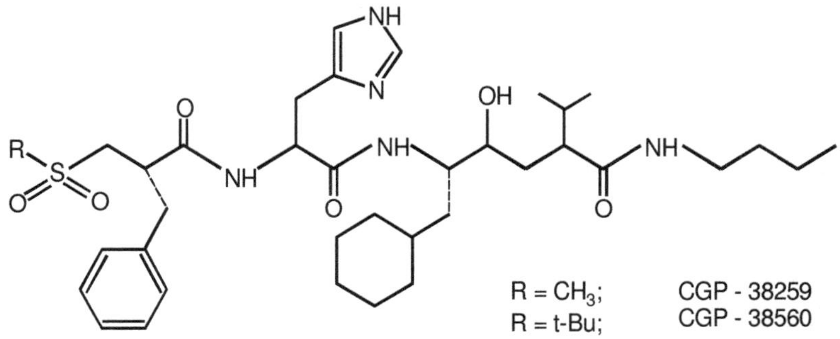

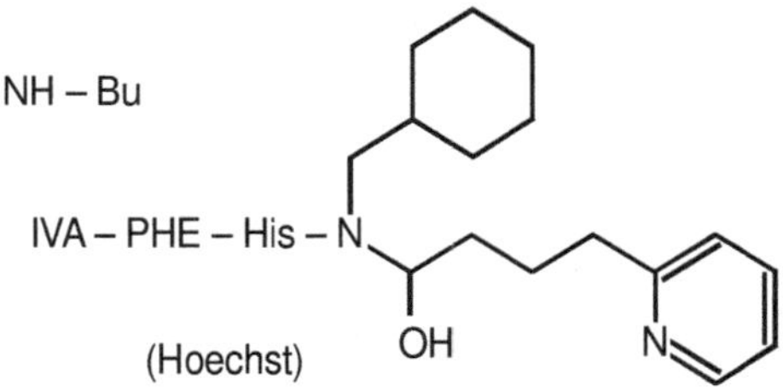

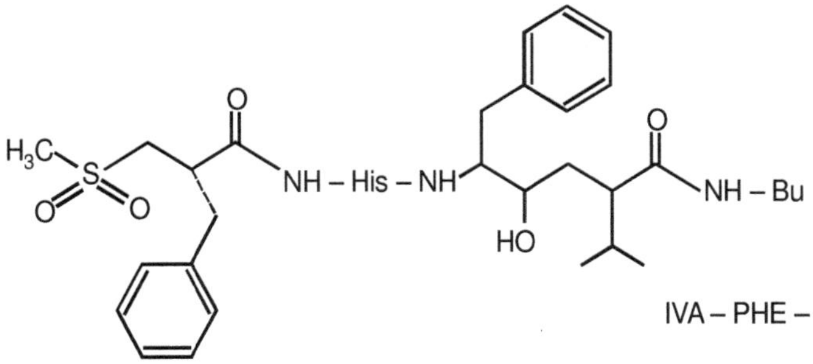

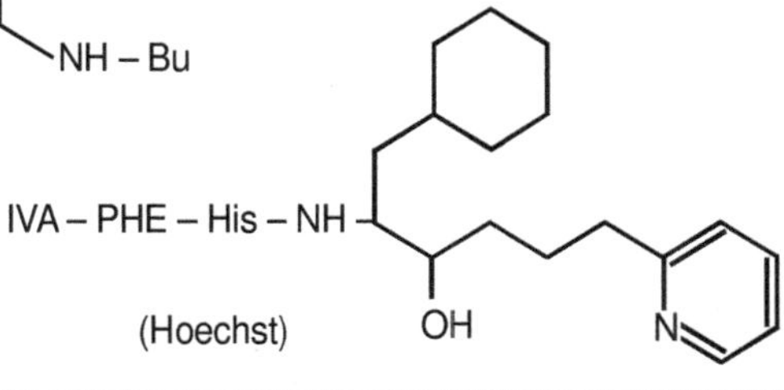

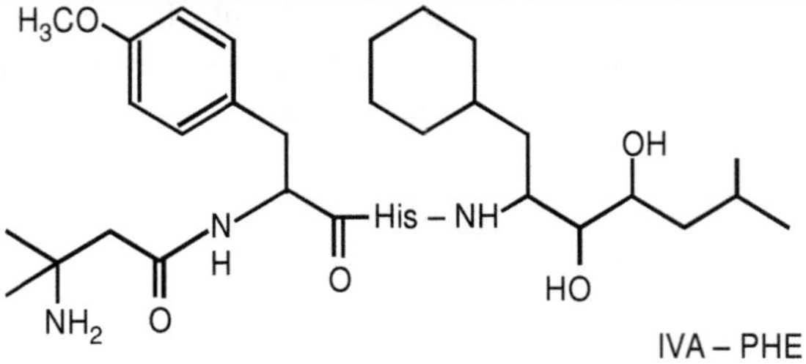

A 64662 (Abbott)

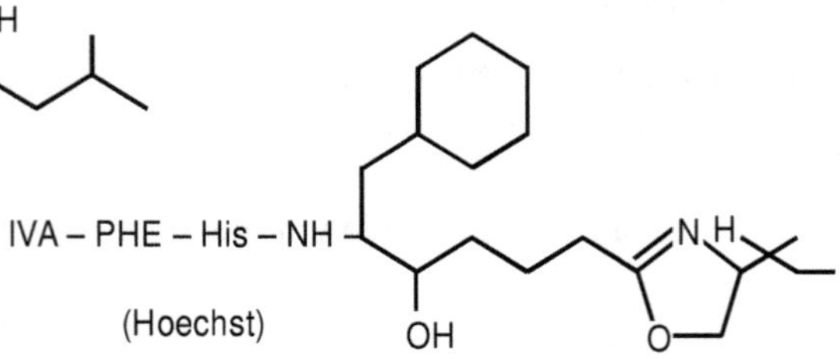

IVA – PHE – His – NH

(Hoechst)

Angiotensin-II (A-II) is a powerful vasopressor peptide produced by the renni-angiotensin system. Angiotensin Converting Enzyme (ACE) inhibitors, which reduce the A-II levels, can be effective antihypertensive agents. The success of captopril and enalapril has been a strong stimulus for continued research and novel ACE-inhibitors continue to appear which include perindolpril, ramipril, cilazapril, spirapril, zofenopril and fosinopril.

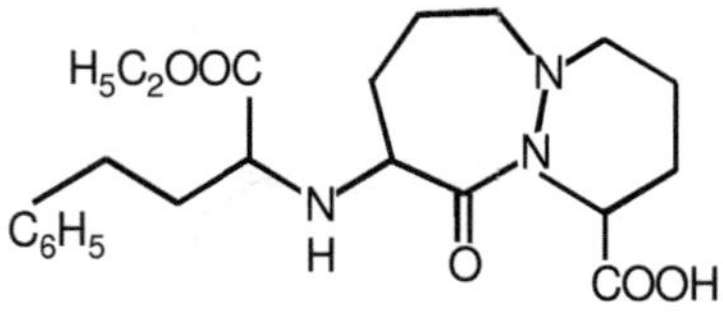

Cilazapril

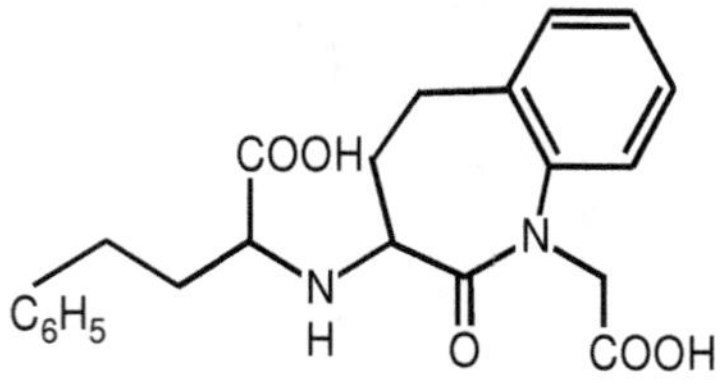

Benzapril

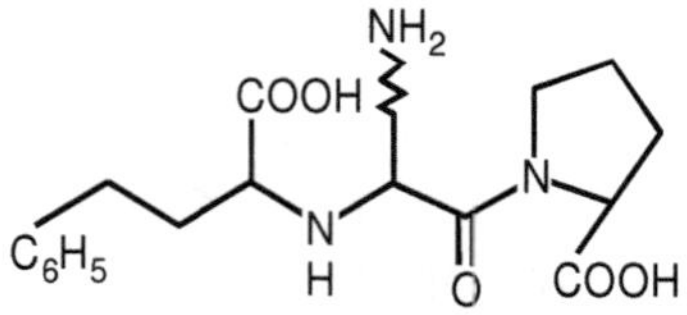

Lisinopril

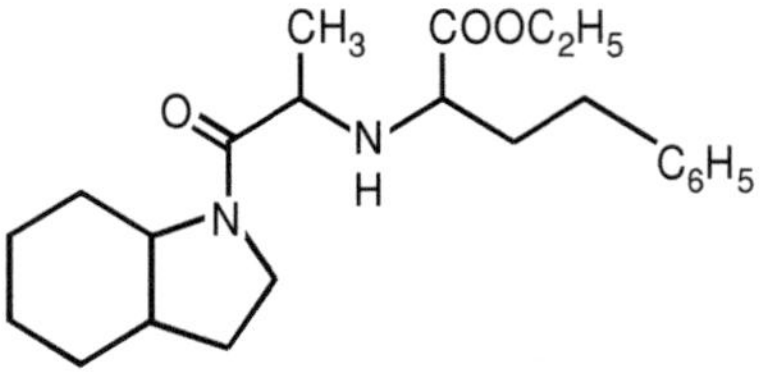

Indolapril

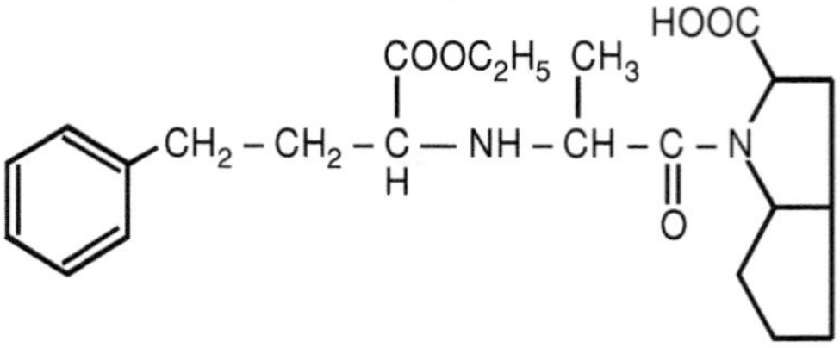

Ramipril

However ACE-inhibitors may produce side-effects such as cough and angioedema probably due to their lack of selectivity, which result in an increase of bradykinin levels. Similarly, A-II can also be formed in-vivo by the action of enzymes other than ACE. Another way to inhibit the A-II effects is to antagonise its action at the receptor level in order to obtain more specific drugs and to avoid side-effects related to bradykinin potentiation. Peptide A-II receptor antagonists were developed by modification of A-II structure with the aim of defining the role of each constituent amino acid and eliminating agonist activity.

Until recently all potent angiotensin-II receptor antagonists reported have been peptide analogues of A-II and have suffered from the problems normally associated with peptides such as poor oral absorption, short plasma half-lives and rapid clearance. In addition many exhibit partial agonism. Recently, potent non-petide A-II antagonists such as DuP 753 (Losartan) L-158809 and SR-47436 have been described as an important advance in the area.

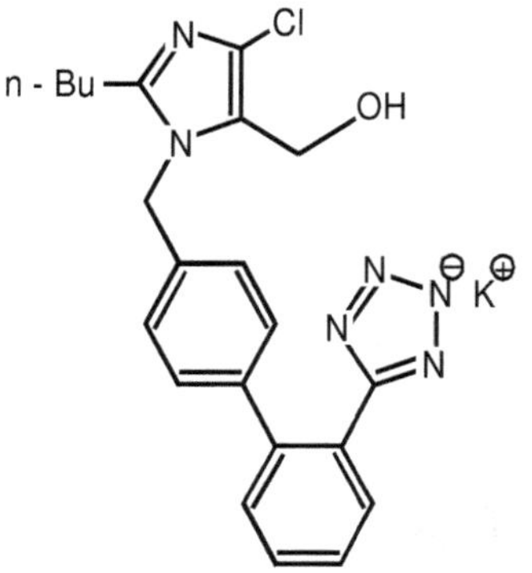

DuP 753

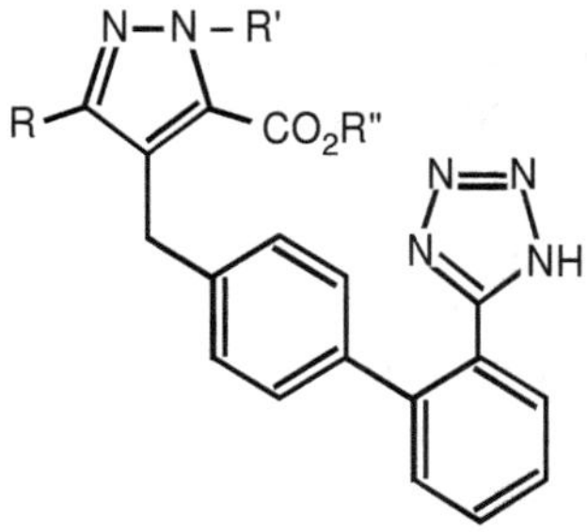

Merck

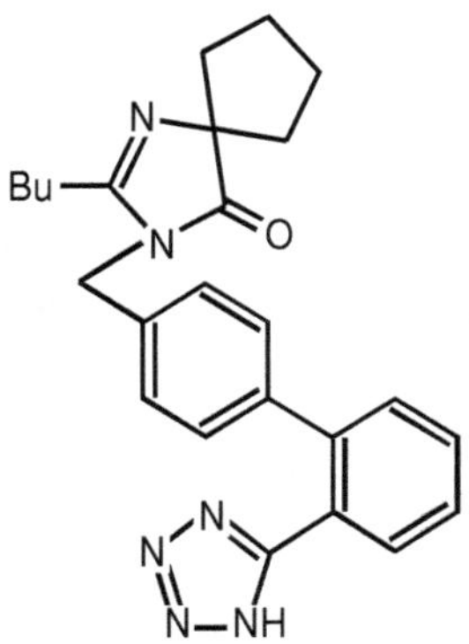

SR - 47436

The great majority of them contain a biphenyltetrazole moiety appended to a five membered or a six membered heterocycle, the biphenyltetrazole being linked to a nitrogen atom.

7.25 DIURETICS

The novel successors of loop diuretic furosemide include piretanide and etozolin which possess high specificity for NaCl transport, minimum potassium ion excretion and prolonged duration of action.

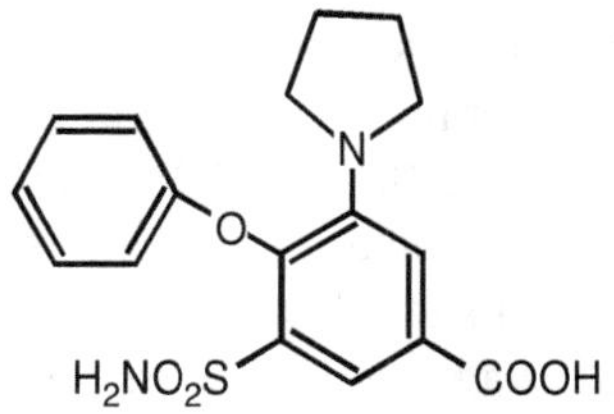

Piretanide

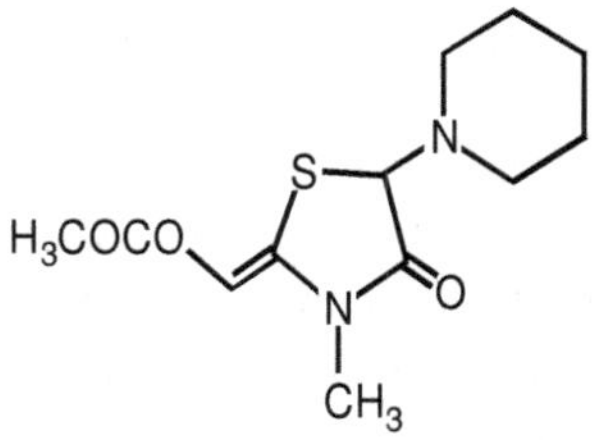

(+) Etozolin

Chronic excessive doses of diuretics can worsen cardiac failure and contribute to symptoms of fatigue through electrolyte disturbances and dehydration. Symptoms of fainting or dizziness on standing may indicate a need to review diuretics or vasodilator therapy.

7.26 CENTRAL DEPRESSANTS

A meprobamate analogue, mebutamate, lowers blood pressure by exerting depressant effect on the vasomotor centers of brain stem.

7.27 ATRIAL NATRIURETIC PEPTIDE (ANP)

Atrial Natriuretic Peptide (ANP) was isolated in 1981 by De Bold, Sonnenberg, et al and was characterized as a factor for the control of hemostasis.

The physiological functions of ANP include,

(a) Vasodilation.

(b) Increased GFR and salt-water excretion (diuretic)

(c) Inhibition of the release of angiotensin-II, aldosterone and vasopression.

ANP is derived from a precursor protein produced by cardiac atrium and at lower levels by other tissues. Since, ANP receptors were found to be located in smooth muscles of vascular, renal and other tissues. ANP may be considered as a potential lead to develop drugs useful in the treatment of heart failure, renal failure and oedematous conditions. The effects are expected to be mediated through guanylate cyclase.

The parent precursor, ANP preprohormone consists of 151 amino acids. ANP molecule consisting of 28 amino acid residues with numbers 99 to 126, is cleaved from the precursor. A 17 membered ring structure, necessary for biological activity is formed due to a disulfide linkage between cysteine - 105 and cysteine 122.

Potassium Channel Modulators :

All the following examples do not share the common parent skeleton. For example, the parent skeleton in BRL 34915 is β-ethanolamine, in nicorandil is nicotinic acid and animopyridine in pinacidil.

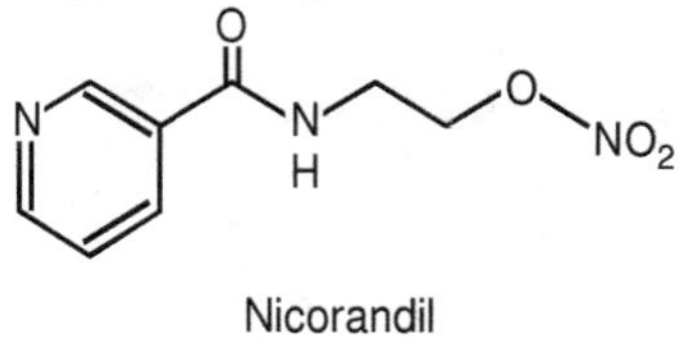

Nicorandil

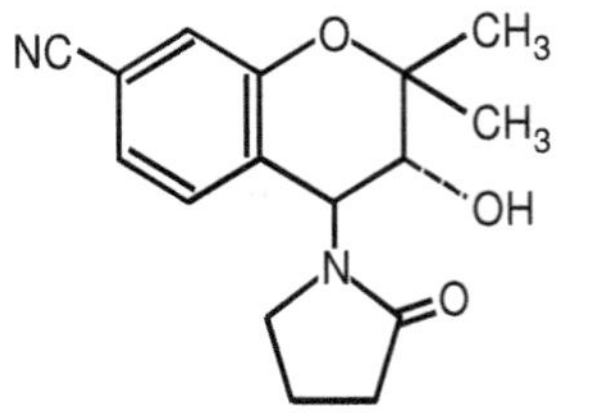

BRL 34915

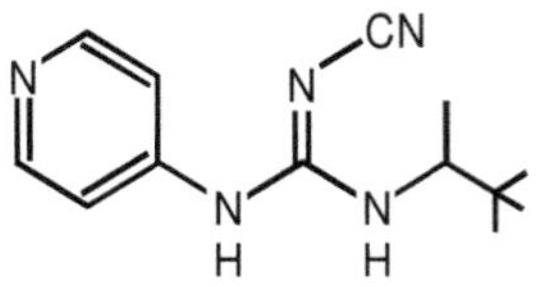

Pinacidil

The potassium channel modulators indicate a possible new direction in the application of ion channel modulators in the therapy of cardiovascular disease.

The recent introduction of new classes of antihypertensive agents has provided the clinician with greater flexibility in the treatment of essential hypertension. A variety of anti-hypertensive agents are available with several mechanisms of action, such as vasodilation, β-blockade, diuresis, inhibition of angiotensin converting enzyme, Ca^{++}-antagonism etc. The usual prescription of anti-hypertensive therapy include combination of drugs acting through different mechanisms. Such combination may often make the prescription costly. Similarly, over-treatment (overloading) with drugs may further aggrevate the severity of the disease. Extensive efforts have been made to find safer and more effective antihypertensive agents. However, the use of two drugs with different characteristics of absorption, metabolism and excretion presents difficulties in synchronizing the two actions. Therefore, the recent trends in designing of antihypertensive agents are directed to develop a single molecule with multiple mechanisms of antihypertensive effect.

Table 7.9 : Recent Trends in Designing of Antihypertensive Agents

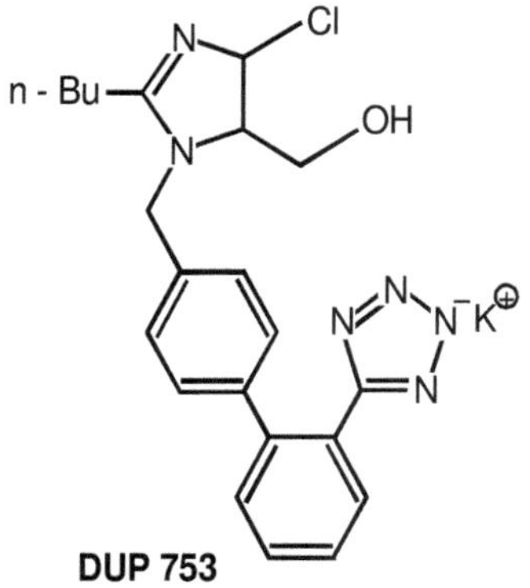

DUP 753
(Losartan)

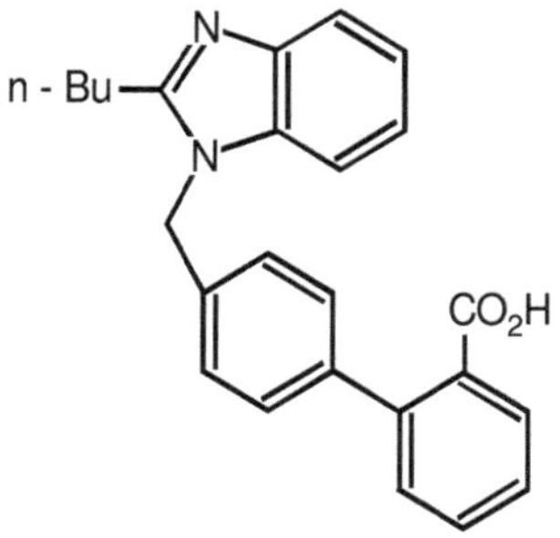

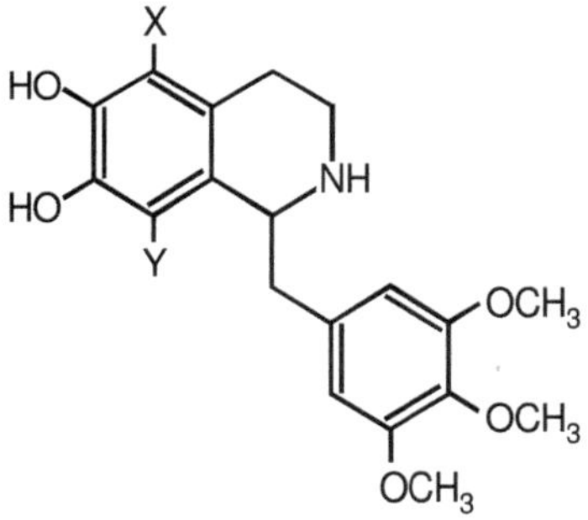

Trimetoquinol; X = Y = H

It is a nonspecific β-adrenergic agonist as well as a competitive inhibitor of human platelet aggregation.

The changes in β-activity were correlated to differences in phenolic pKa attributed to the electronic influence of X and Y.

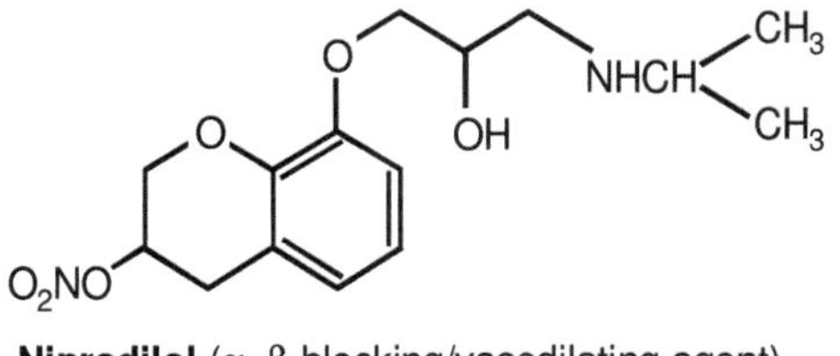

Nipradilol (α, β-blocking/vasodilating agent)

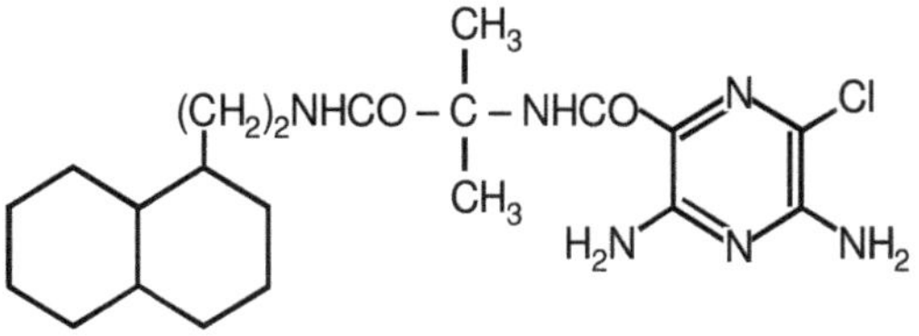

(β-blocker and diuretic)

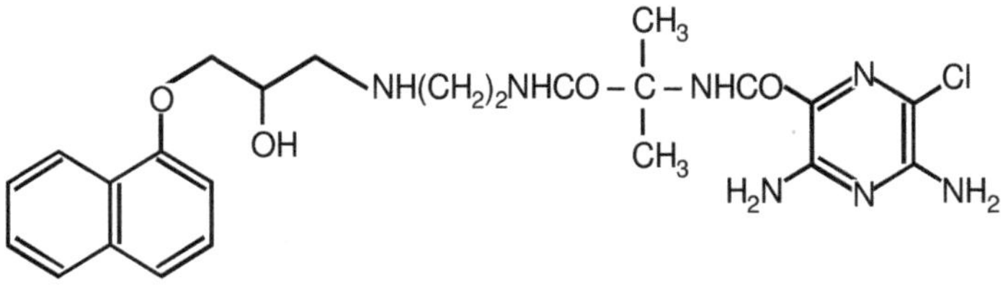

ICI-147 (diuretic and β_1-adrenoceptor blocker)

❖❖❖

8

QUANTITATIVE STRUCTURE ACTIVITY RELATIONSHIP (QSAR)

8.1 INTRODUCTION

The term 'drug design' represents mainly the efforts to develop new drugs on rational basis. The various approaches used in drug design include,

1. Random screening of synthetic compounds or chemicals and natural products by bioassay procedures.
2. Novel compounds preparation based on the known structures of biologically active, natural substances of plant and animal origin, i.e., lead skeleton.
3. Preparation of structural analogues of lead with increasing biological activity and
4. Application of the bioisosteric principle.

Of a number of procedures involved in drug design, the first step is the detection of some biological action in a group of compounds so as to serve as a lead. This is followed by molecular manipulations to increase or modify the activity. Identification of a lead nucleus depends upon the consideration of the following points :

(i) molecular structure of the drug,
(ii) behaviour of the drug in the biophase,
(iii) geometry of the receptor,
(iv) drug-receptor interaction,
(v) changes in the structure on binding, and
(vi) the observed biological response.

After following such a tedious process, only fewer drugs can reach to the level of clinical applicability. Such compounds have to be given extensive trials before they are tried on humans. This adds to the cost of research for new drugs. Broadly, this means that if the development of new drugs is to remain economically feasible, the ratio of output to input must be increased.

The lead is a prototype compound that has the desired biological or pharmacological activity, but may have many undesirable characteristics, e.g., high toxicity, other biological activities, insolubility or metabolic problems. Early SAR studies (prior to 1960s), simply involved the synthesis of as many analogues as possible of the lead and their testing to determine the effects of structure on activity. Attempts were made to interpret chemical structures in terms of physical and chemical properties, transport and distribution of a drug in a biological multicompartment system, the affinity of the drug to a complementary structurally unknown-receptor and the interaction of the drug with its receptor. Corwin Hansch's classic work which appeared in 1964 can be taken as turning point in the study of chemical SARs.

The understanding of structure-activity relationships has developed extensively over the past decades, with very powerful statistical techniques available to predict activities of designed, but yet unsynthesized compounds.

Between 1858 and 1861, three chemists : Archibald, Freidrich August Kekule von Strandonitz and Aleksandr Mikhailovich Butleroy independently introduced the general rules of valence for organic chemistry and the first written structures involving chains of carbon atoms drawn as 'Bonds' to substituent atoms and groups. The term 'Chemical structure' was first used at this time.

The first recorded use of physical molecular model in organic chemistry was done by August Wilhelm Hoffmann in 1865. He used the metaphor of croquet balls joined by sticks to describe methane, chloroform and other compounds. Hoffmann established colour scheme which is still widely used today : white for hydrogen, black for carbon, red for oxygen, blue for nitrogen and green for chlorine.

The introduction of the Hansch model in 1964 enabled medicinal chemists to formulate their hypotheses of structure-activity relationships in quantitative terms and to check these hypotheses by means of statistical methods. From such Quanitative Structure Activity Relationships (QSAR), it is possible to elucidate the influence of various physiological properties on drug potency and to predict activity values for new compounds within certain limits.

QSAR techniques employ powerful computers, molecular graphics and sophisticated softwares; they may be of enormous assistance to those trying to generate the large data bases resulting from the massive efforts in drug research.

The goals of Quantitative Structure Activity Relationship studies were first proposed about 1865 to 1870 by Crum-Brown and Fraser who showed that the gradual chemical modification in the molecular structure of a series of poisons produced some important differences in their action. They observed that a series of quaternized strychnine derivatives could be prepared which, to a varying degree depend on the quaternary substituent, possessed activity similar to curare in paralyzing muscle. In their paper (1868), they proposed the equation shown below, in which **f** is a measure of biological activity (Physiological action) and C is a measure of chemical structure (Chemical constitution). The major problem in obtaining an accurate definition of '**f**' in the equation was attributed to the difficulty of expressing changes in **f** and C with sufficient "Definiteness'.

$$F = f(C)$$

Overton related tadpole narcosis (induced by a series of non-ionized compounds added to the water in which the tadpoles were swimming) to the ability of the compounds to partition between oil and water.

Testing of 51 compounds including alcohols, ethers and amides as narcotics on tadpoles yielded the following equation.

$$\text{Log}\,(1/C) = 0.94 \log P + 0.87$$
$$r = 0.97 \text{ and } n = 51$$

Thus, the strong correlation between the biological activity and partition coefficient supports the proposed mechanism.

Traube found a linear relation between narcosis and surface tension in 1912.

The depressant action of structurally non-specific drugs were rationalized by Fergusson, in 1939, working in ICI laboratories, who formulated a concept linking narcotic activity, partition coefficient and thermodynamics. Relative saturation was termed as thermodynamic activity by Fergusson.

The numerical range of the thermodynamic activity for structurally non-specific drugs is 0.01 to 1.0 indicating that they are active only at relatively high concentrations. Structurally, specific drugs have thermodynamic activities considerably less than 0.01 and normally below 0.001.

Shortly thereafter, Richardson noted that the hypnotic activity of aliphatic alcohols was a function of their molecular weight. These observations are the basis of QSAR.

QSAR is essentially a computerised statistical method which tries to explain the observed variance in the biological effect of certain classes of compounds as a function of molecular changes caused by the substituents. It assumes that the potency of a certain biological activity exerted by a series of congeneric compounds is a function of various physicochemical parameters of the compounds. Once statistical analysis shows that certain physico-chemical properties are favourable to the concerned activity, the latter can be optimised by choosing such substituents which would enhance such physico-chemical properties.

It involves the mathematical and statistical analysis of SAR-data which helps to reduce the number of educated guesses in molecular modification. Description of the molecular structure, electronic orbital reactivity and the role of structural and steric components have been the subject of mathematical and statistical analysis. The ultimate objective of such studies is to understand the forces governing the activity of a particular compound or a class of compounds. QSAR is thus a scientific achievement and an economic necessity to reduce an empiricism in drug design to ensure that every drug synthesized and pharmacologically tested should be as meaningful as possible.

8.2 QSAR-PARAMETERS

Physical organic chemistry deals with characterization of the structure and prediction of the properties, the descriptors for which, are usually found experimentally. If some property depends on the set of selected descriptors, the ordering of the structure will parallel the ordering of the properties. In other words, the structural information is coded in these properties. Therefore, good correlation of physico-chemical properties with a particular set of indices may help in understanding the contribution of these invariants in determining the property.

Table 8.1 : Physico Chemical Parameters used in QSAR

	Physico-chemical parameters	**Symbol**
(I)	**Hydrophobic parameters :**	
	(i) Partition coefficients	$\log P, (\log P)^2$
	(ii) Pi substituent constants	π, π^2
	(iii) R_M - chromatographic parameter	$\log R_M$
	(iv) Solubility	δ
	(v) Elution time in HPLC	$\log K'$
	(vi) Parachor	$[P]$
(II)	**Electronic parameters :**	
(a)	**Experimental parameters :**	
	(i) Ionization constants	$pKa, \Delta pKa$
	(ii) Sigma substituent constants	$\sigma, \sigma^2, \sigma^-, \sigma^+, \sigma I, \sigma^*$
	(iii) Spectroscopic chemical shift	$\Delta Fr, ppm$
	(iv) Resonance effect	R
	(v) Field effect	F
	(vi) Ionization potential	I

(b)	**Theoretical quantum mechanical indices (MO-indices) :**	
	(i) Atomic charge densities	ε
	(ii) Atomic net charge	$q, QT, q^{\sigma}, Q^{\sigma}, q^{\pi}, Q^{\pi}$
	(iii) Super delocalizability	S_r^N, S_r^E, S_r^R
	(iv) Energy of molecular orbit	E_{LEMO}, E_{HOMO}
	(v) Others	$\pi'N, N, \pi'N, NH, F^{[A]}, E^{[A]}$
(III)	**Steric parameters :**	
	(i) Taft's steric substituent constant	Es
	(ii) Van der Waals radii	γ
	(iii) Inter atomic distances	B, L
	(iv) Molar refractivity	MR
	(v) Molar volume	MV

Studies of Meyer and Overton suggested, inter alia, correlations between insecticidal activity and boiling points and narcotic activity with surface tension. This revealed that the biological activity of a drug is a function of chemical features (i.e., lipophilicity, electronic and steric properties) of the substituents and the skeleton of a drug molecule. For example, lipophilicity is the main factor governing transport, distribution and metabolism of drugs in biological systems. Similarly, electron and steric features influence the metabolism and pharmacodynamic processes of a durg. For example, steric crowding of substituents leads to lower the predicted activity and co-operative binding to receptor leads to increase in the predicted activity. An optimum was observed for antibacterial activity and dissociation constant (pKa) in sulphonamide series. Thus, a substituent may affect activity by altering the physical as well as the chemical properties of a skeleton.

Biological activity reflects the fundamental physico-chemical properties of the bioactive compounds. Enantiomers are related physico-chemically very closely. They only differ sterically but are usually identical with respect to lipophilicity, polarity, charge distribution etc. A major problem in QSAR studies arises because the hydrophobic, electronic and steric effects overlap and can not be neatly separated. The parameters which are used to obtain such correlations can be divided into :

(i) Those which describe mainly the physical properties of a skeleton, such as water solubility, partition coefficient, chromatographic R_f values, molecular weight, surface tension etc.

(ii) Those which describe the chemical properties such as dipole moment, charge densities, electron donar-acceptor properties, Hammett's electronic constants, Taft's steric constants etc. (see Table 8.1).

Various QSAR methods are developed with an assumption that the biological properties of organic compounds are a direct consequence of their chemical and physical properties.

8.3 QSAR-METHODS

The introduction of Hansch method in 1964 enabled chemists to describe SAR-studies in quantitative terms. During past decades, QSAR started to develop from a merely intuitive and empirical discipline to more and more advanced state. Various methods used in QSAR analysis can be summarised as follows :

Table 8.2 : QSAR Methods

(I) Free Energy Models :
(a) Hansch Method : linear free energy relationship
(b) Martin and Kubinyi : non-linear free-energy relationship
(c) Free-Wilson Mathematical Model :

(II) Other Statistical Methods :
(a) Discriminant analysis
(b) Principal component analysis
(c) Factor analysis
(d) Cluster analysis
(e) Combined multivariate analysis

(III) Pattern Recognition
(IV) Topological Methods
(V) Quantum Mechanical Methods
(VI) Molecular Modelling

In a given series of compounds, to get a quantitative information about SAR, either of following approaches can be employed :

(a) One may use QSAR methods based on linear free-energy relationships which relate the biological activity of a molecule with contributions from various free-energy related physico-chemical parameters of the substituents, the constants associated with each physico-chemical parameter being generated by regression analysis for the biologically tested compounds.

(b) In other approach mathematical models rather than linear free-energy relationships are used to express the dependence of biological activity on the nature and location of the substituents.

8.4 SUBSTITUENT CONSTANTS

During its journey from the site of administration to the site of action, the drug molecule undergoes continuous changes in conformation. Each conformation has a specific free energy as per its specific environment. Thermodynamically, the extent to which each of the binding, transport and metabolism of the drug occur, is directly thus dependent on the associated change in free energy. The change in free energy is determined from the relative probability of finding the system in a given state.

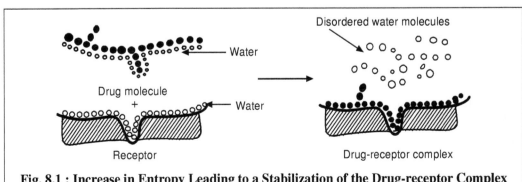

Fig. 8.1 : Increase in Entropy Leading to a Stabilization of the Drug-receptor Complex

The pharmacokinetic and pharmaco-dynamic properties are governed by lipophilic (log P), electronic (σ) and steric feature (Es) of the drug molecule. The Biological Activity (BA) in a given series is influenced by the lipophilicity, electronic and steric properties of the substituent at given position

$$\log (BA) = a \log P + b\sigma + cEs + d$$

where a, b, c and d are the numerical values. A non-polar drug and a hydrophobic region of a receptor are surrounded by a layer of water molecules which are more or less ordered and therefore in a lower state of energy than in free solution. When such a drug molecule contacts receptor, it results in the displacement of water layers and an increase in entropy. This gain in the free energy is proportional to the number of water molecules changed from an ordered to a disordered state, i.e., proportional to the surface area of the non-polar part of the drug and receptor.

Lipophilicity (hydrophobicity) of a drug can be measured readily by disribution of the compound between an aqueous and non-aqueous, water immisible solvent. The non-aqueous solvent usually chosen is 1-octanol. The octanol-water partition coefficient is designated as P and the Hansch value π is the effect of a given substituent on log P of the basic skeleton.

Largely with the initiative of Hansch, n-octanol now seems to be the organic solvent of choice. n-octanol has, a long saturated fatty alkyl chain, hydroxyl group for H-bonding and dissolves water to the extent that saturated octanol contains 1.7 M water. This combination of lipophilic chains, hydrophilic hydroxyl group and water molecules appears to give n-octanol, properties very close to those of natural membranes and macro-molecules. In addition, n-octanol has low vapour pressure

at room temperature and it is well suited for direct measurement of concentrations in the ultraviolet region due to its low absorption over a wide range. n-octanol-water partition coefficients are available from the literature and from the Hansch data bank for a large number of drugs.

Partition coefficient is a free energy related parameter which expresses the relative free energy change occurring on moving a substituent from one phase to another. This is an additive property. It means, with the help of π values of the substituents, the log P value of any molecule may be calculated by simple addition.

$$\log P = \sum_{l}^{m} \pi \ (\text{additive free energy})$$

For example, propranolol.

(i)

OCH$_2$CH(OH)CH$_2$NHCHMe$_2$

$$\log P \ (\text{naphthalene}) = 3.37$$
$$\pi - OCH_2 - \ = \ - 0.02 \ (\text{from anisole})$$
$$\pi - CH - \ = \ 0.50$$
$$\pi - OH \ = - 1.39 \ (\text{from 2-butanol})$$
$$\pi - CH_2 NHCH - \ = \ - 0.17$$
$$(\text{from N} - \text{methylbutylamine})$$
$$2 \times - \pi \ CH_3 \ = \ 1.00$$
$$\Delta \pi \ \text{branch} \ = \ - 0.20$$
$$\log P_{(propranolol)} \ = \ 3.09$$
$$(\log P \ \text{exp.} = 3.33)$$

(ii) $\log P_{C_6H_5CH_2CH_2C_6H_5}$
$$= \ 2 \log P_{C_6H_5} + 2 \ \pi \ CH_3$$
$$= \ 4.26 + 1.00 = 5.26$$
$$\text{Expt. log} \ P \ = \ 4.79$$

Similarly, the hydrophobic substituent constant π of a given substituent X is the difference of log P values of the substituted compound R-X and the unsubstituted compound R-H.

$$\pi_x = \log P_{(R-x)} - \log P_{(R-H)}$$

For example,

(i) $\pi\,CH_3 = \log P_{(toluene)} - \log P_{(benzene)}$

$$= 2.69 \pm 0.01 - 2.13 \pm 0.01$$

$$= 0.56 \pm 0.02$$

(ii) $\pi\,(-CH = CH - CH = CH -) =$

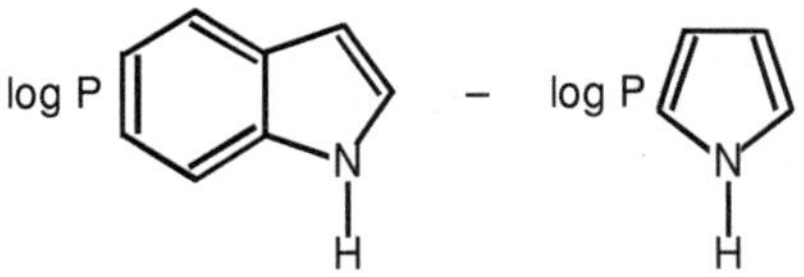

$$= 2.14 - 0.75 = 1.39$$

(iii) $\pi\,NO_2 = \log P_{(nitrobenzene)} - \log P_{(benzene)}$

$$= 1.85 - 2.13 = -0.28$$

(iv) $\pi\,CH_2 = \log P_{(nitroethane)} - \log P_{(nitromethane)}$

$$= 0.18 - (-0.33) = 0.51$$

No differentiation was made between $\pi\,CH_3$ and $\pi\,CH_2$.

(v) $\pi\,CH_2OH = \log P_{(phenyl\ methanol)}$

$$- \log P_{(benzene)}$$

$$= 1.10 - 2.13 = -1.03$$

The environment of a substituent has a significant influence on its chemical properties and therefore different activity contributions may be observed for the same substituent in different positions of a molecule. The values of π are highly position–dependent. It means the π value of a given substituent will not be same for ortho, meta or para position.

Examples :

(a) Calculate log P value for an anticancer drug, diethylstilbestrol (DES).

The structure of DES is as follows :

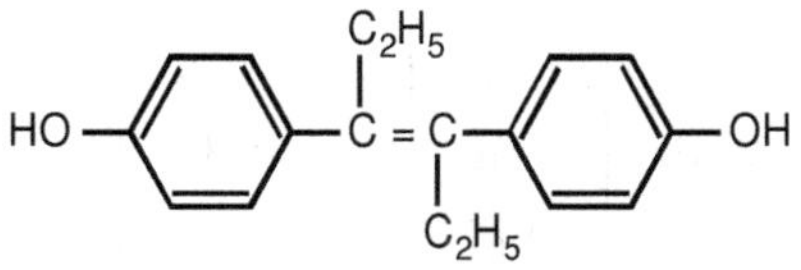

Hence,

$$\log P\ (DES) = 2\pi\,CH_3 + 2\pi\,CH_2 + \pi\,CH_2 = CH$$

$$+ 2\log PhOH - 0.40$$

$$= 2\,(0.50) + 2\,(0.50) + 0.69$$

$$+ 2\,(1.46) - 0.40$$

$$= 5.21\ (Expt.\ \log P = 5.07)$$

Here $\pi\,CH = CH = \dfrac{1}{2}\,(\pi\,CH = CH - CH = CH)$

To account for two branching points, -0.40 is added in the equation.

(b) Calculate log P value for anti-histamine, diphenhydramine.

The structure of diphenhydramine is as follows :

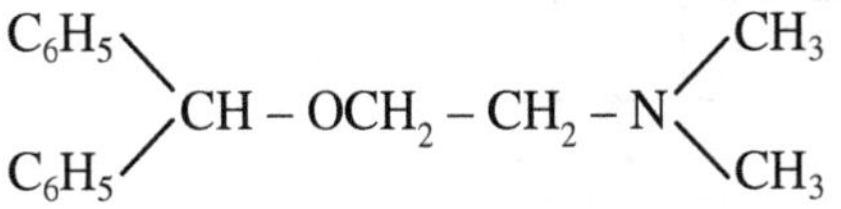

Hence,

$$\log P = 2\pi Ph + \pi CH + \pi OCH_2 + \pi CH_2$$

$$+ \pi NMe_2$$

$$= 2\,(2.13) + 0.30 - 0.73 + 0.50 - 0.95$$

$$= 3.38\ (expt.\ \log P = 3.27)$$

Here 2.13 is log P for benzene; 0.30 is $\pi\,CH\ (0.5 - 0.2$ for branching); -0.73 was obtained by subtracting 1.50 $(2\pi CH_3 + \pi CH_2)$ from log $P_{CH_3CH_2OCH_2CH_3}\ (= 0.77)$; and -0.95 is the value for $\pi\,NMe_2$.

Table 8.3 : π-values of Some Aromatic Substituents

Substituent	π value	Substituent	π value
H	0.00	$2 - OCH_3$	$- 0.02$
$4 - Cl$	0.70	$3, 5 - Cl_2$	1.25
$4 - OCH_3$	$- 0.04$	$4 - CH_3$	0.56
$3 - Cl$	0.76	$3 - N (CH_3)_2$	0.18
$4 - N (CH_3)_2$	0.18	$2 - Cl$	0.71
$3 - CH_3$	0.51	$2 - CH_3$	0.56
$4 - NH_2$	$- 1.23$	$4 - C (CH_3)_3$	1.98
$4 - OH$	$- 0.61$	$3 - CF_3$	0.88
$4 - NO_2$	$- 0.28$		

Table 8.4 : Position Dependent Nature of π Values

Substituent	Ortho	Meta	Para
H	0.00	0.00	0.00
CH_3	0.84	0.52	0.60
C_6H_5	2.13	1.92	1.74
OH	$- 0.41$	$- 0.50$	$- 0.61$
NH_2	$- 1.40$	$- 1.29$	$- 1.30$
NO_2	$-$	0.11	0.22
CHO	$- 0.43$	$- 0.47$	$- 0.47$
F	0.00	0.22	0.15
Cl	0.76	0.77	0.73
Br	0.84	0.96	1.19
I	0.93	1.18	1.43

A negative value of π implies that the substituent prefers an aqueous phase while a positive value implies that an organic (lipoidal) phase is favoured by the drug for distribution.

8.5 LINEAR RELATIONSHIP BETWEEN LOG P AND BIOLOGICAL ACTIVITY

The first linear relationship was observed by Meyer and Overton who found that the narcotic activity of various organic compounds paralleled their oil-water partition coefficients. Exactly linear relationship between lipophilicity and biological activity (log 1/c) is frequently observed, especially for the binding of drugs by proteins, for drugs eliciting unspecific toxic, anaesthetic, bactericidal, fungicidal, narcotic or hemolytic properties. The straight line obtained (y = mx + c) when log P and log 1/c are plotted, can be represented by following equation

$$\log 1/c = a \log P + b$$

In such a linear relationship, the biological activity increases as the lipophilicity increases. Examples include, the antiadrenergic activity of substituted phenethylamines which can be represented by following equation.

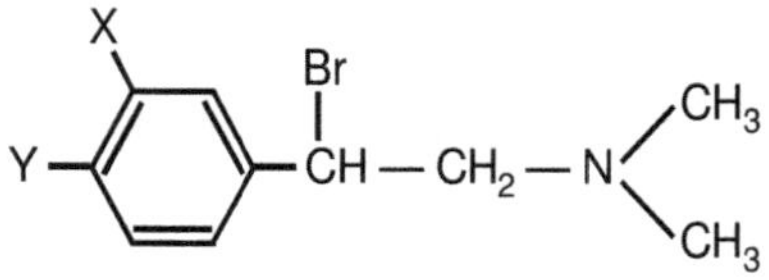

X = H, F, Cl, Br, I, CH_3
Y = H, F, Cl, Br, I, CH_3

$$\log 1/c = 1.15 (\pm 0.19) \pi - 1.47 (\pm 0.38) \sigma + 7.82$$

This is an example of multiparameter linear relationship between activity (log 1/c), lipophilicity (π) and electronic (σ) properties.

Similarly, corrrelation analysis indicated that ascites cell respiration inhibition (pI_{50}) is linearly dependent on π.

$$pI_{50} = 0.46 (\pm 0.11) \pi + 3.22$$

8.6 NON-LINEAR RELATIONSHIP BETWEEN LOG P AND BIOLOGICAL ACTIVITY

Linear relationship between lipophilicity and biological activity only apply to certain range of lipophilicity. If lipophilicity exceeds a definite limit, a more or less sharp decrease of biological activity results for each series of compounds and each type of biological activity. In linear equations, the lipophilicity limits are still beyond the ranges of optimum lipophilicity. If there were no optimum lipophilicity in each series, compounds with infinite biological activity would result if only their lipophilicity were high enough.

In series of compounds, where biological activity is dependent mainly upon lipophilicity, one can not go on increasing the biological activity indefinitely by increasing lipophilicity of the compound. Activity rises to a maximum (log P_o) and then declines.

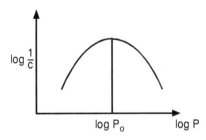

Fig. 8.2 : Parabolic Relationship Between Biological Activity (log 1/c) and Partition Coefficient (log P_o)

P_o = The optimum value for the partition coefficient in the congeneric series under investigation. This remains constant for that particular series.

The main reasons for the decrease in the biological activity beyond a certain range of lipophilicity, include :

(i) Because of the high lipophilicity of the drug molecule, the compound becomes so lipid-soluble that it no longer can circulate in the blood stream but merely becomes 'glued' to the first lipid membrane or macromolecule with which it comes in contact. Highly polar compounds are so insoluble in organic phases that they can not cross lipid membranes and will remain in the first aqueous phase. Hence, only compounds of intermediate lipophilicity will be able to cross lipophilic as well as hydrophilic barriers to reach their target.

(ii) Micelle formation at higher concentration of the drug, may be responsible for non-linear lipophilicity-activity relationships. While drug in dilute aqueous solution is dissolved as monomers, an increase in the concentration may lead to formation of micellar aggregates, consisting of some hundreds or thousands of molecules. Hence, the effective concentration of monomers being capable of interacting with the biological system is significantly lowered down, resulting into a decrease in the biological activity.

(iii) Ariens postulated that hydrophobic interactions between the drug side-chains and a polar amino acids (like leucine, isoleucine and phenylalanine) are responsible for non-linear effects in the protein-binding of drugs. Higher the protein-binding lower will be the effective concentration of the drug.

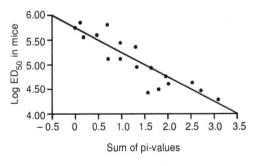

(A)

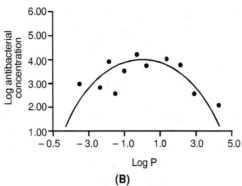

Fig. 8.3 : Linear and Parabolic Hansch Plots

The linear correlation (A) shows the dose of substituted penicillins curing 50% of mice infected with Staphylococcus aureus, versus the sum of the pi values of the substituents. The parabolic curve (B) is the bactericidal concentration of aliphatic fatty acids versus their partition coefficients.

It is interesting to note that a number of non-specific drugs e.g., barbiturates, alcohols, amides share very similar values of log P_o of approximately 2.0. The common log P_o value implies that this group of drugs shares the same site and mechanism of action, assuming that the most important correlation is with partition coefficient. Conversely the series of drugs with significantly different log P_o value (thiobarbiturate; log P_o = 3.1) would be expected to have same biological activity but by different mechanism.

Parabolic dependence of activity upon lipophilicity in many equations is denoted by including π^2 or (log P)^2 term. For example, the hypnosis in the mouse induced by a series of congeneric barbiturates is given by following equation,

$$\log 1/c = -0.44 (\log P)^2 + 1.58 \log P + 1.93 (\pm 0.24)$$

The combination of above type of equation with other physico-chemical parameters accounts for the non-linear dependence of drug transport on lipohilicity as well as for specific hydrophobic, polar, electronic and steric interactions at the receptor.

$\log 1/c = a (\log P)^2 + b$ (lipophilic parameter)
       + c (polar parameter) + d (electronic parameter) + e (steric parameter) + f

Only after reducing the overall lipophilicity of such compounds either by elimination or exchange of substituents or by introduction of additional polar substituents, it will be possible to restore the biological activity.

Other possible reasons for non-linear relationship include steric hindrance, allosteric effects of higher members of a congeneric series, causing conformational distortion of an active site, differences in metabolism of higher homologues, rate control of enzymatic reactions by desorption of reaction products and the principle of minimum receptor occupation. These factors alone or in combination work together.

In general, hydrophobic binding of drugs to a complementary structure will lead to a linear increase in the biological activity as long as the hydrophobic binding site is large enough to bind this part of the molecule. If the size of the molecule surpasses the size of the binding area, no further increase in activity will result from a further increase in lipophilicity.

Schmidt and Sesler evaluated the bacteriostatic activity of various substituted sulphonamides against gram-positive Pneumococcus and gram-negative E.coli. They found that the activity was highly influnced by the position and nature of the substituent present.

The parabolic dependence of biological activity on the electronic and hydrophobic characters of a substituent in a series of substituted sulphonamides was expressed by

$$\log (1/C) = a\pi - b\pi^2 + c\sigma + d$$

where, C is the minimum inhibitory concentration, while a, b, c and d are constants which are determined by the method of least squares.

This equation suggests that the activity increases with the negative character of the SO_2 group. It means that the electron attracting power of the N^1 substituent should be in optimal range for the maximal activity. The ionization constant of the SO_2NH group necessary for optimal biological activity was estimated in the range of 10^{-6} to 10^{-7}. The parabolic dependence may be due to slow rate of transportation of bio-active negative ion to the site of action inside the cell. Thus, the strength of negative charge on the sulphonamido group plays an important role in bacteriostatic activity.

Table 8.5 : Log P Values for Certain Chemicals

Compound	log P	Compound	log P
Ethylamine	– 0.03	1-Propanol	0.38
n-Propylamine	0.47	1-Butanol	0.88
n-Butylamine	0.97	1-Pentanol	1.38
n-Pentylamine	1.47	1-Heptanol	2.38
n-Hexylamine	1.97	1-Octanol	2.88

8.7 CHROMATOGRAPHIC PARAMETERS

Besides π (for a substituent) and log P (for a molecule), other parameters that describe lipophilicity of the drug molecule include, partition coefficient R_M value, molecular connectivity index (it also describes steric properties) and Van der Waals volume V_w.

In 1965, Boyce and Milborrow suggested the use of R_M value from reversed-phase Thin Layer Chromatography (TLC) as alternative lipophilicity parameter in QSAR.

$$R_M = \log\left(\frac{1}{R_f} - 1\right)$$

However, R_M values cannot be regarded as true equilibrium parameters.

Usually silica gel plates are impregnated with liquid paraffin, silicone oil, ethyl oleate or n-octanol as stationary phases. While mobile phase may consist of mixtures of polar solvents like methanol, ethanol or acetone with water or aqueous buffer solutions.

Many advantages are associated with the use of R_M values instead of the use of partition coefficients. These include,

(1) Only minute quantity is required.

(2) Since the impurities do not affect R_f values, the compounds need not to be pure.

(3) Since the determination of R_f value is much quicker and less tedious process, a number of compounds can be investigated simultaneously on the same plate.

(4) No specific quantitative analytical method is involved in the spot localisation.

(5) R_f value can be calculated for both- very polar and very lipophilic substance with equal ease by using a wide range of solvent mixtures.

(6) Log P value can not be calculated in following cases :

    (a) Labile substances may decompose under experimental conditions.

    (b) Mutual electrical interactions may occur between the substituents.

The most prominent disadvantages of chromatographic method are :

(1) The sensitivity of R_f values to the experimental conditions.

(2) Different stationary and mobile phases make it impossible to combine different sets of R_f values due to lack of uniformity.

(3) Chromatographic behaviour of a drug is not identical to the drug partitioning in a biological system.

(4) Fine separation of the small spots between a relatively narrow range of R_f value (0.2 - 0.8) is needed. Hence, the selection of suitable solvent system becomes sometimes problematic.

(5) Large changes due to ionisation or/and H-bonding may cause departure from linearity.

8.8 ORTHO EFFECT

The log P contribution by the substituent at ortho position is difficult to measure due to following reasons :

(i) Mutual electronic interaction may occur between the substituents.

(ii) When there are two substituents 'ortho' to each other, in body fluids both such groups compete for the same layer of water molecules which forms an envelope of ordered structure around the receptor. Therefore, when an ortho disubstituted compound moves from an aqueous phase to lipid phase, the total gain in entropy of aqueous phase is less than its isomeric disubstituted compound. There occurs overall reduction in expected log P and π values. This effect is known as ortho effect.

By subtracting the value of π for para substituent from the value of π of ortho substituent, one may get an approximate estimation of the ortho effect. Thus,

Ortho effect = $\Delta\pi$ ortho = π O-subst – π P-subst

Besides this, the partition coefficient of drug is affected by pH and temperature of the system. In addition to the complications arising from dissociation of acids and bases and from temperature dependence, partition coefficients of charged species can be significantly affected by the formation of ion pairs.

8.9 OTHER PARAMETERS RELATED TO LIPOPHILICITY

Other physico chemical or molecular properties can also be used to express lipophilicity. The use of solubility parameters and dissolution rate constants in QSAR has been proposed. Yalkowsky and Valvani have correlated molecular surface area with the lipophilicity of a polar compounds. Other physico chemical parameters, like molar volume MV, molar refractivity MR, van der Waals volume V_w and parachor PA (all are additive constitutive molecular properties) can also be related to lipophilicity.

$$MV = \frac{MW}{d}$$

where, MW = mol. wt., d = density

$$MR = \frac{n^2 - 1}{n^2 + 2} \frac{MW}{d}$$

where, n = refractive index

$$PA = r^{1/4} \frac{MW}{d}$$

where, d = difference between the density of liquid and the density of vapor in equilibrium with it, essentially constant over wide range.

r = surface tension

Molar refractivity is a volume term, but is also proportional to electron polarisability. Hence, its interpretation in QSAR becomes difficult. If the conformation-dependent steric effects are eliminated, molar refractivity may be used as a measure of dispersion and dipole-induced dipole forces.

Originally it was proposed by Pauling and Pressman as a parameter for the correlation of dispersion forces involved in the binding of haptens to antibodies.

Since, refractive index does not change significantly for organic molecules, the term is dominated by the MW and density. Larger the MW, larger the steric effect, while greater the density, the smaller the steric effect.

A smaller MR for the same MW indicates stronger interactions in the crystal (larger density indicates that the packing is better due to stronger interactions) indicating that molecule may have stronger dispersion interactions with the environment (e.g. a receptor).

Molar refractivity and parachor can be regarded as corrected molar volumes. The lipophilicity can however, not be correlated with molar volume, molar refractivity and parachor if polar compounds are included.

The capacity factor (log k') determined by HPLC is an indicator of lipophilicity.

$$k' = \frac{t_r - t_o}{t_o}$$

where, t_r and t_o are the retention times of the solute and an unretained compound for a series eluted by methanol – H_2O_2 mobile phases on an alkyl-bonded stationary phase.

Partition coefficient may also be measured by centrifugal counter chromatography. Alex-Avdeef devised (1991), a potentiometric instrument which determines log P and ionization constant (pKa) of substance. The instrument consists of 8088/ 8087 and 80552 distributed processors, a pH sensing circuit, a semi-micro combination pH electrode (Orion), a temperature probe, an overhead stirrer, a precision dispenser and a six way valve for distributing reagents and titrants.

From the definition of π values, obviously π_H must be zero. No differentiation was made between πCH_3 and πCH_2. However, the lipophilicity contribution of a hydrogen atom is not zero. Hence, Rekker suggested a new system of hydrophobic fragmental constant f, which indicate absolute contributions of substituents and substructures to the total lipophilicity. There is a hydrophobic fragmental constant of the hydrogen atom, i.e. $f_H = 1.175$.

$$f\,CH_3 = 0.702$$
$$\Delta = 0.172$$
$$f\,CH_2 = 0.530$$
$$\Delta = 0.295$$
$$f\,CH = 0.235$$
$$\Delta = 0.085$$
$$f\,C = 0.15$$
$$f\,H = 0.175$$

Since, there are different values for each type of carbon, no branching corrections are required when hydrophobic constant values are used. The log P value of a compound can be calculated with high accuracy by using f value.

For example,

$\log P_{C_6H_5(CH_2)_3Cl}$

$= \log P_{benzene} + 3\pi CH_3 + \pi\,aliph\,Cl$

$= 2.13 + 1.50 + 0.39$

$= 4.02$

$\log P_{C_6H_5(CH_2)_3Cl}$

$= fC_6H_5 + fCH_2 + f\,aliph\,Cl$

$= 1.886 + 1.590 + 0.061 = 3.537$

Exptl. log P for $C_6H_5(CH_2)_3\,Cl = 3.55$

log P n-pentane

$= 2\,f_{CH_3} + 3f_{CH_2} + 3f_b$

$= 2(0.89) + 3(0.66) + 3(-0.12)$

$= 3.40$ calculated and 3.39 observed

where, f_b = single bond between fragments in rings.

Other examples include,

Compound	Obs.	Calcu-lated	Differ-ence
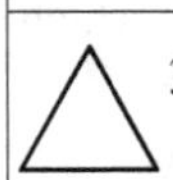 $3f_{CH_2} + 2f_b =$ (0.66) (− 0.09)	1.72	1.80	+ 0.08
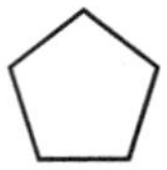 $5f_{CH_2} + 4f_b =$	3.00	2.94	− 0.06
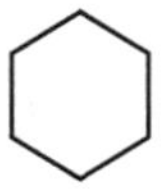 $6f_{CH_2} + 6f_b =$	3.44	3.51	+ 0.07
$C_6H_5CH_2CH_2OH$ $f_{C_6H_5} + 2f_{CH_2} + f_{OH} + 2f_b =$	1.36	1.34	− 0.2
$C_6H_5(CH_2)_3OH$ $f_{C_6H_5} + 3f_{CH_2} + f_{OH} + 3f_b =$	1.88	1.88	0.0
$C_6H_5CH_2CH_2NH_2$ $f_{C_6H_5} + 2f_{CH_2} + f_{NH_2} + 2f_b =$	1.41	1.44	+ 0.03
$C_6H_5CH_2CH_2Cl$ $f_{C_6H_5} + 2f_{CH_2} + f_{Cl} + 2f_b =$	2.95	3.04	+ 0.09
$C_6H_5(CH_2)_3Cl$ $f_{C_6H_5} + 3f_{CH_2} + f_{Cl} + 3f_b =$	3.55	3.58	+ 0.03

Table 8.6 : Hydrophobic Fragmental Constants for Some Substituents

Substituent	Fragmental constant	
	Aromatic	Aliphatic
H	0.175	0.175
CH_3	0.702	0.702
C_6H_5	1.886	1.886
C_6H_4	1.688	1.688
C	0.150	0.150
CH	0.235	0.235
NH_2	− 0.854	− 1.428
NO_2	− 0.078	− 0.939
OH	− 0.343	− 1.491
Cl	0.922	0.061
SH	0.620	0.000
COOH	− 0.093	− 0.954

Single parameters are satisfactory for the quantitative description of unspecific biological activities or for small sets of congeneric compounds. However, a single parameter can not be used to describe the biological effects of a larger group of structurally diversed compounds. In such cases, electronic or steric parameters also may influence the biological activity.

$$\log (1/C) = a \text{ (lipophilic parameters)} +$$
$$b \text{ (electronic parameters)} +$$
$$c \text{ (steric parameters)} + d$$

8.10 ELECTRONIC PARAMETERS

Electronic parameters mainly indicate the influence of polar characters of the drug on its biological activity. They affect (i) metabolism and elimination pattern of the drug, and (ii) the drug receptor interaction. The commonly used electronic parameters are shown in the following Table 8.7. In 1940, L.P. Hammett published his book on "Physical Organic Chemistry" in which he introduced - constants as a quantitative measure of the electronic effects of substituents of aromatic rings on reaction rates and equilibria. Hammett postulated that the electronic effect of a set of substituents on different organic reactions should be similar. He selected substituted benzoic acids X-C_6-H-COOH as the standard system to develop the numerical σ constant scale.

The most commonly used electronic parameter is Hammett substituent constant 'σ' which can be obtained from the dissociation constants KX and KH of the benzoic acids X-Ph-COOH and Ph-COOH respectively.

$$\sigma = \log K_X - \log KH = \log(K_X/K_H)$$
$$= pKa_H - pKa_X$$

The substituent constant σ is linearly dependent on ΔG, the change in the free energy arising due to dissociation of benzoic acids.

The reason for using the logarithm of biological response has thermodynamic origins. Here $\log \dfrac{K_X}{K_H}$ is used instead of free energy change because equilibrium constants are logarithmically related to free energy (ΔG) change through the Van't Hoff equation and therefore additive.

Hammett proposed that an electron withdrawing group, attached to aromatic ring of benzoic acid would increase the acid strength of the carboxyl group and the greater the electron withdrawing power, the greater will be an increase in the strength. Thus electron withdrawing groups have positive values, electron donating groups have negative values and hydrogen has a zero value.

In general, the Hammett equation applies to aromatic systems only for reactions in which substituent (x) and reaction centre (y) are "insulated", so that no resonance interaction occurs between them. That is as long as x affects y in a fashion parallel to the way x affects the ionization constant of the corresponding benzoic acid, the Hammett equation can be expected to hold true.

Table 8.7 : Electronic Parameters

Parameters	Comments
σ_m	Hammett constant for meta substituent derived from ionisation of benzoic acid.
σ_p	Hammett constant for para substituent derived from ionisation of benzoic acid.
σ_p^-	Hammett constant used when there is direct conjugation between substituent and reaction centre; derived from anilines and phenols.
σ_p^+	H.C. Brown constant derived from solvolysis of dimethylphenyl-carbinyl chlorides.
σ_1	Constant describing solely polar effects.
σ_R	Constant describing solely mesomeric effects.
$\sigma*$	Taft's polar substituent constant derived from hydrolysis of aliphatic esters.
σ	Homolytic constant for substituent interacting with a free radical reaction.
F and R	Field and Resonance components derived from linear combination of σ_m and σ_p values.

Such a condition does not prevail, for example, with phenols or aromatic amines. Here a strong resonance interaction can occur with para substituents such as NO_2, CN, $COCH_3$, etc. which can delocalize a pair of non-binding electrons. A special electronic constant σ_p was formulated for phenols and aromatic amines. The same condition appears to hold for π value.

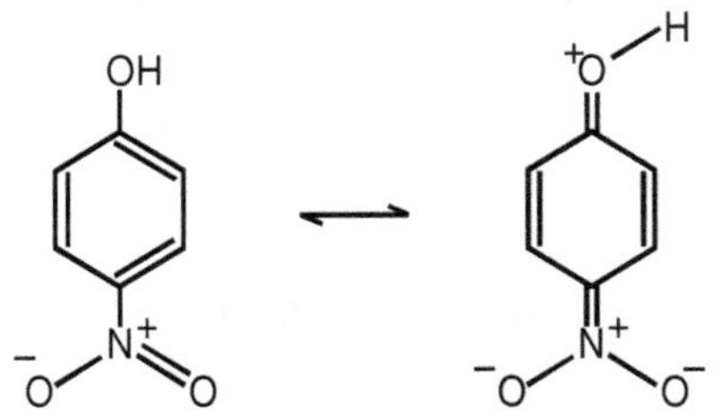

A similar situation occurs when a positive charge is generated in the course of a reaction. Such a charge reacts with many substituents in a different fashion than the partial charge induced by the COOH function of benzoic acid. Hence, Brown formulated the constant σ^+. The standard process for defining σ^+ is the solvolysis of substituted 2-phenyl-2-propyl chlorides in 90% acetone at 25° C.

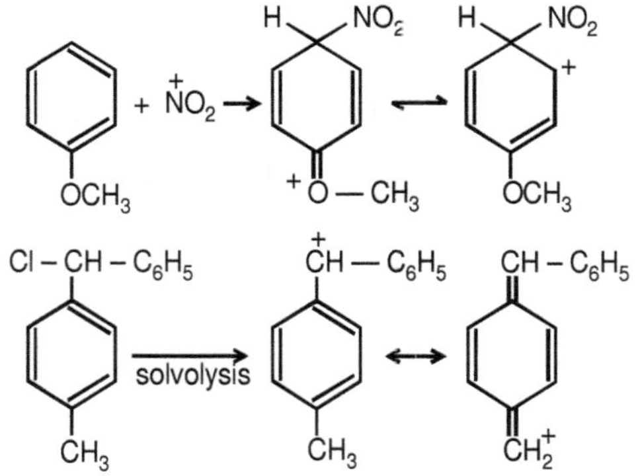

The parameters σ^-, σ^+, E_R have been designed for aromatic systems. They do not apply to non-rigid aliphatic systems. Taft has formulated the parameter σ^* to define the polar effects of substituents when the group in question does not form part of a conjugated system. In this methyl rather than hydrogen, is considered as a standard group, for which σ^* value is equal to zero. It is to be used in aliphatic systems.

This polar constant is defined as :

$$\sigma^* = \left[\log\left(\frac{k}{k_0}\right)_B - \log\left(\frac{k}{k_0}\right)_A \right] \times \frac{1}{2.48}$$

$\left(\frac{k}{k_0}\right)_B$ refers to the hydrolysis rate constants of esters (XCH_2COOR) in basic solution and $\left(\frac{k}{k_0}\right)_A$ to the hydrolysis of the same esters under acid conditions.

The inductive effect of X is quite small in acid hydrolysis but basic hydrolysis is quite sensitive to inductive effects. Thus the difference between $\left(\frac{k}{k_0}\right)_B$ and $\left(\frac{k}{k_0}\right)_A$ is assumed to be only due to the inductive effect of X. Since, steric effects of X are presumably the same in both acidic and basic hydrolysis, they are cancelled. The factor 2.48 is used to place σ^* on about the same scale as σ. The lack of success of σ in biochemical reaction has generally been attributed to unaccountable steric interactions of substrate with enzymes or membranes.

Sigma constants are position dependent. For example, σ value for a substituent at meta position is different from that in the para position. Sigma value for ortho substituent (σ_0) cannot be calculated because of possible steric hindrance. To counteract resonance effect, two new scales have been developed. The σ^- value is used for electron attracting groups where resonance effect lead to an increase in the negative charge of latter (e.g., p-nitro aniline).

The σ^- values are obtained from the pKa values of substituted anilines while in just opposite case the σ^+ values are obtained from the rate constant of solvolysis of substituted cumyl chlorides ($P\text{-}X\text{-}C_6H_4\text{-}CMe_2Cl$). The plain σ value (obtained from the pKa of phenylacetic acids) is used only for such substituents where resonance effect is not possible.

Though Hammett (σ) constant is a measure of both inductive and resonance effect, the p-substituent constant (σ_p) has a greater resonance component than equivalent meta-substituent (σ_m). Hammett's student Taft showed how the electronic effect could be separated into two numerical scales, one for the inductive and other for resonance effects of the substituents. The inductive substituent constants are derived from the dissociation constants of 4-substituted bicyclo (2, 2, 2) octane carboxylic acids (a) and α-substituted acetic acid.

(a)

The constant for inductive effect (σ^+) is used to describe mainly polar effects of substituents on aliphatic system.

$$\sigma^+ = \text{Scal.factor} \, [(\text{inductive} + \text{steric effect}) - (\text{steric effect})]$$

$$= \frac{1}{2.48} \, [\log (kx/kCH_3) \text{ bas. hydr.} - \log (kx/kCH_3) \text{ acid hydr.}]$$

where,

kX = hydrolysis rate constant for esters X – COOR

kCH_3 = hydrolysis rate constant for CH_3COOR

Sometimes the field (F) and resonance (R) effects of the substituent may also be taken into consideration for quantification of its electronic properties. These parameters are not position dependent in nature. Norrington has reported F and R values for the common aromatic substituents at both ortho and para positions, as shown in Table 8.8.

Polarizability (α) plays an important role in the interaction of small molecules with proteins. In 1880, Lorenz-Lorenz derived the following equation from the electro magnetic theory of light.

$$R = \alpha = \frac{(n^2 - 1)\,M}{(n^2 + 2)\,d}$$

where,

n = refractive index of visible light,

M = molecular weight,

d = density (at the temperature quoted for n, usually 20°C).

Since linear correlations are found to exist between σ and NMR shifts (^{1}H, ^{13}C, ^{19}F, ^{15}N etc.), molar IR extinction coefficients or IR frequencies, the latter parameters may also be used as indicators of electronic properties of the substituents instead of σ value. Since, pKa value shows variation with temperature, the standard temperature chosen for determination of pKa value is 37°C. The pKa value is determined by potentiometry.

The pKa values for acids or bases can also be calculated from the σ substituent constant by using following equation, because of its additive nature.

$$pKa = 4.20 - 1.00 \sum \sigma$$

This equation is known as Hammett's equation.

Table 8.8 : F and R Substituent Constants for Some Aromatic Substituents

Substituent	Ortho		Meta		Para	
	F	R	F	R	F	R
H	0	0	0	0	0	0
CH_3	-0.07	-0.12	-0.05	-0.05	-0.05	-0.14
C_2H_5	-0.08	-0.10	-0.06	-0.04	-0.07	-0.11
C_6H_5	$-$	$-$	0.14	-0.03	0.14	-0.09
OH	0.61	-0.56	0.48	-0.22	0.49	0.64
NH_2	0.05	-0.59	0.04	-0.24	0.04	-0.68
NO_2	$-$	$-$	1.09	0.05	1.11	0.16
CHO	0.84	-0.13	0.66	0.05	0.67	-0.15
SO_2NH_2	$-$	$-$	0.67	0.07	0.68	0.19
Cl	0.86	-0.14	0.68	-0.06	0.69	-0.16
Br	0.91	-0.15	0.71	-0.06	0.73	-0.18
CF_3	0.79	0.16	0.62	0.07	0.63	0.19

Problems :

(1) Calculate pKa value for 4-methyl -3, 5-dinitrobenzoic acid using Hammett equation.

$(\sigma_m NO_2 = 0.71; \sigma_p CH_3 = -0.17)$

Ans. :

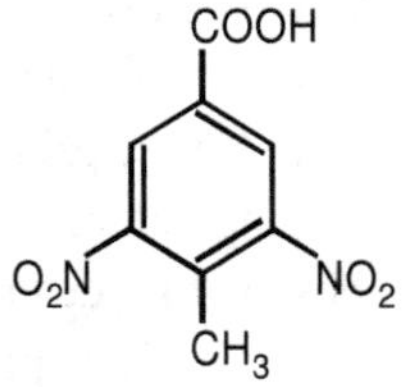

$$pKa = 4.20 - 1.00 \sigma$$
$$= 4.20 - 1.00 (2 \times 0.71 - 0.17)$$
$$= 2.95 \text{ (predicted); } 2.97 \text{ (exptl.)}$$

(2) Predict the pKa value for 3-methoxy -4-hydroxy benzoic acid using Hammett equation.

$(\sigma_m - OCH_3 = 0.14; \sigma_p - OH = -0.37)$

Ans. :

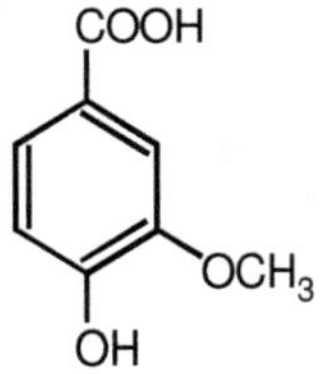

$$pKa = 4.20 - 1.00 \sum \sigma$$
$$= 4.20 - 1.00 (0.14 - 0.37)$$
$$= 4.43 \text{ (predicted); } 4.50 \text{ (exptl.)}.$$

(3) Predict the pKa values using Hammett equation for

(i) p-nitrobenzoic acid

(ii) 3-methyl-4-nitrobenzoic acid

Ans. :

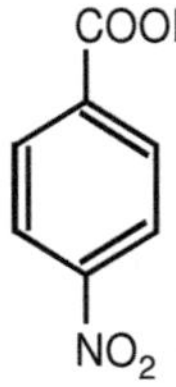

$$pKa = 4.20 - 1.00 \sum \sigma$$
$$pKa = 4.20 - 1.00 (0.71) = 3.49$$

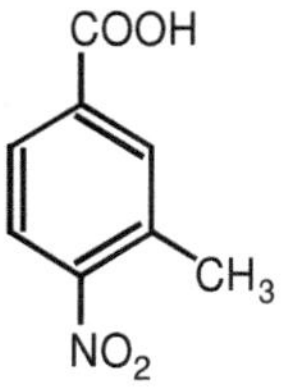

The structure of 4-methyl-3-nitro benzoic acid (COOH at top, CH₃ and NO₂ substituents).

$$pKa = 4.20 - 1.00 \sum \sigma$$
$$= 4.20 - 1.00 \,(0.71 - 0.07)$$
$$= 4.20 - 1.00 \,(0.64) = 3.56$$

(4) Predict the pKa values using Hammett equation for 3-methoxy-5-nitro benzoic acid.

Ans. : The pKa values of some β-adrenoceptor blocking agents available in the literature, are summarised below :

Acebutolol (9.67), Alprenolol (9.7), Atenolol (9.55), Labetalol (8.7), Metoprolol (9.7), Nadolol (9.67), Pindolol (8.8), Propranolol (9.45), Oxprenolol (9.5), Sotalol (9.0) and Timolol (8.8).

The negative σ value indicates, the electron releasing nature of the substituent. The F and R values indicate the sign of the charge which the substituent places on the ring. For example, $- NH_2$ by both resonance and field effects makes the ring more negative and, hence both its F and R values are negative.

8.11 STERIC SUBSTITUENT CONSTANTS

Steric features of the drug markedly affect the drug receptor interactions reflecting the change in the onset and duration of biological action. For example, buprenorphine, a more lipophilic drug than morphine, is expected to enter the CNS rapidly.

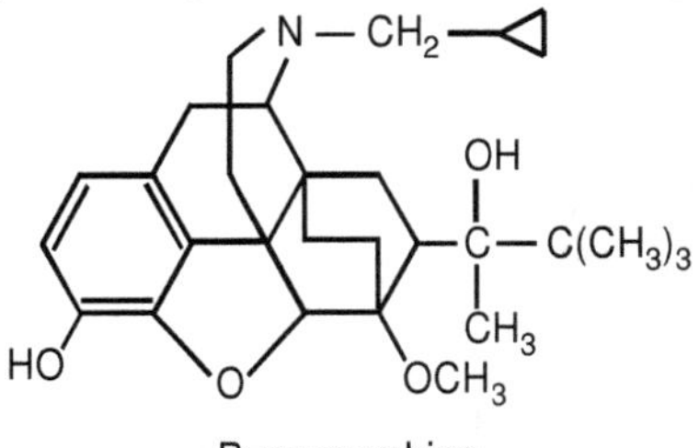

Buprenorphine

Thus, it is expected to exert rapid onset and shorter duration of action. However, because of bulky substituent at nitrogen, it needs time to get oriented in a favourable conformation. The bulky substituent also delays the detachment of drug from the receptor. This leads to late onset and long duration of action.

On the guidelines provided by L.P Hammett, a numerical scale Es for the steric effects of substituents was proposed by Hammett's student, Taft in 1956.

Various parameters are used to describe the steric features of the substituents. The most common is Taft Es constant, which is derived from the acid hydrolysis of aliphatic esters.

$$\log (K/K_0) = Es$$

where,

K = rate of acid hydrolysis of substituted ester

K_0 = rate of hydrolysis of parent ester

This parameter is useful for studying intramolecular steric effects, particularly in reactions where the substituent is near the reaction centre. Other parameters like, molar refractivity (MR), van der Waals radii, molecular weight and molecular connectivity index (χ) can be used to express steric features of the substituents.

Normally, Es is standardised to the methyl group so that Es for CH_3 group is equal to zero. However, it is possible to standardize this parameter to hydrogen i.e. Es (H) = 0.00 and there after adding 1.24 to every additional methyl group. The greater the positive value of Es, the greater is the steric effect affecting intramolecular and/ or inter-molecular hindrance to drug-receptor interactions.

Table 8.9 : Molar Refractivity Values for Some Aromatic Substituents

Substituent	MR value	Substituent	MR value
H	0.0	OH	1.5
CH_3	4.7	NH_2	4.2
C_2H_5	9.4	CHO	5.3
n - C_4H_9	18.7	$CONH_2$	8.8
C_6H_5	24.3	SO_2NH_2	11.3
CF_3	4.0	Cl	4.8

Other steric parameter is molar refractivity. It is expressed by Lorentz-equation.

$$MR = \frac{(n^2 - 1)\,MW}{(n^2 + 2)\,d}$$

where,

n = index of refraction at the sodium D line.

MW = molecular weight of the compound.

d = density of the compound.

Greater the value of the MR, larger is the steric contribution of the substituent. For liquids, the MR value can be calculated in units of volume using the Lorentz-Lorentz equation.

$$MR = \frac{MW\,(n^2 - 1)}{d\,(n^2 + 2)}\ (cm^3/mol)$$

where, MW = molecular weight

n = index of refraction at 20°C

d = density at 20°C

The third steric parameter is molecular connectivity index (χ). It indicates the degree of branching in a given structure. Since, branched isomers of molecule differ in their properties, the arrangement of substructure in the given molecule must be responsible for it. Molecular connectivity describes molecular substructures in topological terms. Correlation of the physical properties with the variation in the structure depends not only on number of atoms in the structure but also upon arrangement of these atoms. Since size and shape of the molecule determines many of the physical parameters that govern the biological activity of drug, molecular connectivity index helps to quantify the effect of size and shape on the biological response.

Table 8.10 : Taft's Steric Substituent Constants for Some Substituents

Aromatic substituent	E_s^c value	Aliphatic substituent	E_s^c value
H	1.28	CH_3	0.00
4 – Cl	0.27	C_2H_5	– 0.07
3 – CF_3	– 0.97	i-C_3H_7	– 0.47
4 – NO_2	– 1.28	CF_3	– 1.16
4 – CH_3	– 0.14	tert-C_4H_9	– 1.54
3 – NO_2	– 1.28	H	1.24
4 – F	0.78	$CHCl_2$	– 1.54
4 – OH	0.69	$CH_2C_6H_5$	– 0.38
4 – NH_2	0.63	Cyclo-C_5H_9	– 0.51
4 – SO_2NH_2	---	Cyclo-C_6H_{11}	– 0.79
4 – CF_3	– 0.98	$(CH_2)_2 - C_6H_5$	– 0.38

The extensive studies on molecular connectivity by Kier and Hall have contributed to the development of quantitative structure property/activity relationships.

Connectivity indices based on hydrogen-suppressed molecular structures are rich in information on branching, 3-atom fragments, the degree of substitution, proximity of substituents and length, and heteroatom of substituted rings.

For calculation of connectivity index, the structural formula of the compound is written as skeletal formula without the hydrogen atoms. It is known as hydrogen suppressed graph. Then the valence number (δi) of atoms attached to each atom is indicated. Such valence numbers of adjacent atoms are multiplied and the bond contribution is calculated by taking the reciprocal square root of the product $\delta i \delta j$.

Thus the molecular connectivity index for the given compound is calculated by using following formula.

$$\chi = \sum (\delta i \delta j)^{-1/2}$$

The following example helps to illustrate the procedure.

Problems :

(1) Calculate the molecular connectivity index for 2, 4–dimethyl pentane.

Ans. :

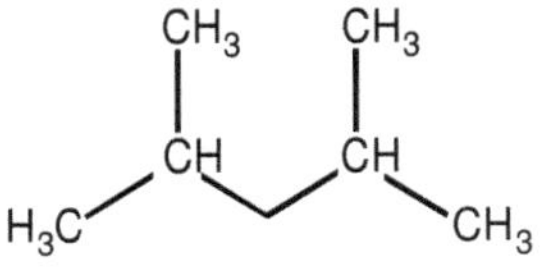

can be written as

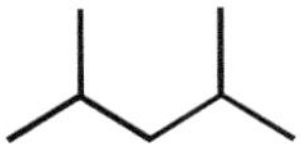

(Hydrogen-suppressed graph)

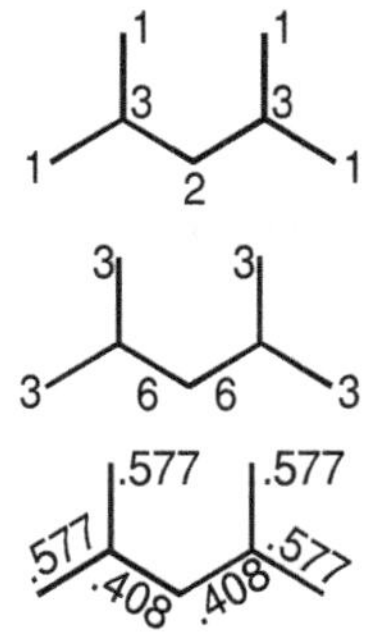

The molecular connectivity index of 2, 4-dimethylpentane is $0.577 + 0.577 + 0.408 + 0.408 + 0.577 + 0.577 = 3.124$.

Exercise :

(1) Calculate the molecular connectivity index for

(i) Methadone (ii) Ibuprofen
(iii) Epinephrine (iv) Atropine
(v) Propranolol.

Table 8.11 : Valence Number (δ values) for Some Atoms

Group	δ value	Group	δ value
CH_3	1	– OH	5
CH_2	2	– O –	6
CH	3	= O	6
C	4	– S –	0.95
– NH_2	3	= S =	3.60
– NH	4		0.15
— N —	5	Br	0.25
— N⁺ —	6	Cl	0.70
= NH	4		
= N⁺ =	6		

Molecular connectivity index represents substructure environment, degree of branching, unsaturation, hetero-atoms and their position and the presence of cyclic structures. The close correlations of molecular connectivity with partition coefficients and molar refractivity shows that connectivity index can be taken as measure of the lipophilic features as well as polar interactions between the molecules. Hence, molecular connectivity index is such a parameter that expresses both, lipophilicity as well as steric features of the drug molecule.

The parachor [P], a steric parameter is defined as a molar volume V which has been corrected for forces of intermolecular attraction by multiplying with the fourth root of surface tension r. MeGowan developed this parameter which principally relates to molecular volume.

$$[P] = V\gamma^{1/4} = \frac{M\gamma^{1/4}}{D}$$

where, M = molecular weight
D = density

He suggested a correction to the parachor as follows :

$P_r^* = 0.012\ P_r$ if to be used for non-polar compounds.

$P_r^* = 0.012\ P_r - 0.6$ if to be used for compounds containing a phenolic OH or phenolic ether function.

$P_r^* = 0.012\ P_r - 1.2$ if to be used for compounds containing carbonyl, ester, amine, nitrile, alcoholic or aliphatic ether functions.

Other parameters (non-additive properties) like boiling point or density were also correlated with steric features within related series with sufficient accuracy. Constitutive indicates that the effect of a substituent may differ depending on the molecule to which it is attached or on its environment.

8.12 EFFECT OF ELECTRONIC AND STERIC PARAMETERS ON LIPOPHILICITY

Inductive effects influence the overall lipophilicity of the molecule. In general, electron withdrawing groups increase π value when a hydrogen bonding group is involved. Thus in an aromatic skeleton having either nitro group or a hydroxyl group, the electron withdrawing inductive effects of the phenyl ring and the nitro group make the non-bonded electrons on the hydroxyl group less available for H-bonding. It leads to a decrease in the affinity of this functional group for the aqueous phase. This then increases the log P or π value. Similarly, delocalization of unbonded electrons (i.e. resonance effect) into aromatic systems decreases their availability for H-bonding with the aqueous phase. It leads to an increase in the log P or π value. That is why, the aromatic π_x values are greater than aliphatic π_x values.

Similarly, if a group sterically shields non-bonded electrons, then aqueous interactions will decrease and the π value will increase. However, crowding of functional groups involved in hydrophobic interactions will have the opposite effect. Conformational effects also can affect the π value.

Problems :

(1) The π_x value for $CH_3(CH_2)_3$ X is usually higher than π_x value for Ph $(CH_2)_3$ X. Explain.

Ans. : In Ph $(CH_2)_3X$, folding of the side-chain occurs on the phenyl ring, thus lowering the polar surface area for solvation. The intramolecular hydrophobic interactions and the interaction of the CH_2-X dipole with the phenyl π electrons are responsible for folding of alkyl chain.

Table 8.12 : Effect of Folding of Alkyl Chains on π Value

X	π_x (aromatic)	π_x (aliphatic)
OH	– 1.80	– 1.16
NH_2	– 1.85	– 1.19
COOH	– 1.26	– 0.67
Cl	– 0.13	0.39
F	– 0.73	– 0.17
Br	0.04	0.60
$CONH_2$	– 2.28	– 1.71

QSAR helps to widen the deeper understanding of the term, bioisosterism. True bioisosters would yield identical (qualitatively and quantitatively) biological responses while partial bioisosters would yield qualitatively the same but quantitatively different responses.

In QSAR the activity is a function of π, σ and Es parameters of the substituents. Hence, compounds having substituents with almost the same values of these parameters may be considered as isometric bioisosters.

For example,

Substituent	π	σ	Es
4 – Cl	0.71	0.23	0.27
4 – Br	0.86	0.23	0.08
$3 – OC_2H_5$	0.62	0.12	

While the following analogues having alcohol dehydrogenase blocking activity illustrate non-isometric bioisosterism.

$$X—\langle\bigcirc\rangle—CONH_2$$

X	Activity	π	σ	Es
4 – F	– 2.6	0.27	0.06	0.78
$4 – NO_2$	– 2.6	0.18	0.78	– 1.28

Non-isometric bioisosterism results when the physico chemical properties of the structure change in altogether different ways but combine additively to produce the same degree of biological activity.

8.13 EXPERIMENTAL DETERMINATION OF PARTITION COEFFICIENTS

The octanol-water partition coefficient (P) represents the drug distribution between an organic phase and aqueous phase.

$$P = \frac{\text{Concentration of drug in n-octanol}}{\text{Concentration of drug in water}}$$

The P value is not independent of concentration and ideally infinite dilutions should be used in the calculations. For very lipophilic molecules, the low concentration (10^{-5} M) below the critical micelle concentration in the aqueous phase, should be used. For easily ionizable drugs, either 0.1 N HCl or 0.1 N NaOH may be used to prevent ionization. If it is not possible to prevent ionization, correction must be made as follows :

$$P = \frac{[C]\ n - \text{octanol}}{(1 - \alpha)\ [C]\ H_2O}$$

where, α is degree of ionization.

Shake-flask method :

A carefully weighed sample of pure compound is dissolved in the phase in which it is most soluble. The sample should be large enough to keep the per cent error under 1%. No loss should occur in transferring the sample to the partitioning bottle. For general use, 250 ml capacity bottles with ground glass stoppers are used. Heating may be employed to aid dissolution of drug. The calculated or equal amount of second phase is added. The phases are usually mixed by inverting the bottles at least 60 times by hand during approximately two minutes.

When high ratios (i.e., 2 ml n-octanol and 200 ml H₂O) are used, longer shaking is required. The bottles are then placed in a centrifuge and turned at about 2000 rpm for 1-2 hours. An aliquot of one phase is removed and analysed.

The commercial n-octanol may be purified by washing it with 10% sodium hydroxide, dilute sulphuric acid and, finally with bicarbonate solution. After drying over MgSO₄, it is distilled under reduced pressure. It is then shaken with distilled water to saturate it. The partition coefficient is not very sensitive to changes (0°C–25°C) in temperatures if the phases employed are quite immiscible in each other. Certain compounds hydrolyze slowly in aqueous solution or are oxidised by air. Such adverse reactions can be minimized by carrying out the work as rapidly as possible in a cold room (4°C). For compounds having higher or lower log P values, the standard deviation can be calculated by

$$S.D. = \sqrt{\frac{\sum (X_i - X)^2}{n-1}}$$

where,

X_i = log P value
X = average log P value
n = number of readings.

8.14 RANDOM WALK MODEL OF DRUG TRANSPORTATION

The simplest example involves someone walking along a sidewalk but unable to decide at each step whether to go forward or back. The direction of each step is random. This is one-dimensional random walk. The two-dimensional random walk is analogous to a dazed football player who may take steps randomly in any direction on the field. On the similar lines it may be generalised to three or more steps.

Lipophilicity is a major factor in governing the passage of a drug across biological membranes within the body for absorption, tissue distribution and elimination. The first step in the overall drug's pharmacokinetic scheme is the random walk process in which the molecule is perfused from a very dilute solution outside the cell to a particular target site in the cell. This may be considered as being a relatively slow process, the rate of which is highly dependent on the molecular structure of the drug. The random passage of the solute in different body compartments is also governed by different pH values (e.g., saliva 5.8 to 7.1, GIT 1.0 to 8.0, plasma 7.4, intracellular fluid 6.4 to 7.5, bile 5.6 to 8.0, urine 4.8 to 7.5 etc.)

Many linear relationship studies have been carried out between log P and the biological activity. However, a biological activity can not run indefinitely parallel with log P value. After some optimum value of lipophilicity (log P_0), the drug is retained in the biological membrane with which it comes in contact first. The random walk model has been suggested to explain the decrease in biological activity, if the lipophilicity of drug is increased beyond log P_0 (i.e., parabolic relationship).

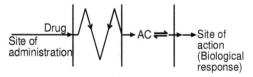

Fig. 8.4

The transport of drug from the site of administration to the site of action is mainly governed by its log P value. This relationship is expressed by Gaussian equation, as

Rate of drug action (A)
= f (log P) = a exp [– (log P–log P_0)²/b]

where a, b = constants.

One such example for transportation of congeneric barbiturates in mice is shown by following equation,

$$\log (1/C) = -0.44 (\log P)^2 + 1.58 \log P + 1.92$$

$$n = 13; r = 0.97; s = 0.098$$

8.15 METHODS USED IN QSAR STUDIES

(I) Linear Free Energy Related (LFER) Method :

Description of the molecular structure, electronic orbital distribution, reactivity, reaction rates and the role of structural and steric components and substituents of chemical compounds have been the subject of mathematical formulation by physical-organic chemistry for half a century. The most promising approach to the quantification of the interaction of drug molecules with biological systems involved the application of established thermodynamic principles. It is known as the Linear Free Energy (LFE) or extra-thermodynamic method which assumes an additive effect of various substituents in electronic, steric, hydrophobic and dispersion data in the non-covalent interactions of a drug and biomacromolecules. This method is expressed as follows :

$$\Delta BA = f (\Delta L/\Delta H, \Delta E, \Delta Es)$$

Depending upon the circumstances, this equation can be modified as,

$$\log BA = b\pi + a$$
$$= c\, pKa + a$$
$$= dEs + a$$
$$= b\pi + c\, pKa + a$$
$$= b\pi + d\, Es + a$$
$$= b\pi + c\, pKa + d\, Es + a$$

Here the variance in the biological activity (ΔBA) is explained by the variance of linear free energy related substituent constants which describe the variance in lopophilic/hydrophilic ($\Delta L/\Delta H$), electronic (ΔE), steric (ΔEs) or other properties of the parent molecule induced by the substituents.

Two important models included in LFE method are :

(a) Hansch model :

Hansch proposed the action of a drug as depending on two processes. Firstly, the journey from the point of entry in the body to the site of action and secondly the interaction with the receptor site. He suggested the linear and non-linear dependence of biological activity on difference parameters.

$$\log BA = a \log P + b\, \sigma + c\, Es + d \quad ...\text{linear}$$

$$\log BA = a \log P \pm b (\log P)^2$$
$$\pm (c\sigma \pm d\, Es + e) \quad ... \text{non-linear}$$

In principle, this method relates the biological activity (BA) within a homologous series of compounds to a set of theoretical molecular parameters which are assumed to describe essential properties of the drug molecule. The coefficients (a, b, c, d, e) are determined by multi-regression analysis. However, the major problem in such analysis is the complexity of the biological effect involving many equilibria. The most significant benefit of this method has been the way it has concentrated the thinking of medicinal chemists on the various additive factors controlling drug activity.

Hansch had applied the ρ - σ - π analysis to various problems in order to correlate the biological activity with chemical structure.

Hansch's ρ - σ - π analysis may serve both to guide the medicinal chemist in future synthesis and testing of other compounds in the series and to untangle the roles of hydrophobic, electronic, and steric factors in drug-receptor interactions.

(b) Free-Wilson model :

The presuppositions made by Bruice et al during study of thyroxine analogues were extended further by Free and Wilson in a more generalised form with a hypothesis that groups make linear contributions either positive or negative to the basic skeleton.

The method of Free and Wilson is based upon an additive mathematical model in which a particular substituent in a specific position is assumed to make an additive and constant contribution to the biological activity of a molecule in a series of chemically related molecules. This method is based on the assumption that the introduction of a particular substituent at a particular molecular position always leads to a quantitatively similar effect on biological potency of the whole molecule, as expressed by the equation,

$$\log BA = \text{contribution of unsubstituted parent compound} + \text{contribution of corresponding substituent}$$

$$= \mu + \sum a_{ij}$$

where, i is the number of the position at which substitution occurs and j is the number of the substituents at that position while μ is the overall average.

By applying symmetry conditions, the equation written for each compound is solved by method of least square. The active molecule is predicted by calculating the group contribution and by number of times a particular group occurs in analysis.

Besides the Hansch approach, another method for the quantitative description between a biological effect and the chemical structure of a drug has been introduced by S. M. Free and J. W. Wilson. This method is preferred when nothing is known about the mode of action or when the physico-chemical properties of the substituents used are unknown. Best results with the Free-Wilson method are obtained in series with several positions available for substitution and only if each substituent at any location is present in at least two compounds of the series.

Based on the Free-Wilson additivity concept, two other modifications were derived, namely the Cammarata model and the Fujita-Ban method.

The principle of Free-Wilson method can be illustrated with the example of acetylenic carbamates having antitumour activity.

where the biological activity (BA) can be expressed as

$$BA = f(R) + f(R_1) + f(R_2) + f(R_3) + \mu$$

where, μ = biological activity of unsubstituted acetylenic carbamate.

This method differs from Hansch analysis, in that substituent constants based on biological activities are used rather than physical properties.

(c) Mixed approach :

Kubinyi has presented the combination of Hansch and Free-Wilson models as "mixed approach".

$$\log 1/c = K_1\pi + K_2\sigma + K_3Es + K\text{- Hansch model.}$$

$$\log 1/c = \mu + \sum a_{ij} \text{ - Free-Wilson approach.}$$

The mixed approach can be written as

$$\log 1/c = \sum a_{ij} + \sum k_j \phi_j + K,$$ where k_j represents the coefficient of different physico-chemical parameters.

In this equation $\sum a_{ij}$ is the Free-Wilson part for the substituents and $\phi_j = \pi$, σ and Es contribution of the parent skeleton. The mixed approach was developed to find possible interactions between Free-Wilson parameters and physico-chemical properties of the substituents used. Another advantage of this equation is that the symmetry equations need not to be develop. The reduction of the matrix is done by setting the increments of the substituents of one chosen reference compound equal to zero.

The basic assumptions for the use of the Free-Wilson approach are :

(a) The approach can be applied to a congeneric series having a common skeleton.

(b) Various derivatives must be prepared by using different substituents at the same distinct positions of the parent skeleton. The substituents contribute to the biological activity additively at the same position.

(c) While choosing derivatives for the synthesis, care has to be taken that every substituent appears at least twice at the same position.

(d) It is stated that the number of derivatives for the solution of the regression analysis must be at least ten, equal to the number of increments. To reduce the number of compounds to be synthesized, Free and Wilson have proposed a symmetry condition where the sum of increments in a substitution position was considered equals to zero.

Advantages of Free-Wilson approach :

(a) It is a simple, fast and cheap method where no substitution constants like, pi, sigma, Es etc. were considered.

(b) The greater complexity of the structure, the larger is the number of possible substituents at desired positions. Hence, the efficiency of this method is high.

(c) At each position, the contribution of each substituent can clearly be identified. The substituents which can or cannot fulfil the principle of additivity, can be recognised.

(d) The Free-Wilson method is effective especially when substituent constants are not available.

Disadvantages of Free-Wilson method :

(a) A prediction of activity increments outside the substituents used in the data set by extrapolation is rather impossible.

(b) The assumed independence of the influence of substituents on the total activity is often not seen in practice.

To overcome above mentioned disadvantages, Fujita and Ban have suggested the modification of Free-Wilson approach.

(II) Cluster Significance Analysis (CSA) :

To evaluate a congeneric series of compounds, if a graph is plotted by taking biological data (e.g.; active/inactive) on Y-axis and physico-chemical parameter on X-axis, sometimes the active compounds tend to cluster in a relatively confined region of the graph. Such clustering suggests that there is a connection between the parameters and the biological activity.

Cluster analysis is used to group the known substituents into groups of similar substituents. Substituents were chosen from the reported clusters based on π, MR, F and R values.

CSA operates by assessing the tightness of the cluster of active compounds and determining the probability that a cluster with the same tightness might have arisen purely by chance. The probability (P) values of that clusters are observed which are at least as tight as the one of the actives. The value $(1 - P)$ is the probability that the physico-chemical parameters used for the calculation are meaningful for the discrimination between the actives and inactives. For practical purpose, value of P < 0.05 should be considered as significant and by inclusion of more parameters, P should decrease to indicate significance.

Advantages of CSA :

(a) It is a simple technique where quantification of the biological activity is not required.

(b) It does not involve any statistical assumptions.

(c) It can be performed in a mono or multidimensional parameter space.

Disadvantages of CSA :

(a) It is difficult to assess with accuracy the contribution made by (i) one parameter in the presence of others and (ii) one substituent in the presence of others.

(b) No significant result will be found by CSA in cases of loose clustering (i.e., large P value) of the actives.

(c) A lot of computer work is required.

(III) Discriminant Analysis :

This method was first introduced by Yvonne Martin in 1974. It is a statistical technique which allows exploration of the significance of correlations between a crude activity parameter (the Group) and either continuous (pi, sigma, Es etc.) or discontinuous indicator variables taking the value 1 or 0 according to the presence or absence of certain molecular features.

Using a congeneric series of 20 compounds, the parameters (i.e. pi, sigma or Es) of these compounds that mainly influence activity can be plotted on the graph as shown in the Fig. 8.5.

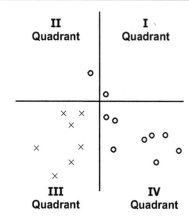

o = Active compound,
× = Inactive compound

Fig. 8.5

Only three out of twenty compounds were misclassified. Then the optimum values for π and σ were calculated for both groups.

Group	π	σ
1 (active)	2.138 ± 1.029	-1.165 ± 0.813
2 (inactive)	-1.613 ± 0.289	-1.513 ± 0.618

Then using a special computerised programme (BMD program), classification functions have been derived.

Group 1 : $\log BA = -2.89\,\sigma + 1.33\,\pi - 1.54$

Group 2 : $\log BA = -10.16\,\sigma - 1.47\,\pi - 3.89$

These equations can be solved by using regression analysis. Sometimes, compounds misclassified may be in fact active or more active than predicted, probably due to in vivo-metabolism to active metabolites.

In summary, discriminate analysis is useful in SAR work where relatively crude data can be applied to a non-linear potency scale. It is useful as a predictive technique or as an analytical tool for crude or poor explanatory data.

(IV) Minimal Topological Difference (MTD) Method :

This method as proposed by Simon and coworkers (1973), is defined as the degree of steric misfit of a drug molecule with respect to the receptor site. Minimal steric differences are obtained by comparing topologically, the shape of newly synthesized drug with the minimum essential parts (i.e. pharmacophore) of the standard clinically used drugs.

The comparison of the molecular shape of the molecules of the drug series under investigation is done by an atom by atom superimposition of the molecular structure yielding a network called hypermolecule. The latter represents partially, the stereochemistry of drug molecules bound to the receptor site.

The basic assumptions in this method include :

(a) Hydrogen atoms are neglected.

(b) Small differences in bond lengths ($\pm$ 0.28 A°) and bond angles ($\pm$ 20°) are neglected.

(c) Molecules may exhibit several low energy conformations. Out of them, such conformation having maximal superimposition with the standard pharmacophore, is chosen.

Disadvantages of MTD Method :

(a) Specific interactions have not been considered.

(b) Sometimes, it becomes difficult to design the hypermolecule in such a way to restrict the maximum molecular size to which MTD method can be applied.

(c) Sometimes finding out the most suitable conformation out of several low energy conformation possible for the molecule, becomes difficult.

(d) Wrong relative orientation of the molecule results because of incorrect definition of the pharmacophore.

(V) Molecular Orbital Method :

This method is one of the most important method among several semi-empirical approaches used in drug-design. As per the basic assumption of this theory, the electrons are considered as being associated with the molecule as a whole rather than with a particular sub-structure. The MO wave functions (ψ) constructed from atomic orbital provide information about the physical properties of a molecule. This in turn, helps to get information about ionization potential, electron affinity etc.

The important MO-techniques used in drug-design include,

(a) Huckel (HMO) or Pariser-Pople-Parr (PPP) method which is used for the study of unsaturated molecules. Hence, it is also known as pi-electron theory.

(b) Huckel theory was further extended (i.e., Extended Huckel Theory, EHT) to study all valency (sigma as well as pi) electrons.

(c) Del Re Method was extended further to study Perturbative Configuration Interactions using Localized Orbitals (PCILO).

(d) INDO, MINDO and CNDO (Complete Neglect of Differential Overlap) methods.

(e) The ab initio method.

The above mentioned MO-techniques help to provide the information regarding conformational features, dipole moments, charge distribution, hydrogen bonding and charge-transfer interactions of drug molecules. The stereochemical information obtained by these methods provides a better understanding of drug-receptor interactions at molecular level.

(VI) Principal Component Analysis (PCA):

When compounds have been evaluated in several biological tests, it is not possible to apply normal multiparameter regression analysis because of its limitations of analysing only one dependent variable at one time. In such cases, the parameter space may be reduced by a few significant components known as Principal Components (PCs) which may then be correlated with certain molecular properties.

Factor or principal component analysis is a mathematical method which is used to study the relationship between several properties which are associated with a series of observations. Factor analysis has been used to study the relationships (or lack of) between the physical properties of a set of substituents. To determine the degree of relationship between variables, the first step is the calculation of the correlation matrix.

The basic assumption of the PCA is that variation of different observable parameters depends linearly on few basic unobservable properties or parameters that affect the biological response. It is the aim of PCA to trace out these basic properties in the form of principal components.

This method is based upon the data set obtained from a series of compounds evaluated for biological activity in several test systems. Individual physico-chemical parameters can then be correlated with these quantitative activity variables. It has a wide role in analyzing the multivariate data both in chemical and biological systems.

(VII) Molecular Modelling:

Currently available techniques (NMR or crystallography) define the shape of the molecule present in the biophase. The QSAR calculations will fail if the shape of the molecule in the biophase is different from the shape of the molecule when it actually interacts with the receptor. Molecular modelling helps to predict the conformational effects of proposed modification in order to maximise the probability to generate an active and more site-specific analogue.

It is a science of Computer Assisted Drug Design (CADD) that utilizes the three dimensional molecular structures (i.e., molecular graphics), computational chemistry or conformational analysis to correlate physico-chemical parameters with the biological activity. Various molecular modelling softwares (AMBER, CAMSEQ, FRODO, HYDRA, SYBL, etc.) are available which can be used to calculate molecular properties for the search of new lead nuclei, for arriving at the best fit model or to design target molecules.

(VIII) Topliss Decision Tree Method (Operational Scheme):

A very common problem in drug design is to find the optimum substitution on a benzene ring or on the benzenoid portion of a fused ring system in an active lead compound for maximization of potency of the drug. Since, there are many possible substituents and several ring positions open for attack, this method helps to select a limited number of substituents which will give good discrimination between π, σ and Es for the series under consideration. This approach is completely a non-mathematical and non-statistical and does not need computerization of the data. An initial group of 6-12 compounds is synthesized and a regression analysis is carried out to determine which parameters are influencing the activity and to what extent. This maximizes the chances of finding the most potent compounds as early as possible.

The basic assumption in 'Topliss decision tree' approach is that the lead nucleus contains an unsubstituted phenyl ring in its structure. The p-chloro analogue is first to be prepared because :

    (i) Ease of synthesis, and

    (ii) To check the dependence of biological activity on lipophilicity.

If the potency increases, this can be attributed to positive values of π and σ or to a combination of $+ \pi$ and $+ \sigma$. Since, both the π and σ values for chlorine atom are positive, naturally then the activity can further be increased by incorporating substituents (e.g., 3, 4-Cl_2) which will contribute to increase the lipophilic and electronic features of the molecule. If 3, 4-dichloro analogue was found to be more active, then 3-CF_3, 4-Cl analogue would be the next choice for synthesis, since again both $\sum\pi$ and $\sum\sigma$ would be larger.

In certain conditions, lipophilic character is often a positive factor while a simultaneous increase in steric features may prove to be a negative factor in drug-design.

Cycloalkyl groups have the advantage of maximizing the possibility of hydrophobic bonding while minimizing unfavourable steric influences. If enhanced potency is noted with the cyclopentyl compound, the cyclohexyl, benzyl, and phenethyl analogues, in sequence, would be prime candidates for synthesis with their progressively larger π values and moderate Es values.

The failure of cyclopentyl to show a potency increase would indicate that the optimum π value had been exceeded thus suggesting cyclobutyl which has the advantage of a very low Es value in addition to having about the right π value. A suitable alternative choice would be cyclopropylmethyl. A second possibility is that activity is increasing with increasing $- \sigma$ values and π is not as important, in which case tertbutyl should be a favourable substituent.

Table 8.13 : Substituents with $+ \pi$ and $+ \sigma$ Values

Substituent	π value	σ value
4 – Cl	0.70	0.23
3 – Cl	0.76	0.37
2 – Cl	0.71	0.23
4 – F	0.14	0.06
3 – CF_3	0.88	0.43

Table 8.14 : Substituents with $- \pi$ and $- \sigma$ Values

Substituent	π value	σ value
4 – OCH_3	– 0.04	– 0.27
4 – NH_2	– 1.23	– 0.66
4 – OH	– 0.61	– 0.37
2 – OCH_3	– 0.02	– 0.27

Table 8.15 : Substituents with $+ \pi$ and $- \sigma$ Values

Substituent	π value	σ value
4 – $N(CH_3)_2$	0.18	– 0.83
3 – CH_3	0.51	– 0.07
4 – CH_3	0.56	– 0.17
3 – $N(CH_3)_2$	0.18	– 0.15
2 – CH_3	0.56	– 0.17
4 – $C(CH_3)_3$	1.98	– 0.20

Table 8.16 : Substituents with $- \pi$ and $+ \sigma$ Values

Substituent	π value	σ value
4 – NO_2	– 0.28	0.78
4 – CN	– 0.32	0.66
4 – $COCH_3$	– 0.37	0.38
4 – SO_2CH_3	– 1.26	0.72
4 – $CONH_2$	– 1.49	0.40
4 – SO_2NH_2	– 1.82	0.57

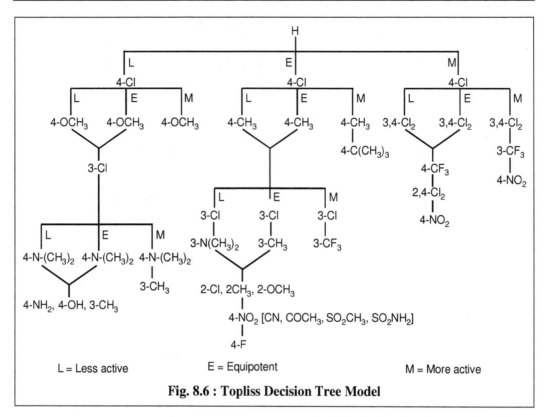

Fig. 8.6 : Topliss Decision Tree Model

Above tables provide the substituents with varying combinations of π and σ values. Through regression analysis, the nature of parameters influencing the activity can be predicted. Based upon this prediction, substituents from any of the above tables can be selected to optimize potency. The detailed scheme of Topliss approach has been shown in Fig. 8.6.

Depending upon the effect of 4–Cl substituent on the biological activity, one can predict the parameters (π, σ or Es) and their nature (either positive or negative) that increase the biological activity. Once it is known, substituents from foregoing tables can be used to optimize the activity.

Besides studying the effect of substituents on the unfused benzene ring, the study on side–chain optimization can also be done using Topliss method. It can be applied to the side–chain when the group is adjacent to a carbonyl (– OR), amino (– NHR) or amide (– CONHR, – NHCOR) function; where R is the variable substituent. Tailor-made schemes may also be constructed for special situations. When the most favourable type of substituent has been identified by working through operational scheme, a detailed examination of similar substituents would be a logical procedure. When data on enough compounds have been obtained, the option to perform a multiple regression analysis is open.

Thus Topliss approach is stepwise where the next compound is determined on the basis of the results obtained with the previous one. Three other stepwise methods include, Craig plot, Fibonacci search method and sequential simplex strategy.

Table 8.17 : Side-chain Substituent Constant Values

Substituent	π	σ	E_s
H	0.00	0.49	1.24
CH_3	0.50	0.00	0.00
C_2H_5	1.00	– 0.10	– 0.07
$i – C_3H_7$	1.30	– 0.19	– 0.47
tert. – C_4H_9	1.98	– 0.30	– 1.54
Cyclo – C_4H_7	1.80	– 0.20	– 0.06
CH_2–cyclo–C_3H_5	1.80	– 0.13	–
Cyclo – C_5H_9	2.14	– 0.20	– 0.51
Cyclo – C_6H_{11}	2.51	– 0.15	– 0.79
C_6H_5	2.13	0.60	–
$CH_2C_6H_5$	2.63	0.22	– 0.38
CF_3	1.07	2.76	– 1.16
$CHCl_2$	1.15	1.92	– 1.54
$(CH_2)_2 C_6H_5$	3.13	0.08	– 0.38
CH_2CF_3	1.57	0.92	–
CH_2SCH_3	0.77	0.44	– 0.34
CH_2OCH_3	0.02	0.64	– 0.19
$CH_2SO_2CH_3$	– 0.76	1.32	–

Since, about 40% of all reported medicinally active compounds incorporate an unfused benzene ring, it is essential to search out the optimum substitution on a benzene ring or on the benzenoid portion in the lead nucleus to maximize the drug potency. The presence of even a single phenyl ring in a drug structure offers many positions for a variety of substituents. All these possible analogs might not really be worth synthesizing. Hence, a more rational approach need to be developed which will help to select a limited number of substituents having good discrimination between π, σ and Es values. In order to overcome the problem of synthetic difficulty, Topliss has suggested a useful strategy for the stepwise selection of substituents for synthesis of new analogues of an active lead to maximize the chances of synthesizing the most potent compounds in the given series as early as possible.

The stepwise selection takes the form of decision tree and does not require multiple regression analysis. The initial group of analogues for synthesis consists of the first five compounds as shown in following table.

Table 8.17

Sub-stituents	Parameters					
	π	$2\pi– \pi^2$	σ	$2\pi–\sigma$	$\pi– 2\sigma$	Es
H	4 - 5	4 - 5	3	5	5	1
4 – Cl	2	1 - 2	2	2 - 3	3 - 4	2 – 5
4 – CH_3	3	3	4	2 - 3	1	2 – 5
4 – OCH_3	4 - 5	4 - 5	5	4	2	2 - 5
3, 4 – Cl_2	1	1 - 2	1	1	3 - 4	2 - 5

The unsubstituted, 4–Cl, 3, 4–Cl_2, 4–CH_3 and 4–OCH_3 analogues are considered to be easy to synthesize and having wide differences in their π, σ and Es values. This helps to get a sufficient spread in the biological activities of this initial set of compounds. Application of this method would be particularly advantageous when analogue synthesis is difficult and slow.

The substituents for the second small set of analogues are then selected on the basis of the apparent relationships between potency and physical properties which are revealed in the first set of analogues. One can easily predict the influence of a particular parameter (π, σ, Es) on biological activity after evaluating the potencies of compounds from second set. Depending on the relationship, one may synthesize still more potent compounds by referring following table.

It may sometimes happen that significant increase in activity may not be observed even after synthesizing the second set of compound. In such cases, an examination of 2-substituents is suggested as a next step. Thus the examination of 2-substituents is to be made after first exploring the potential of 4- and 3-substituents. In following table, the substituents listed under designation 'other' may be checked if even compounds with 2-substitution do not show substantial increase in potency. For example, the 4–F derivative does not differ from unsubstituted compound in the effects of π and σ but would be advantageous if the unsubstitued compound is essentially optimal in terms of π and σ and suffers from unwanted 4-hydroxylation as metabolic transformation.

Table 8.19

Probable operative parameters	New substituent selection
π, $\pi + \sigma$, σ	$3-CF_3$, $4-Cl$; $3-CF_3$, $4-NO_2$; $4-CF_3$; 2, $4-Cl_2$; $4-C-C_5H_9$; $4-C-C_6H_{11}$
π, $2\pi - \sigma$, $\pi - \sigma$	$4-CH(CH_3)_2$; $4-C(CH_3)_3$; 3, $4-(CH_3)_2$; $4-O(CH_2)_3\ CH_3$; $4-OCH_2Ph$; $4-N(C_2H_5)_2$
$\pi - 2\sigma$, $\pi - 3\sigma$, $-\sigma$	$4-N(C_2H_5)_2$; $4-N(CH_3)_2$; $4-NH_2$; $4-NHC_4H_9$; $4-OH$; $4-OCH(CH_3)_2$; $3-CH_3$, $4-OCH_3$
$2\pi - \pi^2$	$4-Br$; $3-CF_3$; 3, $4-(CH_3)_2$; $4-C_2H_5$; $4-O(CH_2)_2CH_3$; $3-CH_3$, $4-Cl$
	$3-Cl$; $3-CH_3$; $3-OCH_3$; $3-N(CH_3)_2$; $3-CF_3$; 3, $5-Cl_2$

Ortho effect	$2-Cl$; $2-CH_3$; $2-OCH_3$; $2-F$
Other	$4-F$; $4-NHCOCH_3$; $4-NHSO_2CH_3$; $4-NO_2$; $4-COCH_3$; $4-SO_2CH_3$; $4-CONH_2$; $4-SO_2NH_2$

Topliss has illustrated the application of this method to find the most potent derivatives as early as possible by taking following examples.

(a) The initial set of five compounds was synthesized in a series of 5-aryltetrazolylpropionic acids in order to apply Topliss method. The anti-inflammatory activity values of these compounds revealed that the unsubstituted parent is more potent than others. The activity drop in other analogues may be due to the steric hindrance of 4-substituent. Hence, a second group of compounds was synthesized having substituents at 3 or 3, 5–positions. Out of them the 3–Cl and 3, 5–Cl$_2$ possess increased activity.

The remaining listed substituents 4-NHSO$_2$CH$_3$, 4-NO$_2$, 4-COCH$_3$, 4-SO$_2$CH$_3$, 4-CONH$_2$, and 4-SO$_2$NH$_2$, are all examples of $- \pi + \sigma$ type substituents which should prove fruitful if increased potency is related to reduced lipophilicity or reduced lipophilicity combined with $+ \sigma$ effect. Alternatively, these substituents may be employed at the 3 position. Cases benefiting from the $- \pi - \sigma$ effect have been detected through the 4–NH$_2$ and 4–OH substituents.

Table 8.20 : Anti–inflammatory Activity of 5–aryltetrazolylpropionic Acids

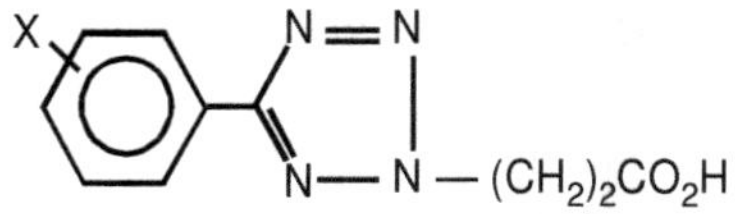

X	Activity
Initial compound group	
3, 4–Cl$_2$	6.2
4–Cl	5.9
4–CH$_3$	3.1
4–OCH$_3$	4.9
H	8.2
Second compound group	
3–Cl	11.2
3–CH$_3$	7.9
3–CF$_3$	5.7
3, 5–Cl$_2$	11.2
Other compounds	
3–Br	11.2
3–NH$_2$	0.3

In another example, the preparation of initial set of five compounds in a series of substituted sulphonamides revealed the dependence of carbonic anhydrase inhibitor activity on π or $\pi + \sigma$ relationship. This observation led to synthesis of only one member, the 3–CF$_3$, 4–NO$_2$ analogue which was found to be most potent in the entire series.

Table 8.21 : Sulphonamide Carbonic Anhydrase Inhibitor

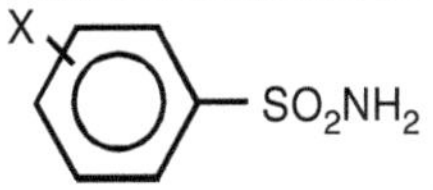

X	Log activity
Initial compound group	
3, 4–Cl$_2$	1.40
4–Cl	0.72
4–CH$_3$	0.42
4–OCH$_3$	0.35
H	0.22
Second compound group	
3–CF$_3$, 4–NO$_2$	1.85

The third illustration was provided by a series of 2–phenyl–8–azapurin–6–ones showing antiallergic activity. The higher activity associated with unsubstituted compound in the initial set suggested an examination of 3–substituents.

Table 8.22 : Anti–allergic activity of 2–phenyl–8–azapurin–6–ones

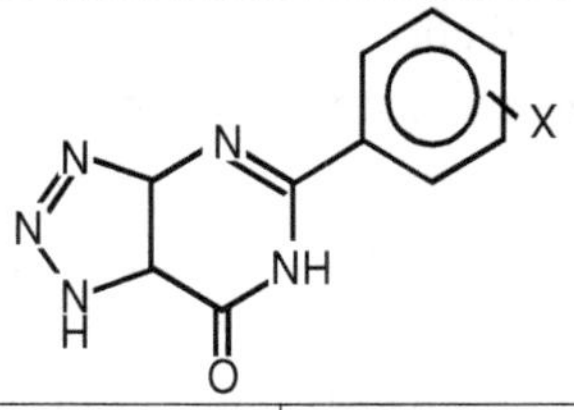

X	Activity
Initial compound group	
4–Cl	2
4–CH$_3$	0.8
4–OCH$_3$	1
H	4
Second compound group	
H	4
3–CH$_3$	4
3–OCH$_3$	2
3–N(CH$_3$)$_2$	0.5
3–CF$_3$	4
Third compound group	
H	4.0
2–Cl	0.2
2–CH$_3$	0.04
2–OCH$_3$	10.0
2–F	0.5

Since, the second set of compounds prepared employing 3–substituents did not offer any advantage in activity over parent compound, a third set of 2–substituted compounds was synthesized.

In this set, the 2–OCH$_3$ compound exhibited exceptionally high activity, probably due to a strong influence of the hydrogen bonding capability of the ortho–OCH$_3$ functional group.

(IX) Pattern Recognition :

This is the method of data analysis which derive model that gives qualitative results. There are two conditions :

(1) Model should reproduce biological activity for compounds on which they are based.

(2) Prediction should be done with few parameters compared to number of degree of freedom data.

e.g. the change in methyl or chloro group changes pKa value of p-benzoic acid. It causes change in coefficient in 1-octanol/water of p substituted benzoic acid. This change can be described numerically in different physicochemical variables corresponding pKa and log p.

It gives four levels of information :

Level I : Predict assignment of unknown and untested substance of class.

Level II : The resulting test compound may belong to undiscussed loss equivalent to autlier at level I and level II.

Level III : Involve prediction of qualitative class assignment of autlier.

Level IV : Prediction of several biological responses and it is natural level of classification. e.g. linear learning machine for classification of toxic vs. non-toxic and carcinogenic vs. non-carcinogenic.

ALLOC is a new method of supervised pattern recognition which is under development by Coomans et al. It uses the cumulative potential of object in its position with the training compounds to make a class assignment. The cumulative potential is calculated from Gaussian function.

Disadvantages : Non-parametric about shape and homogenisity of class, when applied to medical diagnostic data on hyperthyroid and hypothyroid patients.

8.16 TERMS COMMONLY USED IN REGRESSION ANALYSIS

To express a correlation quantitatively, graph is usually a preferred method over regression analysis. In regression analysis to show how representative of the results the correlation is, additional data is to be given in terms of the correlation coefficient (r), number of compounds utilised (n), standard deviation (S) and statistical validity (F). When the number of variables exceeds 3, the results can not be expressed in the form of either a graph or a model. A regression equation therefore remains the only method of expression which can be used in such situation.

(a) Correlation coefficient (r) :

High value of regression coefficient $(r > 0.90)$ indicates that the statistical significance of the regression equation is high, while the low value of 'r' indicates that the substituents constant is not important for the process under consideration.

If the 'r' value does not decrease significantly when a particular substituent (coefficient) constant is omitted from the equation, it means that process represented by equation is least affected by the factor symbolised by that particular substituent coefficient.

For example, inhibition constant (K) of alkyl phosphoric acid esters against cholinesterase enzymes is expressed by the following equations :

	r	s
$\log K = 2.576 \, Es^c + 7.941$	0.927	0.648 ... (1)
$\log K = 5.678 \, \sigma^* + 6.310$	0.410	1.581 ... (2)
$\log K = -0.230 \, \pi + 6.151$	0.107	1.711 ... (3)
$\log K = 2.965 \, Es^c + 0.182\pi - 3.052\sigma^* + 7.558$	0.944	0.641 ... (4)

Conclusions :

(a) The low values of π in equations (3) and (4) indicate that hydrophobic binding contributes little towards inhibitory activity. This is supported by low value of 'r' in equation (3).

(b) Similarly low value of r in equation (2) suggests that electronic parameter is also not important.

(c) Equation (1) does not contain the terms π or σ but still r value is higher and does not decrease significantly from equation (4) to equation (1) and hence only steric effects are of prime importance for inhibitory activity.

(b) Number of compounds utilised (n) :

For a good correlation, large number of compounds must be used. The value of 'r' must be assessed with reference to 'n'. For example,

r = 0.89 for n = 10 is a better correlation than r = 0.98 for n = 3.

(c) Standard deviation (S) :

This value gives us an idea about precision of that equation. Greater the value of 'S', large will be the accuracy with which the expected potency of a new compound may be guessed.

(d) r^2 :

The term explains about percent data represented by that particular equation. For example, if r = 0.7 then r^2 = 0.49 or 49% data is accounted by regression of that parameter/s, still leaving 51% data yet unaccounted. Thus the value of 'r' can be improved by inclusion of another parameter. Thus the term, r^2 helps us to understand whether other parameters should be sought for or not. Greater the value of r^2, lesser is the variance (data) that remains unaccounted by the equation.

(e) F :

It evaluates, the statistical validity of a particular equation. For example, for 1% probability level of statistical invalidity or insignificance, F = 13.74. Hence, for a particular equation if, F std (i.e., 13.74) < F calculated then the relationship represented by that equation is statistically significant.

Formulae for Calculation of Terms :

The linear regression single parameter dependent equation is represented by

$$Y = mX + c$$

where, m = slope of the line, c = constant, X and Y represent variables.

(i) $\quad m = \dfrac{n \cdot \sum xy - \sum x \cdot \sum y}{n \sum x^2 - (\sum x)^2}$

(ii) $\quad c = \dfrac{\sum y - m \sum x}{n}$

(iii) $\quad r = \dfrac{n \sum xy - \sum x \cdot \sum y}{\sqrt{[n \cdot \sum x^2 - (\sum x)^2]\,[n \cdot \sum y^2 - (\sum y)^2]}}$

(iv) $\quad F = (n - 1)\,\dfrac{r^2}{1 - r^2}$

(v) $\quad t = r \sqrt{\dfrac{n - 2}{1 - r^2 \, m}}$

(vi) $\quad S = \sqrt{\dfrac{\sum y^2 - 2m \sum xy - 2c \sum y + m^2 \sum x^2 + 2mc \sum x + nc^2}{n - 1}}$

The linear regression multiparameter dependent equation can be written as

$$\log BA = b_1 X_1 + b_2 X_2 + c$$

where b_1 and b_2 are the coefficients of parameters X_1 and X_2, while c is a constant.

(i) $\quad b_2 = \dfrac{(\sum x_1^2)\,(\sum x_2 y) - (\sum x_1 x_2)\,(\sum x_1 y)}{D}$

(ii) $\quad b_1 = \dfrac{(\sum x_2^2)\,(\sum x_1 y) - (\sum x_1 y)\,(\sum x_2 y)}{D}$

(iii) $\quad D = (\sum x_1^2)\,(\sum x_2)^2 - (\sum x_1 x_2)^2$

(iv) $F = \dfrac{\text{Regression SS}/2}{\text{Error SS}/(n-3)}$

where,

Regression SS = Total SS − Error SS

$$\text{Total SS} = \sum_{i=1}^{n}(y_i - \bar{y})^2; \quad \bar{y} = \dfrac{\sum y_i}{n}$$

$$= \sum y_i^2 - n(\bar{y})^2$$

$$\text{Error SS} = \sum_{i=1}^{n}(y_i - \hat{y_i})^2$$

8.17 CRAIG PLOT

The Topliss decision tree approach has emerged from the work of Craig who pointed out the utility of a simple graphical plot of π versus σ or any such two parameters to guide the selection of next substituent.

Through regression analysis, the sign and magnitude of coefficients of substituent constant (π or σ) can be found out. Thus, if both the π and σ terms have negative coefficients, then the substituents like OH or NH_2 can be selected for further analogues.

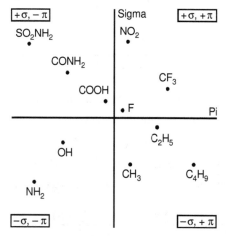

Fig. 8.7 : Craig Plot

Pattern recognition methods attempt to define the set of parameter values which will result in clustering compounds of similar activity into regions of n-dimensional space.

8.18 BATCHWISE TOPLISS OPERATIONAL SCHEME

It involves a batchwise analysis of small groups of compounds.

The substituents were categorized by Topliss according to π, σ, π^2 and a variety of $\pi - \sigma$ or $\pi - \pi^2$ combinations (like $\pi - \sigma$, $2\pi - \sigma$, $\pi - 3\sigma$, $\pi + \sigma$, $2\pi - \pi^2$ etc.). The approach begins with the synthesis of five basic analogues namely, 4–H; 4–Cl; 3, 4–dichloro; 4–CH_3 and 4–OCH_3. These analogues could be ranked in order of decreasing potency. The most active analogue helps to predict the parameter that influences the activity. Once the parameter dependence is identified, substituents with proper $\pi + \sigma$ combinations can be selected.

8.19 CLUSTER ANALYSIS

In this method, substituents are grouped into clusters with similar properties according to their σ, π, π^2, Es, r, F, MR and MW values. For example, Cluster 3a contains CN, NO_2, COOH and $COCH_3$, while cluster 1 contains Br, OCF_3, CF_3, NCS, SO_2F etc.

One member of each cluster is selected for substitution into lead nucleus. If a substituent from a particular cluster showed increase in potency, then other substituents from the same cluster would be selected for synthesizing further analogues.

It is surprising to note that in cluster analysis, the appearance of Cl, F and Br, and I are in different groups while F and $N(CH_3)_2$ and Br and SO_2F appear in the same group. A still advanced computerised programme developed by Norrington, uses a more restricted set of substituents. The computer is programmed to respond by giving the next analogue which differs from the starting compound by more than a specified amount. Both these approaches have an advantage that the initial batch of analogues selected for synthesis has the widest possible range of non-inter-related parameters.

Example :

About 10 new analogues of propranolol, a β-adrenergic blocking drug were prepared by making substitution at ortho position of naphthalene ring. The ED_{50} of these compounds were correlated with physico-chemical properties and regression equations were developed. Interpret the equation.

$$O-CH_2-\overset{\overset{\displaystyle OH}{|}}{CH}-CH_2-NH-CH(CH_3)_2$$
$$CONH--R$$

The regression analysis results into following equation :

$$\log ED_{50} = -3.21\,R - 0.22\,MR + 1.36$$

$$n = 10;\ r = 0.92;\ S = 0.45;\ F = 13$$

Conclusions :

(i) The values of r, S and F suggest that the equation is statistically valid.

(ii) It means that both, steric and electronic parameters play an important role in influencing the activity.

(iii) The coefficients of both parameters (R and MR) carry a negative sign. It means a less bulky substituent of electron releasing nature increases the activity.

Exercise :

Interpret the following equations :

(a) $\log K = 0.512\,(\pm 0.05)\log P + 1.881$
$$(\pm 0.23)$$
$$n = 40;\ r = 0.96;\ S = 0.159;\ F = 30$$

(b) $\log 1/c = 1.028\,(\pm 0.12)\,\sigma m - 0.13$
$$(\pm 0.03)\log P + 3.298$$
$$n = 14;\ r = 0.998;\ S = 0.071;\ F = 41$$

8.20 QUANTITATIVE STRUCTURE PHARMACOKINETIC RELATIONSHIP (QSPR) IN DRUG-DESIGN

Pharmacokinetics deal with the processes concerned with drug absorption, distribution, metabolism and elimination. The knowledge of the rate constants for these pharmacokinetic parameters has been used and is essential for :

(a) calculation of dose and dose interval,

(b) estimation of bioavailability,

(c) correlation of pharmacokinetics to pharmacodynamics,

(d) detection of effect of metabolism on kidney function,

(e) prediction of toxic effects of drugs.

In order to evoke a biological response, the drug must reach to the receptor site in active form in high concentration. In its journey from the site of administration to the site of action, drug is subjected to the attack of various processes involved in absorption, distribution, metabolism, binding and excretion. Because of influences of various body processes, the in-vitro results need not be reproduced in the in-vivo testing of drugs. QSPR can also be used to predict the parameters which quantitatively govern the pharmacokinetic behaviour of the drug. These parameters include :

(i) Absorption rate constant, Ka

(ii) Metabolism rate constant, Km

(iii) Elimination rate constant K_{el}

(iv) Volume of distribution, V_d

(v) Degree of plasma–protein binding, K_A. It influences all the above four parameters.

Absorption rate depends upon lipophilicity, polarity, degree of ionization and molecular size. It governs the bio–availability of drug. Through QSAR work, it was recognized that for penetration into the CNS, the drug should have $\log P_0 = 2.0$. Metabolism rate depends upon the lipophilicity and ionization. The rate of elimination depends upon lipophilicity, ionization and degree of plasma–protein binding. Same factors also affect volume of distribution. The plasma-protein binding increases with an increase in lipophilicity and ionization (pKa) of the drug molecule. Thus with the help of QSPR, it is possible to design a drug with better pharmacokinetic properties like, long biological half–life and low plasma–protein binding. Both in prodrug design and in straight analogue modification, QSPR would be helpful to have an estimate of the type of metabolic transformations the compound might undergo.

The most important condition for selection of compounds for QSPR studies, is all the compounds should have common structural skeleton (i.e. congeneric series) so that scatterness in pharmacokinetic processes can be restricted. Similarly, the complexity of the in–vivo system and individual body's internal environment may create problems to arrive at conclusions in QSPR analysis.

It was a long–lasting assumption that the various processes of gastrointestinal absorption, distribution, metabolism and excretion are less sensitive to the specific molecular structure than in true interaction with a receptor. Yet another generalisation is absorption, brain penetration and metabolism by liver increase with increasing log P whereas urinary excretion decreases with increasing log P.

8.21 ACHIEVEMENTS OF QSAR

QSAR helps to understand the forces that govern the activity in a congeneric series of compounds. It thus helps to reduce the empiricism in drug-design and ensures that every drug synthesized and pharmacologically tested is as meaningful as possible. The main area where QSAR provides insight include :

(a) Forcasting of Biological Activity :

Innumerable applications of QSAR have been reported where successful prediction of biological activity played an important role. Through the regression analysis, parameters or nature and position of substituent which may increase the activity can be guessed. The advanced techniques using computerised programmes even give the structural features of the most possible active compound from the series. However, QSAR is not the final answer to drug discovery. It may be considered as one of the refined tools for drug development.

(b) Selection of Proper Substituents :

Proper selection of substituents to develop a series leads to a decrease in the average number of analogues required to investigate the relationship between substituent parameters and the biological activity. Batch selection and cluster analysis are the examples of QSAR–techniques that help in proper design of series. Such a planning gives a good chance of finding out what combinations of parameters will optimise the potency. The analogues should vary substantially in each of the properties proposed to be important in the determination of potency. If the minimum number of analogues represent all possible combinations of parameter, decision to terminate synthesis can be taken at early state in a series that does not show promising results.

(c) Bioisosterism :

With the introduction of QSAR, the qualitative concept of bioisosterism has turned to be more quantitative and constitutive. QSAR also helps to decide an isoster which will give better pharmacokinetic and/or pharmacodynamic properties to lead nucleus.

(d) Drug–receptor interactions :

In a congeneric series of compounds, QSAR studies help to predict in quantitative terms, the forces involved in the drug-receptor interactions if the substitutions are made in non-essential part of the drug molecule. Such studies have been reported for the drugs that inhibit mammalian and bacterial dihydrofolate reductase. It is possible to derive a quantitative correlation between the strength of binding and the number and types of bonds possible. If selection of parameters is proper, QSAR may also suggest at which positions of the receptor, increased lipophilicity of drug increases binding, how changes in the strength of potential H-bonds affect binding, etc. The three dimensional feature of receptor and minimum energy active conformational forms of the drug molecules can also be predicted through QSAR-studies.

(e) Pharmacokinetic information :

The correlation between various types of parameters and the pharmacokinetic features of the drug can be done using QSAR. The passive reabsorption of substances from the urinary filtrate to decrease the total amount of drug, excreted in the urine has also been studied by QSAR.

Other recent developments in QSAR include approaches such as HQSAR, Inverse QSAR and Binary QSAR. Improved statistical tools such as Partial Least Square (PLS) can handle situations where the number of variables overwhelms the number of molecules in a data set, which may have collinear X-variables.

Environmental toxicology is also a field in which QSAR has been applied in the study of bio-concentration, toxicity of chemicals and movement through soils. QSAR has provided insight into the structure - activity pattern of taste and olfactory compounds. Drug metabolism and distribution and anesthesiology are also fields for QSAR application. QSAR also finds use in rationalizing the relative lethality of certain classes of drugs in forensic toxicology.

Synthesis of molecules in a combinatorial fashion can quickly lead to large numbers of molecules. For example, a molecule with three points of diversity $(R_1, R_2$ and $R_3)$ can generate $NR_1 \times NR_2 \times NR_3$ possible structures, where NR_1, NR_2 and NR_3 are the number of different substituents utilized.

In order to handle the vast number of structural possibilities, researchers often create a 'virtual library', a computational enumeration of all possible structures of a given pharmacophore with all available reactants. Such a library can consist of thousand to millions of 'virtual' compounds. The researcher will select a subset of the 'virtual library' for actual synthesis, based upon various calculations and criteria (ADME, Docking etc.)

8.22 LIMITATIONS OF QSAR

Even though the applications of QSAR analysis may result in statistically valid equations, it is often difficult to interpret the relationship in biochemical terms. Failure of regression analysis in the prediction of biological activity of analogues results mainly due to :

(a) A poorly designed series or ambiguous regression analysis.

(b) An extrapolation outside the range of the physical properties represented by original substituents.

(c) Improper conditions of the biological testing and

(d) Multiple modes of action.

The most serious problem in QSAR is the lack of fundamental understanding of how to quantitatively describe substituent effects on noncovalent intermolecular (e.g., drug-receptor) interactions. Hence, the knowledge about the sort of interactions and quantification of substituents effect (parameter) on the interactions is essential.

A successful QSAR can provide only indirect (in terms of Es, MV or MR) information about the three dimensional aspects of drug-receptor interactions. However, mutual conformational adaptation of drug and receptor may also occur after interactions. Since, no specific parameter has yet been developed for the description of the variation in conformation, conformational flexibility or three dimensional aspects of the drug, it imposes limitations on the success of QSAR analysis.

Other effects (like electronic or steric) have their own influences on the overall lipophilicity of the molecule. This may result in the wrong correlation and interpretation of activity in a series that mainly depends upon lipophilicity for biological action. Electronic effects of a substituent may change both, the degree of ionization and the charge distribution. The former may affect the amount of active species available to the receptor while the latter may affect the strength of the drug-receptor interaction.

Since, the biological activity determination process is susceptible to considerable experimental variations, a non-linear scatter may be observed during correlation of biological activity with physico-chemical parameters. QSAR fails to explain this built-in scatter mathematically.

Although a variety of linear parameters (about 41) descriptors of electronic features of a substituent are available, several workers have found that quite often in a particular case one electronic parameter has worked while others did not.

Similarly, physiologically active compounds on their way from the site of administration to the target sites, are known to undergo diverse chemical and biochemical transformations. It is likely that they act differently on different bio-targets to exert same kind of activity.

In summary, if the problem is to learn more about the mechanism of action of a congeneric series of compounds or to design a more active drug from the information available, Hansch or Free-Wilson approach may be useful. Best results with the Free-Wilson approach are obtained in a series with several positions available for substitution and only if, each substituent at any location appears in atleast two compounds of the series.

The first published use of a computer for empirical force field calculations of molecular structure was in 1961 by Hendrickson, who examined the conformations of medium-sized rings. Hendrickson applied his technique widely to the conformational analysis. The use of classical QSAR was expanded during the 1960's as a mean of correlating observed activity to chemical properties; however there are much areas where these techniques could not be used or where they failed to provide useful correlations. There are cases where biological activity values could not be determined accurately for a variety of reasons.

Alternative statistical techniques can be used in these cases. The problem is simplified to a classification scheme in which compounds are labelled as active, partially active, inactive etc. The resulting data set is then searched for patterns which predict these categories. The methods which have been used for this type of analysis include SIMCA (Soft Independent Modelling of Class Analogy), ADAPT (Automated Data Analysis by Pattern Recognition Techniques), CASE (Computer Automated Structure Evaluation) and CSA (Cluster Significance Analysis).

If the problem is to screen structurally diverse compounds for a specific biological activity such as sedative action, then pattern recognition or probabilistic methods with substructural fragments may be more valuable approaches. These methods may be helpful in setting testing priorities by determining which compounds are more likely to possess a specific activity and which compounds have substructural components that have not been tested.

Over the years, a number of non-mathematical and relatively simple novel approaches have been sketched out to optimize the activity of the lead compound. Of these, Topliss approach appears to be most interesting and of practical utility in medicinal chemistry.

8.23 MOLECULAR MODELLING IN DRUG DESIGN

All molecules have a range of conformations produced by the vibrations of all the bonds and the torsional rotations about the single bonds.

Drug receptors are macromolecules, but not all macromolecules are drug receptors. As discussed above, a macromolecule should be "Worthy and capable of being targeted for drug design". Such a macromolecule is typically a protein that is intimately connected with a disease process but is not crucial to a wide range of other normal biochemical processes.

There are several physical and chemical forces that interact between the two molecules. These forces are used to define various docking scores that measure how good is each interactions. Different contributions to molecular interactions can be divided into two types. Bonded interactions include bond stretching, bond angle bending and torsion angle rotation. Non-bonded interactions include London-Van der Waals and Coulomb interactions. Sometimes all of the non-bonded interactions are simply called Van der Waals interactions. This force is very significant when the molecules are close and their contact surface is large. The formula for this force is $A/(r^6)-B/(r^{12})$, where A and B are constants and r is the distance between them. Note that when the distance is very small there is a significant rejection force driving them apart. The total energy is simply the sum of all of the bonded and non-bonded interactions. These interactions can be used to calculate low energy conformations of a molecule. Energy minimization is routinely used to improve approximate structures obtained from X-ray diffraction of crystals or molecular magnetic resonance data of solutions.

Non-covalent Reactions :

Interactions between a charged ion and a neutral molecule with a dipole moment are called ion-dipole interactions. Ions can also interact with neutral moelcules with zero dipole moment. For example, the permanent dipole moment of CCl_4 molecule is zero because of symmetrical location of all four chlorine atoms at the four corners of a tetrahedron. However, a charge if placed near a CCl_4 molecule, will distort the electronic distribution and the CCl_4 molecule becomes polarized. Interactions between a charged ion and such polarized molecules are called charge-induced dipole interactions.

A molecule with no permanent dipole moment may acquire an instantaneous dipole moment due to fluctuations in the electronic distributions. This instantaneous dipole may induce a dipole in a neighbouring neutral molecule. Interactions between such dipole-induced dipoles are called London interactions. London interaction is always present in all kinds of molecules and is the only attractive force acting between identical rare gas atoms.

Van der Waals interactions are another most common type of interactions. It includes permanent dipole-permanent dipole interactions, permanent dipole-induced dipole attractions and steric repulsions. The London-Van der Waals interactions are usually non-specific forces which contribute to the energies of all reactions.

A hydrogen atom while remaining covalently bonded to one oxygen or nitrogen may form a weak hydrogen bond to another oxygen or nitrogen. The hydrogen bond plays an important role in governing the three-dimensional structures of proteins and nucleic acids.

These bonds could significantly strengthen the bonding between two molecules and occurs when one molecule has a hydrogen atom close to the docking surface that interacts with an electro negative atom from the second molecule when the docking occurs. Water molecules have a strong attraction for each other, primarily as a consequence of hydrogen-bond formation.

Hydrophobic (fear-of-water) Interactions :

The molecules of water form a mobile network through hydrogen bonds with four tetrahedrally oriented neighbours. The network is not a rigid one and change of neighbours occurs rapidly because of thermal motions. A hole is created due to insertion of any other molecule into this network. Some hydrogen bonds in the original network are broken.

When two such hydrocarbon groups are inserted into water, each will lead to an unfavourable free energy change. If the two groups cluster together, the disruptive effect on the solvent network will be less than the combined effects of two separate groups. Hence, the clsutering of such groups will be thermodynamically favoured. The clustering of the groups is not because they like each other but because they are both disliked by water. The clustered arrangement results in a decrease in the overall free energy of the system in comparison with the separate dispersion of unlike molecules. Hydrophobic interactions are characterised by low enthalpy (energy) changes and are entropy (conformations) driven.

Partial Charges and Dipole Moments :

A molecule is an arrangement of nuclei surrounded by electrons. The electron distribution determines the partial charge on each atom. The electron wave function for all of the electrons in a molecule tells us the electron density at every point in space. The interactions of the assigned bond dipoles produce a net dipole for a molecule. Then, by using the co-ordinates of the nuclei of the atoms, one can estimate the dipole moment.

Thermodynamics deals with interchange among different forms of energy. Interactions between ligand and receptor involve physical contact which if exceeds for a certain time period, results in an attractive force. In general, these interactions mainly depend on the concentration of reactants and salt in the solution.

Bond Stretching and Bond Angle Bending :

Bond stretching and bond angle bending can be treated as if the atoms were connected by springs. The energy of moving the atoms so as to stretch or compress a bond or to change a bond angle depends on the square of the change in bond length or the square of the change in bond angle.

$$u = K_r (r - r_{eq})^2$$
$$u = K_b (\theta - \theta_{eq})^2$$

Here, $r - r_{eq}$ is the difference between the perturbed bond length and the equilibrium bond length, and $\theta - \theta_{eq}$ is the difference between the perturbed bond angle and the equilibrium bond angle. The constants K_r and K_b are positive which means the energy increases when the bonds are perturbed from their equilibrium positions.

Stretching and compressing a bond requires a large amount of energy. For example, changing the bond length of a single bond by 0.1 A° requires about 10 kJ mol^{-1} while a double bond requires about twice as much energy.

Rotation around single bonds can cause large changes in the conformation of a molecule but it does not require much energy. The energy necessary to rotate around a C – C single bond will have maxima and minima corresponding to different orientations of the substitutents on the carbon atoms. It takes a large amount of energy to rotate around a double bond as one has to break the pi bond.

Lead discovery is basically a search process. The search can proceed through a variety of computational methods both in the presence or absence of structural information of the target. De Novo Ligand Design or structure-based design highlights the usefulness of structural information in drug discovery. It involves the use of structural information of ligand/receptor and computational methods to facilitate the process of introducing compounds into the clinic. The structure is known either through X-ray or NMR based methods or it can be modelled using computational methods. The more commonly used database include the Cambridge Structural File, the Available Chemical Directory, the National Institute of Cancer Database and sections of the Chemical Abstracts Registry.

Molecular geometry is a source of information about the molecular architecture, its electronic structure and interaction mechanisms. It helps us to understand many biological or chemical processes at the molecular level. Various spectroscopic techniques like NMR and X-ray diffraction can give valuable insight of molecular geometry. X-ray diffraction is useful when the sample is in crystal state. X-ray scattering is almost entirely due to external electrons and the intensity of the scattered radiation depends upon the electron distribution within the atoms. From electron densities, a density map may be drawn where peaks indicate the location of the atoms. There are about 125000 well resolved experimentally determined crystal structures in the Cambridge structural database. The crystal structure reveals much of the conformational information of the flexible molecule. The success of Cambridge Database or the Brookhaven Protein Data Bank, are the examples of commercial application of geometrical data about organic compounds and protein derived from X-ray diffraction.

NMR derived information directly concerns with conformations of the molecules in solution.

Computer-aided drug design may either ligand-based design or the de novo design relying on the 3D structure of the macromolecular target site. The latter are usually derived by X-ray crystallography. Solved structures are available free of charge on the Brookhaven Protein Data Bank (PDB, http:// www.pdb.bnl.gox) site financed by the US government. This site also contains a number of structures obtained by 2D-NMR spectroscopy. These NMR measurements are useful to derive solution structures or structures of proteins which can not be crystallized for X-ray analysis. As the membrane bound proteins are difficult to crystallize, structural information on these proteins can be obtained using electron diffraction techniques or electron cryomicroscopy. In the absence of experimental data, macromolecular structures can be explored by homology modelling. This method utilizes the knowledge of certain degree of similarity between the primary sequences of unknown protein and the protein whose 3D structure is known. The primary sequence of all the structurally known proteins may be derived from Genbank at ncbi.nlm.nih.gox, the EMBL server at ftp.embl.heidelberg.de and the Swiss Prot server at www.expasy.ch.

Substrate conformations can also be obtained using X-ray diffraction studies and NMR experiments. The Cambridge Structural Database is the most relevant source of 3D structures of small molecules derived from neutron and X-ray diffraction data. The conformational space of the substrate can be explored by the theoretical methods as well.

Site-directed de novo drug design is based on the complementarity between the generated ligand and its site. It can be achieved by searching for the possible structure from a database of structure fragments which will maximally fit and satisfy the local constraints of the site. Three-dimensional database searching enables the identification of compounds that match the pharmacophoric distances or shape and electrostatic complementarity. Alignments are generated by random rotations and translations of one structure relative to the other, followed by minimization of the alignment function for each overlay. If we have n fragments and each fragment can be connected to its neighbour by m different ways, there is a possibility of m^n different combinations of fragments. Ranking according to an energy of interaction between the ligand structure and receptor site may then be used as a basis to pick up the final few combinations. Softwares commonly used in De Novo Drug Design methods include DOCK, GRID, CAVEAT, LEGEND, LUDI, SPROUT, NEWLEAD etc.

In general, for larger sites, structure generation is so diverse that detailed inspection of each structure becomes impracticable. In order to reduce the number of combinations and to potentiate the specificity of resulting combinations, larger target sites may be divided into subsets. These subsets include hydrophobic regions, hydrogen-bonding region and dividing the electrostatic potential to regions of maxima and minima. These subsets can also be surveyed energetically by a program such as GRID to identify favourable interaction sites for a large variety of functional polar groups. The software DISCO allows automatic computation of hydrogen bond accepting and bond donating sites. The combinations developed at each subset, then can be connected to generate the drug structure.

Structure-based Lead Generation :

The de novo structure-based design is also possible where the structure of the target enzyme or receptor is known. In this case, lead generation may be done both through the application of 3D searches to identify existing compounds and by the de novo design of novel structures including automated structure generation. Various element, substructure or distance range keys (based on single atoms from the functional groups or centroids, lines, planes or excluded volumes derived from the functional groups) are used in 3D searching to screen out rapidly unsuitable structures. These keys act as a very fast filter to eliminate all structures that could not possibly fill the query.

Modelling describes the generation, manipulation, and/or representation of three-dimensional structures of molecules and associated physico-chemical properties. As computers are becoming even more powerful, new methods enabling the modelling of molecular realities have been described.

(a) Molecular structure building :

One of the simplest and most reliable ways is to use libraries of typical organic fragments and the Cambridge X-ray Crystallographic Data Base, which contains about 1,25,000 structures. Several common building functions were involved in these operations. make-bond, break-bond, fuse-rings, delete-atom, add-atom-hydrogens, invert chiral center etc. The molecular structures are generated in a 3-step process. First, molecular connectivities and atom information is entered using either an interactive computer graphics template program or a user written non-graphics program. Second, EMBED, a distance geometry program is used to obtain three-dimensional co-ordinates. A novel feature of distance geometry is the use of random number generator with a uniform distribution to select the internal distances so that they lie between the upper and lower bound values. Finally, these co-ordinates are refined with molecular programs MM2 or AMBER, CONCORD has been also used to generate three-dimensional structures from two-dimensional structures stored in large industrial databases to provide confor-mations for newly developing three-dimen-sional based techniques.

(b) Molecular mechanics :

With the invent of computers in 1950s, early molecular mechanics programs were developed in 1960s for certain specific compounds. Molecular mechanics deals more with the number of atoms while quantum mechanics is concerned more with the number of orbitals.

Computational chemistry techniques are now used routinely to simulate chemical and physical properties on a computer prior to synthesis. The accuracy of these calculations is highly dependent on the accuracy of the parameters employed, the solvation model used or the completeness of the conformational search.

The traditional force fields used for structural predictions, are formulated on the basis of vast experimental data (i.e. bond lengths, bond angles and other structural/energetic data) available for organic and inorganic molecules in the form of typical small fragments.

Emperical molecular mechanics calculations utilize force fields to reproduce molecular geometries, conformational energies, torsional barriers, inter- and intramolecular interaction energies, vibrational frequencies, heats of formation and other gas-phase and condensed (i.e., solid and liquid) phase properties.

Molecular mechanics consists of a series of mathematical steps used to calculate molecular geometry, energy, vibrational spectra and other chemical (e.g. electronegativity, anomeric and Bohlmann effects) properties.

Molecular mechanics (emperical force field) expresses the potential energy mainly in terms of three main groups : non-bonded energy, electrostatic energy and intramolecular energy. The potential energy reflects the energy necessary to stretch bonds, to distort bond angles and to generate strain in the torsion angles by twisting around the bonds.

Energy terms (Parameters) of molecular mechanics can be classified as follows :

(a) **Bonding interactions :** Stretching, bending, and torsional.

(b) **Non-bonding interactions :** Dispersive attractions (Van der Waal's), dipole-dipole and charge-charge interactions.

Bonding parameters can be further subdivided into equilibrium type and force constant type parameters. Equilibrium type parameters (bond length, bond angles, etc.) can be obtained easily from X-ray, neutron or electron diffraction; parameters belonging to the force constant type can be measured by microwave and IR spectroscopy. X-ray structures are suitable for the evaluation of bond lengths and bond angles. Microwave and IR spectroscopy provide stretching and bending force constants while NMR measurements are helpful to describe torsional profiles. Among non-bonding interactions, atomic radii and E values characteristics of hardness/softness are typical van der Waal's parameters, while electrostatic interactions are usually represented by atomic charges or bond dipoles.

(A) Non-bonded energy describes the energy of interaction between two non-bonded atoms. At long distance the atoms attract each other owing to dispersion forces, whereas at short distances, there is a strong repulsion due to overlap of the atom's electronic clouds. Between the two regions there is a minimum.

Restricted rotations of molecular fragments connected through covalent bonds are qualified by torsional barriers. Dispersive attraction is usually formed between particles which do not have a dipole moment or a charge. Here the induced dipole moments are created by the distortion of electron distribution.

The electrostatic interactions depend mainly on atomic charges, the interatomic distance and a dielectric constant accounting for environmental effects. Atomic charges can be calculated by ab initio or semiempirical calculation. In addition to charges obtained from Mulliken population analysis or natural bond orbital analysis (NBO), ESP charges derived from electrostatic potential are also available. Conformational dependence of atomic charges, however, would make the calculation of electrostatics rather complicated and therefore in most force fields, this conformational effect is neglected.

In the long-range region, even electroneutral molecules exert attractive forces on each other. These forces are function of the intermolecular distances as well as of the elecronic structures. London proposed this theory of attractive forces in 1930. At any given moment, instantaneous dipoles are created because of nuclear and electronic fluctuations. These fluctuating dipoles induce dipoles in other atoms and the interaction of these two dipoles creates a net attraction.

The short-range forces are repulsive forces. When atoms are close, there is considerable overlap of their electronic clouds and these clouds are distorted owing to the Pauli exclusion principle. The net effect is a repulsion between the two atoms.

(B) Electrostatic energy mainly exists, due to the presence of highly polar groups. In such groups, the Coulomb or dipole-dipole forces are more important. They must be taken into account in conformational calculations where dielectric constant is used to explain the effect of solvent in attenuating the electrostatic interactions of charged groups in an aqueous environment.

The most widely used method for obtaining partial atomic charges is by performing a quantum mechanical calculation and doing a Mulliken population analysis. Partial atomic charges are derived by fitting to quantum mechanically calculated electrostatic potentials.

Consider a molecular force as a collection of atoms held together by elastic or harmonic forces. These forces can be described by potential energy functions of structural feature like bond length, bond angles, non-bonded interaction and so on. The combination of these potential energy function is the 'force field'. Molecular force fields help to calculate interaction energies. These equations describe both intra and inter-molecular forces including bonding, Van der Waals interactions and coulombic interactions. The energy, E, of the molecule in the force field arises from deviations from 'ideal' structural features and can be approximated by a sum of energy contributions.

$$E_{total} = E_s + E_b + E_{(w)} + E_{nb} + \ldots\ldots$$

E is sometimes called as the 'steric energy'. It is the difference in energy between the real molecule and a hypothetical molecule where all the structural values like bond lengths and bond angles are exactly at their 'ideal' or 'natural' values. E_s is the energy of a bond being stretched or compressed from its natural bond length, E_b is the energy of bending bond angles from their natural values, $E_{(w)}$ is the torsional energy due to twisting about bonds, and E_{nb} is the energy of the non-bonded interaction. If there are other intramolecular mechanisms affecting the energy, such as electrostatic (coulombic) repulsions or H-bonding, these too may be added to force field. The most extensively tested force fields are MM2 (hydrocarbons plus a limited selection of simple heteroatom functional groups), AMBER and CHARMM (peptides and nucleic acids) and ECEPP (peptides). MM2 is current standard for small-molecule work, AMBER and CHARMM force fields are similar and are the standard for macromolecules.

Since the development of MM2, the first high-performance molecular mechanics force field in 1977, several general and specialized force fields have been published.

MM4 was obtained by the complete reparameterisation of MM3 to reduce the error that comes from the neglect of inductive and hyperconjugative effect.

General force fields are meant for handling a structurally diverse set of molecules and are therefore of limited accuracy as it would require careful parameterisation based on a very large set of reference molecules. Designing of specialized force fields is promoted for the accurate calculation of a chemical limited class of compounds. The limited diversity of structural units allows precise parameterisation for structural building blocks. This concept has been used in the development of the AMBER force filed by Kollman et al in 1985.

CHARMM is parameterized for high-quality computations of a limited set of molecules on the similar lines of AMBER. Although the first version was only parameterized for amino acids and proteins, CHARMM was finally reparameterized in Hyperchem package to yield the BIO + force field. The other force field include, OPLS, ECEPP and the Merck force field (MMFF 94). The MMFF 94 is one of the most recent molecular mechanics force field developed by Tom Halgren at Merck to handle most types of structures represented in the Merck Index.

The concept of the force field originated in the first half of the twentieth century from vibrational spectroscopy, which considered the forces acting between every pair of atoms in the molecule, or in a lattice in the case of ionic crystals. A formulation which later had a significant effect on molecular modelling was that of Urey and Bradley, in which they wrote quadratic **Hooke's Law** potential equations to describe some of the harmonic vibrations in simple molecules, but found the **Morse potential** give the best fit to empirical data for bond stretching.

Class 2 Force Fields, which contain anharmonic potentials, and utilize explicit off-diagonal terms form the force constant matrix.

The **Class 3 Force Fields** will be able to model the influence of chemical effects, electronegativity, and hyperconjugation on molecular structure and properties.

(c) Molecular dynamics :

Originated in 1957, molecular dynamics simulations were first used for the study of a simple fluid made of two-dimensional hard disks and to evaluate relaxation phenomena and transport properties in liquids.

Molecular dynamics is a method of studying the motions and the configurational space of the molecule in which the time evolution or trajectory of a molecule is described by the classical Newtonian equations of motion.

The molecular dynamics method directly simulates the motions of all the molecules in the system. The system is started in an arbitrary arrangement at a temperature near absolute zero; the atoms are nearly stationary. The velocities of the atoms are then allowed to increase so that the average kinetic energy of the system is increased to correspond to the temperature of interest, such as 300 K. At this temperature, the motion of all the atoms in the system is simulated. A great deal of computer power is needed to simulate the motion even for a few nanoseconds. The simulation studies help us to understand fluctuations in the shape of the molecule and molecule-solvent rearrangements occuring to facilitate binding of a substrate. The analysis of the motions of all the molecules can provide the free energy of the system.

Molecular dynamics aims to reproudce the time-dependent motional behaviour of a molecule. In molecular dynamics simulations, the system is first partially minimized to relieve strain in the system. Then by taking small time steps and integrating the equations of motion, new forces and accelerations are calculated.

The interactions of large molecules may be understood by simulating their motions on a computer. The entropy requires knowledge of how many ways the system can change without affecting the energy; the more rearrangements (conformations) that are possible for the system, the higher the entropy and the lower the free energy. There are two methods for calculating entropy and free energy for a system by simulating the motion of the molecules : Monte Carlo and Molecular dynamics. Both are effective methods used to calculate the energies of different possible conformations of the molecule. Consider two molecules having same minimum energy. If changes in the conformations do not raise the energy much, it is flexible molecule. On the other hand, if any change in the conformation raises the energy greatly, the molecule is said to be rigid. It means the rigid molecule will have always a higher free energy than the flexible molecule.

Two kinds of molecular simulations (behaviour of molecule model as a function of time) may be performed.

(a) Monte Carlo Method.

(b) Molecular dynamics method : It produces trajectories in the configurational space and leading to both static and dynamic properties.

Monte Carlo :

In 1950 with the publication of Barton's short note on how the conformations of steroids affect their chemistry which laid the foundation of the concept, conformational analysis.

From then onward, an appreciation of the 3-D aspect became crucial for understanding of the structure, stability, conformation and reactivity. In the year 1953, a group of scientists from Los Alamos published their studies of, "equation of state calculations by fast computing machines". This work carried out on the advanced MANICAC computer, laid the ground work for computer based Monte Carlo methods, established Metropolis algorithm for simulated annealing and was the ancestor of molecular dynamics calculations.

The Monte Carlo method is named after the famous gambling city in Europe. It starts with perturbating slightly the whole conformation or a part of conformation of a large molecule step by step. After each step, calculate the change in energy. If the energy has decreased, you continue the move. If energy is higher, an algorithm is used to determine whether the new configuration is to be accepted. By repeating such moves several times, you will eventually find the lowest free energy for the molecule. The number of perturbations that do not increase the system near the minimum is a measure of the entropy. The Monte Carlo search followed by energy minimization may be used to generate pharmacophore which is further refined by energy minimization of all compounds simultaneously using the Multifit program.

In Monte Carlo technique, several million configurations are generated. Using these configurations, the average of some desired property can be calculated using following equation.

$$x = \frac{\sum_i x_i \exp(-E_i/kT)}{\sum_i \exp(-E_i/kT)}$$

where, x is the desired property, x_i is the value of the property in the configuration i, E_i is the energy of the configuration, k is the Boltzmann constant and T is the temperature.

The knowledge of the accessible structures and insight into accessible spatial relationships is gained through structures of minimum energy, dynamic trajectories of analogues (molecular dynamics) or a series of Monte Carlo configurations. This allows the chemist to judge the importance of a given conformation in interacting with the receptor. New analogues with certain conformation to enhance the stability or potency then may be synthesized.

In principle, molecular dynamics simulations can be used to describe many of the kinds of events involved in drug-receptor interactions, including the solvation and conformational changes required for initial complex formation, and any conformational or covalent rearrangements that may occur subsequent to binding. Molecular dynamics is used simply as a powerful method for generating the samples of thermally accessible molecular configurations that are needed in calculations of entropies, enthalpies and other thermodynamic quantities. The molecular dynamic calculations can be used, for example, to predict how changes in the chemical structure of a drug will change the equilibrium constant for binding to a receptor if a high resolution structure of the original drug-receptor complex is available.

Molecular dynamics produces a great many molecular conformations. Through docking studies, one can know about the number of unfavourable conformations of the drug which do not fit the receptor. This number may be drastically reduced by inserting a methyl "blocking" group or a ring constraint in the structure to prevent too much conformational freedom. The most favourable drug conformation chosen through the results of a dynamics may be subjected to molecular mechanics.

(d) Quantum mechanics :

Molecules are made of electrons and nuclei. The nuclei attract the electrons but, of course, the electrons repel each other and the nuclei repel each other. The electrons move relative to the nuclei. The balance of the forces determines the structure and the chemical reactivity of each molecule. The nuclei and electrons arrange themselves to obtain the lowest-energy possible. This produces the bonding and the electron distribution of the molecule in its most stable form. Higher energies correspond to excited states of the molecule caused by molecular collisions or by photoexcitation; these states are important in the reactions of molecules. The energies of molecules are quantized.

Quantum mechanics is necessary to describe quantized energy levels and to understand bonding and electronic orbitals of atoms and molecules. Quantum mechanics was introduced during 1930s to describe molecular and subatomic behaviour.

To understand reaction mechanisms and molecular interactions, one should know in detail about bonding, orbitals, electron distribution and charge densities. Quantum mechanics explain molecular interactions in terms of electron distribution and motion.

The nuclei of atoms may be treated as particles with wavelengths that are very much shorter than those of the lighter and faster electrons. The Schrodinger equation may be solved by using widely available ab initio programs and an ever increasing computation power. The Schrodinger equation assigns an amplitude ψ to the electron wave which is known as the wavefunction of the system. It helps to calculate the average position of the electron and its energy in each electronic state. The energy of the electron tells us whether the

molecule is stable and what is stable bond distance is. From the wavefunctions, measurable properties can be calculated. These properties are functions of the positions and moments of the electrons and nuclei in the molecule. The electron distribution determines what is the most stable configuration or geometry of the molecule besides bond lengths, force constants and bond angles.

Calculation of electronic properties implicated in physical and chemical reactions of drugs with their biological environment can only be done using quantum mechanical methods. In addition, calculation of energy conformational profiles and intermolecular interactions in a variety of contexts are best done using quantum mechanical methods. In principle, the exact solution of the Schrodinger equation, where H is the Hamilltonian operator, y is the wave function and E is the energy of the system, would yield a complete description of a molecular system.

$$H_y = E_y$$

The Schrodinger equation of a given molecular system can be solved either with no approximations at all (ab initio) or with the introduction of some approximations (semi-empirical). In most ab initio methods, all electrons are explicitly included. Ab initio method has the advantage of not requiring any parameterization and therefore can be used for all type of systems.

It is also much easier to identify failings of these methods and improve them in a conceptually consistent and even-handed way. In Semi-empirical method, only valence electrons are explicitly included, some integrals are neglected and others are approximated by parameters derived from experiment. The selection of the most appropriate method depends not only on the size of molecule but also on the type of molecular property (e.g. conformation, electron density, electrostatic potential, frontier orbitals etc.) that is derived.

Quantum mechanics defines the behaviour of nuclei and electrons. The quantum mechanics is based on the Schrodinger equation. The wavefunction derived from Schrodinger equation, contains all the information needed to describe the properties of atomic and molecular systems.

Besides the classical Schrodinger equation method, certain semi-empirical methods may also be used to calculate the wavefunctions of valence electrons only. These include,

(a) Extended Huckel Method.

(b) Complete Neglect of Differential Overlap (CNDO) Method.

(c) Intermediate Neglect of Differential Overlap (INDO) Method.

(d) Modified Intermediate Neglect of Differential Overlap (MINDO) Method.

(e) Neglect of Diatomic Differential Overlap (NDDO) Method.

(f) Modified NDDO (MNDO) Method.

Semi-empirical treatments such as AMI, MNDO, CNDO, INDO, EHT, MINDO, PRDDO and PCILO are some of the most popular semi-empirical programs, whereas the GAUSSIAN and HONDO series are typical ab initio programs. AMPAC and MOPAC are QCPE packages that include the AMI, MNDO and MINDO programs. Along with GAUSSIAN series these are among the most popular programs for quantum mechanical calculations. Quantum chemical calculations can provide detail insight into the electronic nature of the molecular structure.

Quantum mechanics offers a much better description of electronic structure than molecular mechanics can ever do. Energy of the highest occupied molecular orbital represents charge distributions in a molecule. Quantum mechanics helps in the electrostatic potential energy evaluation directly using the wave function as opposed to using the point charges extracted from the wave function. If one computes this energy at the points generated from a molecular surface calculations, the resulting colour-coded surface can be displayed. The surfaces of drug and receptor protein can be visually compared and evaluated. The optimal docked orientation will be that in which the two surfaces are optimally complementary in shape and charge distribution.

(e) Conformational analysis :

The energy treatment in this approach to QSAR resembles a linear free energy model or Free-Wilson analysis; the added feature is the geometric constraints during the fitting of the data so that the ultimate outcome is a geometric interpretation of the biological activity. In the distance geometry approach, one constructs a geometry of the receptor site from the drug molecular structure and subsequently evaluates the interaction energy matrix so that the given binding mode for each molecule is its optimal binding mode. The method generally focus on the comparison of chemically similar analogues, where it is clear that a substantial subset of the atoms of one drug molecule match corresponding subsets in the other molecule. In reality, however drug molecules bind in whatever orientation and internal conformation will minimize the drug-receptor-solvent system. The distance geometry calculations directly simulate this search for the most favorable binding mode and rather similar compounds may bind quite differently.

Starting from an arbitrary initial conformation, a specified number of attempts, N, are made to generate a random ligand conformation. In each attempt, all rotatable bonds are subjected to a quasi-random change in torsion angle. The possible values for change in torsion angle about a bond are based on the total number of rotating atoms.

The initial docking of the ligand is obtained by alignment of the principal axes of the ligand to the principal axes of the site. There are four possible orientations to be considered. There are two energy terms in the expression for the dock energy, internal energy of the ligand and the interaction energy of the ligand with the protein. The interaction energy is taken as the sum of the Van der Waals energy and elecrostatic energy.

The RMS calculation takes topological symmetry into account and automatically associates atom pairs between the X-ray structure and the docked structure to report the best RMS for all possible topologically equivalent pairings.

(f) Physical properties :

Theoretical calculations can provide a number of indices that may not be directly related to experimental data but that can be very useful since they carry high physical information content. For example, electron densities are useful because they provide a good basis for the stereoelectronic properties of either isolated or interacting molecules. Molecular electrostatic potentials are usually generated from the partial atomic charges derived from a quantum mechanical calculation. Other properties can be calculated by empirical methods; the most popular are the prediction of log P (octanol/water partition coefficient) and molar refractivity.

(g) Distance Geometry :

Distance geometry refers to the study of geometric problems with an emphasis on distance between points. The use of interatomic distances or atomic co-ordinates as representative of molecular shape is common in 3D QSAR. Distance geometry permits both, the projection of important interatomic distances in the ligand molecule and postulates the critical intermolecular binding distances in ligand-receptor interaction. It has been used extensively to generate molecular structurs from NMR data, for NOESY cross-peaks can be translated into distance constraints. Distance geometry is also used to search the conformational space of the ligand by specifying artificial constraints.

Approaches to Molecular Docking
Shape Complementarity Methods :

Geometric matching/shape comple-mentarity methods include molecular surface/complementary surface descriptors. In this case, the receptor's molecular surface is described in terms of its solvent-accessible surface area and the ligand's molecular surface is described in terms of its matching surface description. Another approach is to describe the hydrophobic features of the protein using turns in the main-chain atoms. Whereas, the shape complementarity based approaches are typically fast and robust, they cannot usually model the movements or dynamic changes in the ligand/protein conformations accurately, although complementarity methods are much more amenable to pharmacophore based approaches, since they use geometric descriptions of the ligands to find optimal binding.

Simulation Processes :

In this approach, the protein and the ligand are separated by some physical distance, and the ligand finds its position into the protein's active site after a certain number of "moves" in its conformational space. The moves incorporate rigid body transformations such as translations and rotations, as well as internal changes to the ligand's structure including torsion angle rotations. Each of these moves in the conformation space of the ligand induces a total energetic cost of the system, and hence after every move the total energy of the system is calculated. This process is physically closer to what happens in reality, when the protein and ligand approach each other after molecular recognition.

The success of a docking program depends on two components; the search algorithm and the scoring function.

The Search Algorithm :

The search space consists of all possible orientations and conformations of the protein paired with the ligand. This would involve enumerating all possible distortions of each molecule and all possible rotational and translational orientations of the ligand relative to the protein. Each "snapshot" of the pair is referred to as **Pose.**

The Scoring Function :

The scoring function takes a pose as input and returns a number indicating the likelihood that the pose represents a favourable binding interaction.

Most scoring functions are physics based molecular mechanics force fields that estimate the energy of the pose, a low (negative) energy indicates a stable system and thus a likely binding interaction.

Global energy optimization can be accomplished using simulated annealing, the Metropolis algorithm and other Monte Carlo methods or using different deterministic methods of discrete or continuous optimization. The main aim of optimization methods is finding the lowest energy conformation of a molecule or identifying a set of low-energy comformers that are in equilibrium with each other. The force field represents only the enthalpic component of free energy, and only this component is included during energy minimization.

Other applications of MM include potential energy mapping and ligand docking simulations.

MM implements more 'static' energy minimization methods to study the potential energy surfaces of different molecular system. However, MM can also provide important dynamic parameters, such as energy barriers between different conformers or steepness of a potential energy surface around a local minimum. MD and MM are usually based on the same classical force fields. But MD may also be based on quantum chemical methods like DFT.

Modelling Drug-Receptor Interactions

The interactions of macromolecular receptors and their small molecule ligands is an essential step in many biological process: regulatory mechanisms, the pharmacological action of drugs, the toxic effect of certain chemicals etc. Drug-receptor 'docking' is typically done interactively with molecular surface displays (e.g. 'extra radius' surface) used to guide the fit, based on hydrophobic or electrostatic potential colour coding.

The contact surface is defined as the surface where the distance between the molecules is smaller than a given threshold.

Note that, we shall usually try to achieve a contact surface which is 'large enough' instead of `maximal' and that we usually try to maximize not the size of the contact surface but a score measuring the quality of the proposed docking solutions.

Molecular docking can be thought of as a problem of *"lock-and-key"*. There can be potentially multiple "keys" (ligands of various sizes including may be other proteins themselves) that can bind to the same protein. Molecular docking describe the "best-fit" ligand that binds to a particular protein of interest.

The optimization problem for molecular docking is twofold; finding an optimal geometry (shape complementarity) in which the protein and ligand fit together and finding an optimal energy which minimizes the energy, while maximizing the entropy of the overall system.

While detailed structural information about the receptor is not available, a model must be deduced from the ligands that bind it. A number of statistical methods like Hansch analysis and distance geometry, are commonly used to predict characteristics of a site by relating the selected structural properties of active compounds to their biological activities. For example, the shape of a binding site on a macro-molecular receptor is represented as a set of over-lapping spheres. Each ligand is divided into small set of large rigid fragments that are docked separately into the binding site and then rejoined later in the calculation. The division of ligands into separate fragments allows a degree of flexibility at the position that joins them. The rejoined fragments are then energy minimized in the receptor site. In addition, free energy perturbation methods offer the exciting possibility of calculating accurate differences in binding free energies between related ligands, which could make it possible to predict the binding affinity of new compounds prior to synthesis.

Designing Ligands to Fit a Specific Macromolecule Site :

As far as direct drug design is concerned, full interactive control over the position (translation and rotation along the x, y and z co-ordinate axes) and conformation (adjustment of torsion angles) in both the macromolecule and the ligand(s) should be simultaneously available. Good torsion angle adjustments are essential, specially where most of the time is spent in interactive modelling. The system should be capable of handling several molecules simultaneously to enable the comparison of different ligands in the binding site or different fits of the same ligand. The system should also include the option to calculate fast Van der Walls surfaces, which are useful for surfacing small molecules and small portions of a macromolecule. The other approach is usually to design and build the ligand piece by piece in the binding site by combining three-dimensional fragments from a library. Small molecules can be built very rapidly in this way and the resulting structures are usually accurate enough for initial fitting or 'docking' into the site model.

Plausible docking sites are cavities in the surface of the receptor. Computer graphics enables us to qualitatively visualize drug receptor-interactions and molecular mechanics can provide rough estimates of the interaction energy, which allows to design molecules that are apparently complementary to a binding site.

An enumeration on the rotations of one of the molecules (usually smaller one) is performed. For each rotations :

- Calculate the surface and volume cells of the molecule.

- Assuming that there is at least one pair of surface cells (one from each molecule) that are matched during the transformation, an enumeration on all of these pairs is performed. For each pair the transformation is calculated and it is evaluated by checking the directions of the normals, the number of surface-to-surface matches and the number of penetrations.

- The good transformations are those who have a small number of penetrations and a lot of surface-to-surface matches.

This is done first in low resolution and the best results are calculated again in fine resolution with the addition of an approximated energetic score. The approximated energetic score is calculated according to the number of "favourable"' and "unfavourable" interactions.

For example, it is unfavourable that an atom with positive charge is placed near another atom with positive charge, but it is favourable if two atoms are adjacent if one of them is an H-donor and the other is an H-acceptor.

The main goal of the Molecular Modelling Facility is to provide investigators advanced tools and services regarding sequence analysis, protein structure prediction, molecular docking and graphics.

The facility provides the following services :

- Protein sequence analysis, including database search, simple sequence alignment, profile-profile sequence alignment, multiple sequence alignment, phylogenetic trees, secondary structure prediction, transmembrane segment prediction.

- Sequence-structure alignment editing, using an integrative approach that takes into account the secondary structure prediction and the secondary structure of the template protein.

- Homology modelling resulting in the building of three-dimensional models for the proteins of interest, including side-chain and loop conformation prediction.

- This technique is also used in the identification of unknown binding sites when the ligand is known or to search for small inhibitory molecules against a known binding site.

- Advanced molecular graphics for an effective representation of complicated three-dimensional structural information.

- Model interpretation and experiment design contributes to the interpretation of the experimental data in terms of structure-function relationship and also to the design of experiments involving loss of function and changes in the affinity and specificity of binding sites.

Molecular Similarity in Drug Design :

Drug Design is a multifaceted discipline where molecular similarity is one important tool to dig out new ideas for design. Molecular similarity involves the process of searching the features of similarity in a set of flexible and dissimilar active molecules and use that informtion to design novel drug molecules. Similarity, may be searched for bonding patterns, atomic positions, conformations, electrostatic potential, shape and spatial display of molecule or molecular properties. The result is usually expressed by a similarity coefficient. A least-square fit method is used to find the optimal superimposition for each acceptable combination. Apparently a lower root mean square (rms) deviation between the structures so matched, reveals the better correspondence. The superimpositions so generated by matching programs can be used directly to predict pharmacophore. This pharmacophore with a distance matrix between pharmacophoric points, then can be used to search a 3D structural database for novel structures that fit the query.

The shape of a molecule is represented by its Van der Waals volume. The degree of molecular shape change, that is possible if a molecule is related to the number and position of the rotatable bonds. Rotation and translation of one molecule relative to the other is performed. Many softwares are developed that allow electrostatic potential comparisons of conformationally frozen structures of drugs containing bioisosters.

The atom correspondences or functional group similarities revealed through similarity studies, are usually expressed as points in space with associated properties. A distance matrix is constructed between the points. Alternatively, a novel structure with similar shape may be constructed through a space filling network of bonds with appropriate angles and bond lengths to create molecular skeletons without atomic identities. Rotation and translation of one molecule relative to the other is performed. This matrix we call an envelope in which structurally diverse ligands can be generated. Automated structure generation is also possible if the matrix with complementary shape and electrostatic properties is generated. Atoms may then be incorporated into this network to create molecules with the desired similar

properties. The optimization can be achieved by annealing an atom placement procedure from a small library of acyclic and aromatic pieces of combinations of atoms from the set. Not all the molecular surface of the ligand is involved in activation of the receptor site. Hence, optimization of the 'active' surface is critical to yield a novel drug structure.

The properties of a molecule are intimately linked to the 3D structures or conformations that it can adopt. Consideration of the conformational properties (i.e. the energy of a given conformation) of a molecule is therefore essential in any drug design method.

The hypothesis, 'similarity in behaviour implies similarity in structure' highlights the importance of the comparison of structural characteristics in QSAR. Computer graphics allows automated detection of the degree of overlap between given molecular shapes and the common patterns. If molecules to be compared are not closely related, it sometimes becomes difficult to decide how to superimose such ligands to identify common binding interactions with the receptor involved. Molecular similarity studies are also useful to screen large 3D databases in the search of leads containing desired structural features.

Detection and evaluation of the similarity between "structural shapes" (steric complimentarity) and "electronic shapes" (electronic characteristics such as electrostatic potential or electron distribution) are more useful than structural similarity in realistic comparison of chemical or biological activity.

Steric fit plays an important role in recognizing "lock-and-key" models of molecular interactions involved in pharmacophore identification. Encoded or coloured surfaces with reference to the value of property such as electrostatic potential and hydrophobicity may be used to obtain a better insight to judge chemical complementarity. The Van der Waals contour (or volume) gives a good estimate of the molecular shape for small molecules.

Feature-based Docking and Shape or Similarity-based Docking :

Ligand feature - based docking works by analyzing the active site of a protein to obtain a representation of the optimal locations of ligand features. Such as hydrogen bond donors, acceptors and hydrophobic regions. You may just look only docking poses that overlay the ligand features onto the optimal positions in the active site. In general, shape-based docking methods involve characterizing the shape of the active site and generating ligand poses that are complementary to the shape of the receptor surface. The Ligand Fit docking procedure consists of two parts : (1) cavity detection to identify and select the region of the protein as the active site for docking; and (2) docking ligands to a selected site. Three-dimensional regular grids of points are employed for site detection and also for estimating the interaction energy of the ligand with the protein during docking.

Electronic Properties :

Electronic properties are used to predict the chemical behaviour of the compound. These properties include molecular orbitals, electron densities, electrostatic potentials and electric fields. Electrostatic potential can be determined experimentally by X-rays diffraction or electron diffraction techniques. It can be used to predict the regions and sites of the substrate which are most reactive towards protonation or an electrophilic attack. The sites of addition will be those having electrostatic potential minima. Similarly, a nucleophile will be

added in the region having electrostatic potential maxima. Various ways of representation of electrostatic potential on computer include :

(i) Contour levels in selected planes.

(ii) Coloured area maps where areas between successive contour levels in a plane are coloured as a function of the electrostatic potential.

(iii) Colour coded dots on the Connally molecular surface.

(iv) Mapping of electrostatic potential value onto solid models of electron density isosurfaces or of molecular surfaces.

(v) Isoenergy surfaces represented as wire-frame or solid models.

Besides these, other useful molecular properties derived from the ground state wavefunction of a given compound include, superdelocalizability and average local ionization energy. The former defines how tightly the electrons are held by the molecule at any point. While the latter defines the average energy needed to ionize an electron at any point. Both properties may be used as alternatives to electrostatic potential to correlate with pKa values or ring aromaticity.

Simulated Annealing :

Simulated annealing is a method used for exploring the conformational space of the given drug structure to identify minimum energy conformations. Annealing is a widely used technique by which a substance is first heated until it melts and then the temperature is slowly lowered until it crystallizes into a perfect lattice. A careful control during the temperature lowering spread over a long time-interval is required at the phase transition from liquid to solid. This is essential to produce a crystal free of any defect. The perfect lattice corresponds to the minimum of the global free energy. Simulated annealing is the computer aided annealing used to find out a global minimum energy conformation for molecules having considerable degrees of torsional freedom. Thus, it can be treated as a serial optimization procedure which is thermodynamically motivated. Representative conformers for each compound can be obtained from a cluster analysis of thousands of conformers generated by simulated annealing. Recently two new improved techniques have been introduced. These include very fast simulated annealing, VFSA and annealing with simplex optimization.

Kinetic energy is directly related to the temperature of the system. High temperature moelcular dynamics based on simulated annealing is a commonly used technique to find a small set of very different conformers to represent conformational space of each molecule in the given set.

Neural Networks :

Many of the similarity tools are used in drug design to express similarity; the most useful being pattern recognition techniques. Neural networks are the outcome of artificial intelligence research. In recent years, neural networks have received a great deal of attention and are being explored as one of the greatest computational tools for similarity ranking.

Silicon chip or a single microprocessor may be used as an artificial equivalent to a biological neuron. Using such a set of artificial neurons, neuronal networks are constructed and connected with each other through their input and output connections. As the biological neuronal networks learn from input (information) received from their environment, similar learning patterns are induced in artificial neuronal networks to train them to respond to surrounding environment. Networks trained in this way are often referred to as supervised network. The type of network used in similarity and structure activity relationship studies is known as back-propagation networks or multilayer feed forward networks.

Comparative Molecular Field Analysis (CoMFA) :

Biological activity of any molecule is a consequence of its 3D shape, size and geometry. However, the 3D structures of drugs are not given adequate representation in the classical QSAR methods developed by Hansch, Free Wilson, Martin, Topliss etc. As both the drug and the receptor has 3D structures, the use of 3D-QSAR approaches would furnish better information about the drug-receptor interactions. Comparative Molecular Field Analysis (CoMFA) is one of such 3D-QSAR method developed by Dick Crammer et al in 1988.

Biological activity is especially sensitive to spatially localized differences in molecular field intensities. The concept of identifying those critical local differences by sampling field intensities on a Cartesian lattice is the main basis of CoMFA.

Bioactive conformations of each compound in the given series are superimposed to define the orientation and binding mode. When all the compounds are superimposed, they are located in a grid box for calculating interaction energies with various probes at each lattice point. The probe may be any chemical unit like, small molecule such as water or a functional group like methyl. Computer-assisted modelling of solvation effects helps us to investigate the ionization state and intermolecular H-bonding ability of the drug molecules which in turn affects conformational preferences. CoMFA then identifies the important regions in three-dimensional space by calculating and comparing the steric and electrostatic fields around the molecules. Thus, each CoMFA descriptor column in data table contains the magnitude of either steric or electrostatic field exerted by the atoms in the tabulated molecules on a probe atom located at a point in Cartesian space. Thus, when all compounds have been processed, each row of the resulting table will describe the fields exerted by a particular conformation of a molecule on any surrounding atoms. Because this table usually has many more CoMFA steric and electrostatic descriptors than compounds, standard multiple regression is not possible. Hence, the important features related to the biological activity are extracted by partial least-suares statistical analysis. Interpretation of the results of statistical analysis will help in design and forecasting the actvity of unknown compounds.

In CoMFA, molecular fields are used as descriptors in regression models. Lennard-Jones potentials and electrostatic potentials against simple probe ions are used as steric fields and electrostatic fields respectively. Hydrophobic fields, intersection volume field, molecular lipophilic potential etc. may also be used.

The results of CoMFA are in equation showing the contribution of energy fields at each lattice point.

All the compounds in the series under consideration should share the same binding mode and mechanism of action. Similarly, possible conformational changes of the receptor are presumed to be equivalent among all the compounds. The compounds chosen should have maximum variance and minimum colinearity (interdependence) in their hydrophobic, electrostatic and steric properties. In practice minimum three probes are employed : a steric probe, a positive-charge probe and a negative charge probe. Although there is no restriction on the number of probes to be chosen, the probes so selected should atleast reflect the field characteristics at the major binding sites present on the receptor. Lastly, the success of CoMFA approach depends on the establishment of the bioactive conformations which can be obtained from X-ray crystallography or NMR spectroscopy. However, since the bioactive conformation is not necessarily the same as that in the crystal state (X-ray crystallography), in solution (NMR spectroscopy) or at the energy minimum, many conformations near the global minimum energy conformation may be considered as a possible bioactive conformation. DISCO, CATALYST and APEX-3D are some of the software programs used to find the bioactive conformation of molecules. DISCO has been integrated into the SYBYL molecular modelling program. All these softwares attempt to find sets of features common to low energy conformations of each compound. These features include ring centers, hydrophobic regions, and hydrogen-bonding sites.

Comparative Molecular Field Analysis (CoMFA) is currently the method of choice in 3D-QSAR studies as it correlates the two major interactions, i.e., electrostatic and steric interactions, with bioactivity through a Partial Least Square (PLS) analysis (Cramer et al., 1988). Comparative Molecular Similarity Index Analysis (CoMSIA) is a similar technique, in that it only replaces the original interaction field calculation function with Gaussian type functions to avoid extreme values in interaction fields (Klebe et al., 1994). GOLPE (Baroni et al., 1993) is an alternative method that performs multivariate analysis based on interaction fields generated by GRID (Pastor et al., 2000).

It explains the gradual changes in observed biological properties by evaluating the electrostatic (Coulombic interactions) and steric (Van der Walls interactions) fields at regularly spaced grid points surrounding a set of mutually aligned ligands for a specific target protein.

The colour scheme which he established is still widely used today, with occasional variations: white for hydrogen, black for carbon, red for oxygen, blue for nitrogen and green for chlorine.

Yellowish-green for fluorine, light green for chlorine, midgreen for bromine, dark green for iodine, yellow for sulfur, purple for phosphours, black or gray for silicon, and brown, silver or gold for metals.

Contour Plots :

The results of CoMFA may also be displayed as contour plots showing the regions in space where specific molecular properties increase or decrease the potency. The contours are coloured in green and yellow for positive and negative steric effects respectively while blue and red for positive and negative electrostatic effects respectively. Positive steric contours define the region where substituent size is proportional to biological activity and the negative steric contours highlight the area where substituents decrease the potency. The positive electrostatic contours show the regions where positive charges increase the potency whereas in negative electrostatic contours regions, negative charges increase the potency.

Pharmacophore Mapping :

The pharmacophore is often described only by a set of distance constraints between atom centers or centroids of a defined environment (normally hydrogen bond acceptor/donar, acidic, basic, aromatic ring / hydrophobic centroid). A pharmacophore highlights the set of "features" a compound must have to elicit a certain biological activity.

The program DOCK, developed at the University of California, San Francisco identifies molecules that are complementary in shape and chemical interactions to a user-supplied receptor structure.

The hardest task to ask of a docking computation is to predict the best binding geometry of a ligand, for this involves assessing the relative free energy of several alternative binding modes.

Many structure based approaches involve the combination of developing a phamacophore hypothesis and then searching 2D or 3D databases. The pharmacophore may be derived from crystallographic information of the binding site or from superimposition of a lead molecule on the NMR structures of peptides in solution. Variety of programs including Chem DBS-3D, ALLADIN UNITY, MACCS-3D, CATALYST, CAVEAT, CSD (Cambridge Structural Database), etc. are used for quick searching of a database of 3D structures.

Both known and novel binding sites can be identified through automated procedures, such as negative imaging approach used with DOCK. The potential pharmacophore points such as hydrogen bond acceptors or donars, positively charged atoms and aromatic ring centroids may be identified. The distances between pairs of these points (distance keys) and data on the number, types and interpoint connectivity (formula keys) may be used as guidelines for pharmacophore mapping. Pharmacophore mapping attempts to find features important for receptor binding. Tracing of pharmacophore pattern in large, more complicated structure can be done by investigating the full structure part by part. Alternatively, the use of structurally rigid molecules (i.e. conformationally restrained analogues) is preferred to probe requirements for receptor binding. Occassionally, there may be several binding modes with similar energy that may be difficult to distinguish.

Pharmacophore mapping may be used for de novo compound design. In the program, NEWLEAD, key fragments from bioactive conformations are joined with spacers to generate new structure to fit the model. While the program SPROUT helps to join the templates, such as five and six-membered rings and acyclic fragments to mimic pharmacophore model.

QSAR analysis is applied to structure-activity data sets only in such cases where molecular geometry of a common receptor is unknown. If the receptor geometry is known, intermolecular locking is usually performed to the exclusion of a QSAR analysis.

Through multiple linear regression analysis, QSAR helps to develop functional relations between biological activity and 2D/3D physico-chemical molecular properties.

The affinity of two molecules that form a non-covalent complex is described by the overall change in the free energy of the system. The system consists of the molecules and solvent (before complex formation) and the complex and solvent. Free energy is the total energy of the system and includes both enthalpy and entropy.

The types of interaction energies important in drug (ligand)-receptor interactions include,

(a) Intramolecular ligand conformational energy.

(b) Ligand solvation energy.

(c) Intramolecular receptor conformational energy.

(d) Receptor solvation energy.

(e) Solvent reorganization energy.

(f) Intermolecular ligand-receptor energy.

All above contributions to free energy of binding can be calculated separately and they are additive.

Any 2D/3D QSAR will not be meaningful unless it accommodates or represents all above types of interaction energies.

Molecular Shape Analysis (MSA) :

When bioactive conformation of each compound in the series is superimposed on one another, the resulting Common Overlap Steric Volume (COSV) is the basis of measuring molecular shape similarity. Attempts were also made to include the thermodynamic and electronic descriptor in conjunction with COSV to develop QSAR equations.

The combination of the equations and parameters in the mathematical formulation that define the potential energy surface of a molecule is referred to as the force field (molecular mechanics). MM_1 was developed in 1970 and MM_2 was developed in the 1980. The MM_3 hydrocarbon force field is introduced in 1989 with an additional ability to calculate vibrational frequencies over MM_2. Many mechanical and chemical properties of molecules have been incorporated in the new MM_4 program introduced in 1996 by Allinger and coworkers.

Summary : In cases where a known X-ray ligand-protein complex is available, the docked ligand structure may also be used to define the active site. A Monte Carlo conformational search procedure is used for generating candidate ligand docking conformations. A shape comparison filter is then used to evaluate each ligand conformation against the active site shape. Ligand conformations satisfying the shape comparison filter are initially docked into the active site via a shape alignment protocol based on principal axes and moments. These intial poses are further refined via a grid-based energy calculation which rapidly evaluates protein-ligand interaction energies.

Theoretical prediction of the association of flexible ligands with protein receptors requires efficient sampling of the conformational space of a flexible ligand, a sufficiently accurate energy function and an efficient way to account for the receptor flexibility. Monte Carlo methods allow to increase the sampling efficiency by making larger conformational rearrangements.

Deformations of the backbone may still be crucial to docking with detailed atomic models. An adequate simulation of the backbone flexibility simultaneously with the ligand docking is still out of reach for the current computational approach. To some extent, softening the potential or using an approximate grid potential, which is less steep than the realistic Van der Waals repulsion, may be a practical way of overcoming this problem.

Discovering new lead compounds through virtual screening of chemical databases targeting protein structures has shown great promise. Several virtual screening programs have been developed with primarily two parts varying : scoring functions and searching (optimizing) methods. Of the available docking programs, the most widely used are GOLD FlexX, AutoDock, and DOCK. For any docking method, the primary criteria are docking accuracy (RMSD i.e.; Root Mean Square Displacement to known pose), scoring accuracy (prediction of the absolute binding free energy), screening efficiency (discrimination of active hits from random compounds), and computational speed (full conformation and orientation searching time).

'There are two parts to the docking problem : developing a scoring function / energy function that can discriminate correctly or near-correctly docked orientations from incorrectly docked and developing a search method that will be able to find a near-correctly docked orientation with reasonable likelihood. The simplest, yet still powerful, scoring function is shape complementarity. To use this, it is necessary to describe the surface shape of the protein. This may be done by discretising the molecule onto a grid in space and considering which cells ('voxels') are occupied, or by using some sort of 'surfacing algorithm', which calculates the solvent-accessible or solvent-excluded surface and a point set that triangulates it. The triangulation reflects the geometry of the surface : surface critical points (extrema), normals and curvature.

Some 'softening' of the energy function is required otherwise, even in near-native dockings these overwhelm the complementarity that remains. However, this softening necessarily reduces the capacity of the energy function to discriminate the correctly docked orientation from incorrect dockings, producing the many false positives that bedevil docking algorithms.

One widely used technique in the first stage of docking is the Fast Fourier Transform (FFT) method. This approach was first used in molecular docking by Katchalsik-Katzir, Vakser and co-workers. It has proved successful in blind trials of protein docking. More recently, it has been used in the program DOT and in work on identifying binding sites.

Docking algorithms, first suggested in 1978, operate on the atomic co-ordinates of two individual proteins usually considered as rigid bodies and generate a large number of candidate association modes between them. These candidates are then ranked by using various criteria, used independently or in combination. The criteria generally include geometric and chemical complementarity measures, electrostatics, H-bonding interactions and solvation, and use empirical potentials or database derived functions.

A sizeable fraction of the procedures uses a cubic grid representation of the protein surface and fast Fourier transform search algorithms. Another involves alternative representations of the protein models and different algorithms for sampling interaction modes, which include geometric hashing, Monte Carlo, genetic algorithm and Molecular or Brownian-type, mechanics procedures.

More recent methods make increasing use of composite scoring functions, which involve contributions from H-bonds, electrostatics and solvation.

Hardware

The purpose of Computer Aided Drug Design is mainly to propose models displaying the three dimensional structure of drug molecules and the target site. Evaluating shape or electronic complemantarity, conformational flexibility and adaptation processes in molecular recognition allow us to simulate the complex and intimate interaction mechanisms leading to receptor recognition and its activation.

Energy calculations can predict the interaction between the drug and its target site. This procedure is called locking. The interaction energies are calculated as the molecules are brought near each other. The molecules are rotated and moved relative to each other to find a minimum energy orientation. The interaction energy is the net difference between the energy when the two molecules are locked together and the energy of each molecule separately.

Molecular docking defines the binding modes of two interacting molecules depending upon their topographic (3D) features or energy based consideration.

Ligand docking has become a typical computational task where a series of small molecules from a 3D database are docked into the active site of an enzyme. Ligand docking is usually carried out in two or three stages : quick, preliminary docking using one of the fast docking algorithms such as DOCK, followed by simple energy minimization or a full conformational search to find the most favourable binding conformations.

The objective of molecular docking is to obtain the lowest free energy structure(s) for the receptor-ligand complex. The most systematic approach is to search through all binding orientations of all conformations of the ligand and receptor. Sometimes the largest rigid fragment in a molecule is docked and the rest of the molecule is attached while exploring conformational choices.

The activity of a drug molecule is directly linked with the stability of its complex with the target protein. The stability of this complex is measured by the binding free energy.

For chemical information systems the choice of a computer is generally larger and many packages run on VAX, IBM or PRIME machines. Generally, IBM proves to have larger disk spaces and faster input output (I/O) operations on disks. The response time is a key point hence to avoid bad response times due to computer overload there is tendency to use dedicated computers. This is the case with molecular modelling, which needs batch runs for several hours (if not days), with few I/O interruptions, for which fast response time is a must. Stand alone workstations (SUN, APOLLO, SILICON GRAPHICS) running with the UNIX operating systems, are now providing impressive graphics possibilities and computational power.

Wiberg employed computer force field calculations to address conformational analysis in 1965. He developed a steepest descent algorithm as a scheme for geometry optimization.

In 1971, Lee and Richards described the molecular surface in the context of protein structure and provided an algorithm to derive it. In 1972, Wiberg and Boyd presented an algorithm for exploring conformational interconversions based on systematic modifications of torsional angle.

The 1974 saw the first report of computer aided molecular modelling of oligosaccharides from the Lemieux group.

In 1979, Marshall extended the 2-D approach to QSAR by explicitly considering the conformational flexibility of a series as reflected by their 3-D shape. The first step of the Active Analogue Approach was to exhaustively search the conformations of a compound which was highly active in a particular biological assay.

Once the, "Active conformation" was determined, molecular volume for each molecule was calculated and superimposed. Regression analysis of the volumes was used to establish a relationship to biological activity. Marshall and co-workers commercialized the Active Analogue Approach along with other drug design techniques in the SYBYL molecular modelling program.

Hopfinger and co-workers also used 3-D shape in QSAR. In molecular shape analysis of the Baker Triazines, the common space shared by all molecules of a series and the differences in their potential energy fields were computed. When these calculations were combined with a set of rules for overlapping the series, comparative indicies of the shape of different molecules were obtained. Inclusion of these shape descriptors in standard Hansch analysis schemes lead to improve descriptions relating computed parameters to biological activity such that no compounds in the original data set had to be eliminated from the calculations. The techniques developed by Hopfinger and co-workers were made available in the CAMSEQ, CAMSEQ-II, CHEMLAB and CAMSEQ-M computer programms. The early 1980's saw the beginning of the personal computer industry and the consequent increase in the accessibility of computers in general, and the use of the Graphical User Interface (GUI). At about same time, the development of high quality real-time colour graphics and Connolly's molecular surface program contributed to the rapid evolution of this technique.

In 1988, Richard Cramer proposed that biological activity could be analyzed by relating the shape-dependent steric and electrostatic fields for molecules to their biological activity. Additionally, rather than limiting the analysis to fitting data to a regression line, CoMFA (Comparative Molecular Field Analysis) utilized new methods of data analysis, PLS (Partial Least Squares) and crossvalidation, to develop models for activity predictions.

In 1985, Peter Good ford has reported an energy based grid approach for compound design. The GRID program is a computational procedure for detecting energetically favorable binding sites on molecules of known structure. GRID has also been used to distinguish between selective binding sites for different probes.

ExtHuckel is a semi-empirical quantum mechanical computation that solves the Schroedinger equation to predict the distribution of electrons in a molecule.

Results are added to the molecule file and can be converted to generate molecular orbitals, electron density or electrostatic potential. MOPAC is a comprehensive semi-empirical quantum mechanical computational tool. It can search for an optimized geometry and compute molecular properties such as bond order, partial charges, orbital energies, and vibrational spectra. MOPAC also has interesting options that find and characterize transition states and reaction pathways.

ZINDO is a semi-empirical tool that includes a method for computing spectroscopic properties (UV-visible spectra) and a method of computing molecular geometries. ZINDO is unique in that it includes the transition metals in its parameterized elements. Like MOPAC, the more computing power you have, the better ZINDO perform.

Within the past 10 years, so much has occurred that it is difficult to sort out which advances will truly stand out overtime. It has been predicted that the class 3 Force Fields will be able to model the influence of chemical effects, electro negativity and hyper conjugation on molecular structure and properties.

Another ongoing trend is the development and implementation of virtual reality for molecular modelling.

In one recent report stereo lithography is used to translate computer-designed structures into physical models. Another recent patent claims the preparation by stereo lithography of a physical model of an inhibitor plus part of receptor, guided by use of modelling software.

Molecular Modelling :

- 1860-Structural stereochemistry first considered (structural formulae used)
- 1874-Tetrahedral carbon discovered by Van't Hoff.
- 1953-Barton introduces conformational analysis.
- 1958-3D structure of myoglobin solved by X-ray crystallography.
- 1959-Drieding stick models developed.
- 1965-CPK space-filling models developed.
- 1970-Computer models began to be used. They are basically mathematically representations / models of molecules and properties such as :
  - Atomic positions (cartesian co-ordinates, internal co-ordinates - bond lengths, angles, and torsions).
  - Molecular surfaces are mathematical functions based on atomic position and atomic radii.
  - Energies are sets of equations involving atomic distances, atom type, bonding arrangement etc.

Typical Modelling Exercises can Involve :

- Prediction and visualization of shape/properties.
- Comparison of shape/properties.
- Examination/prediction of molecular interactions and reactions
- Investigation of unstable or excited molecules
- Modelling of dynamic systems (vibrations, diffusion, conformational changes, reactions)

Examples of (Simple) Model Types :

- Stick
- Ball and stick
- Space filled
- VDW surfaces
- Dot surfaces
- Ribbon structures.

Table 8.23 : Commonly Used Molecular Modelling Softwares

Sr. No.	Program	Functions
1.	Amber	M, MM, MD, FE
2.	Biograf	G, S, M, CA, MM, MD, MO
3.	Chem X	G, S, M, C, A, MM, STAT, MO
4.	Grid	PR
5.	Insight/Discover	G, S, M, CA, MM, MD, MO
6.	Macromodel	G, S, M, CA, MM, MD, MO
7.	Midas	G, M
8.	MM^2	MM, CA
9.	Quanta/Charm	G, S, M, CA, MM, MD, FE, PR, STAT
10.	Sybyl/Alchemy/Nitro	G, S, M, CA, MM, MD, STAT, MO

G : graphic display and manipulations

S : small molecule structure building

M : macromolecule structure building

CA : conformational analysis

MM : Molecular mechanics

MD : molecular dynamics

FE : free energy perturbation methods

DG : distance geometry

PR : probe interaction energies

STAT : statistical tools

MO : molecular orbital methods

Table 8.24 : Various Drug - Design Softwares Available in the Market

Sr. No.	Company and Address	Software	Application in Drug Design
1.	Synopsys Scientific Systems Ltd., 175, Woodhouse Lane Leeds LS2 3AR, U.K. www. Synopsys. CO. UK	Accord for Access Biocatalysis Methods* in organic Synthesis Solid-Phase Synthesis Metabolism Bioster	Interface for visualisation of chemical structure access to over 20,000 reactions. Over 5000 reaction data base structural database for analogue design.
2.	Interactive Simulations, Inc. 5330 Carroll Canyon Rd., Suite 203, San Diego, CA 92121 http://www. instsim.com	Sculpt	Building of 3D structures superimpose flexible molecules through conformational analysis, identify pharmacophore, visualise properties of drug.
* Identifies best catalyst (chiroscreen, peptiscreen). It focus on synthetic use of enzyme and micro-organisms for a particular transformation, followed by a kit for rapid optimization of (chiro tool, pepti tool) the reacting, scale up and manufacturing e.g. (1) It provides a quick, simple and cost effective way to identify the best catalyst for the resolution of racemic mixtures, optimize the reaction for enantio selectivity, product yield and scale up. (2) Coupling both natural and unnatural amino acids or peptide fragments, the database identify the best catalyst.			
3.	Gaussian Inc., Carnegie Office Park, Bld., 6., Pitsburgh, PA 1506 USA www:http//www.gaussian.com	Gauss view Gaussian 97 W	Graphical interface to Gaussian molecule building, advanced 3D visualisation graphically display-molecular orbital, electron density surfaces, electrostatic potential structures, atomic charges, ionization potential, dipole moment.
4.	Oxford Molecular Ltd., Medawar Center, Oxford Science Park, Oxford OX 4 46 A, U.K. http://www.oxmol.co.UK/	Cameleon	Predictive tool - to generate DNA and protein as per your own sequence in 3 D - to correlate sequence with residue properties (i.e. antigenicity hydropathy and flexibility) - Gives structural characteristics.
		Amber V 4.1	Molecular modelling and modular simulation studies. It uncovers loops, interactions and active site and examines structural similarity with pharmacophore families data base and PDB.

		Tsar	QSAR analysis - data import, data calculations, analysis and interpretation, automatically. Genetic information about intrinsic molecular properties - lipophilic 2-D and 3-D topological indices, electrostatics.
		Asp	Predicts binding affinity of a potential drug where structure of binding site is unknown. By comparing shape and properties of novel compound with known active drugs, the comparative interactions with the active site can be inferred. (Quantitative property - based molecular similarity applies to 3D QSAR).
		Cobra	Automated conformational analysis to generate a set of low energy conformations. Rapid 2-D to 3-D conversion tool.
		Anaconda	Identifies pharmacophore by visual quantitative comparison of molecular surface properties in a set of compounds having same activity, superimpose flexible molecules.
		Unichem	Electronic structure computations to visualise charge densities, electrostatic potential, IR frequencies and intensities, NMR chemical shifts polarizability, Van der Waals surfaces and interactions.

No.			
5.	Health Designs, Inc., 183, East Main Street Rochester New York 14604, USA	Topkat	Predicts various toxic effects of organic chemicals by means of statistically significant Quantitative Structure Toxicity Relationship (QSTR) models, e.g. Rodent carcinogenicity, Rat oral LD50, teratogenicity, skin sensitization.
6.	Cambridge Soft Corporation, 875, Massachusetts Avenue Cambridge, MA 02139 USA. www.camsoft.com	CS Chem Draw CS Chem 3D	Drawing structure, reactions and mechanisms rotate 3D molecule in any view (wireframe through ribbons) and perform MM2 calculations, compute physical properties and show transition state geometris.
		CS Chem Finder **Chem office**	Electronic features and SAR, Docking studies.
7.	Advanced Chemistry Development, 141 Adelaide St. West, #1501, Toronto, ON M5H 3L5 Canada http://www.acdlabs.com	ACD/CNMR ACD/HNMR ACD.LogP	Calculates accurate 13C NMR spectra and interpretes Calculates accurate proton NMR and interpretes Calculate log P for organic molecule
8.	Brookhaven National Lab. http://www.pdb.bnl.gow	Protein Data Bank	Contains thousands of protein.
9.	VCH Publishers http://www.vchgroup.dc	Antibase	Database of natural compounds with stereochemistry, source, spectral data, biological activity and literature references.
10.	Institute for Scientific Information http://www.isinet.com	Index Chemicus	Over 200,000 new compounds from more than 17000 articles each year.
11.	Synergy software, 2457 Perkiomen Avenue, Reading PA 19606. http://www.synergy.com	Kaleida Graph	Graphing and data analysis of huge and complex data into meaningful visual displays. Contains 256 columns and 32000 rows in each data window. Over 8 million total values.
12.	Hypermedia, 2500 N. Lakeview Avenue, Suite 1902 Chicago, IL 60614.	Spec Tool	Database on most important classes of organic compounds for spectral studies. Prediction of 1H- and 13C-NMR chemical shift, UV absorption maxmima.

Table 8.25 : Current Drugs Discovered through Modern Techniques

Sr. No.	Name of Drug	Category	Outcome of
01.	Captopril (1981)	ACE inhibitor	Structure based drug design
02.	Norfloxacin (1986)	UTI	Lead optimization by QSAR
03.	Dorzolamide (1994)	Glaucoma	Structure based drug design
04.	Saquinavir (1995)	Anti HIV	Structure based drug design
05.	Donepizil (1996)	Alzheimer's disease	Lead optimization by QSAR
06.	Nelfinavir (1997)	Anti HIV	Structure based drug design
07.	Zanarnivir (1999)	Swine Flue H1N1	Structure based drug design
08.	Dasatinib (2006)	Chronic mylogenous leukemia	Structure based drug design
09.	Aliskiren (2007)	Hypertension	Pharmacophore modelling
10.	Raltegravir (2007)	Anti HIV	Pharmacophore modelling
11.	Boceprevir (2011)	Hepatitis C	Structure based drug design
12.	Nolatrexed (Phase III trials)	Liver cancer	Structure based drug design

9

PROTEOMICS AND HOMOLOGY MODELLING

9.1 INTRODUCTION

The majority of drugs available today were discovered either from chance observations or from the screening of synthetic or natural product libraries. The protein structure-based approach relies on an iterative procedure of the initial determination of the structure of the target protein, followed by the prediction of hypothetical legands for the target protein from molecular modelling and the subsequent chemical synthesis and biological testing of specific compounds (the structure-based drug design cycle)

Although the Protein Data Bank (PDB; http://www.rcsb.org/pdb) is growing rapidly (~ 13 new entries daily), the 3D structure of only 1-2% of all known proteins have yet been experimentally characterized.

9.2 HOMOLOGY MODELLING TECHNIQUES

Homology, or comparative modelling uses experimentally determined protein structures to predict the conformation of another protein that has a similar amino acid sequence. The method relies on the observation that in nature the structural conformation of a protein is more highly conserved than its amino acid sequence and that small or medium changes in sequence typically result in only small changes in the 3D structure.

Generally, the process of homology modelling involves four steps - fold assignment, sequence alignment, model building and model refinement. The assignment process identifies proteins of known structure (template structures) that are related to the polypeptide sequence of unknown structure (the target sequence; this is not to be mistaken with drug target). Next,

a sequence database of proteins with known structures (e.g. the PDB-sequence database) is searched with the target sequence using sequence similarity search algorithms or threading techniques. Following identification of a distinct correlation between the target protein and a protein of known 3D structure, the two protein sequences are aligned to identify the optimum correlation between the residues in the template and target sequences. The next stage in the homology modelling process is the model-building phase. Here, a model of the target protein is constructed from the substitution of amino acids in the 3D structure of the template protein and the insertion and/or deletion of amino acids according to the sequence alignment. Finally, the constructed model is checked with regard to conformational aspects and is corrected or energy minimized using force-field approaches. Homology modelling techniques are dependent on the high-resolution experimental protein structure data.

9.3 APPLICATIONS OF HOMOLOGY MODELS IN THE DRUG DISCOVERY PROCESS

Structure-based assessment of target drug ability :

Based on the total numbers of known genes, disease modifying genes and drugable proteins, the number of drug target proteins for humans, has been estimated as approximately between 600-1500.

In the absence of experimental structures of drug target proteins, homology-models have supported the design of several potent pharmacological agents. **Homology modelling,** also known as **comparative modelling,** is a class of methods for constructing an atomic-resolution model of a protein from its amino acid sequence (the "query sequence" or "target"). Almost all homology modelling techniques rely on the identification of one or more known protein structures (known as "templates" or "parent structures") likely to resemble the structure of the query sequence, and on the production of an alignment that maps residues in the query sequence to residues in the template sequence. The sequence alignment and template structure are then used to produce a structural model of the target. Because protein structures are more conserved than protein sequences, detectable levels of sequence similarity usually imply significant structural similarity.

Regions of the model that were constructed without a template, usually by loop modelling, are generally much less accurate than the rest of the model, particularly if the loop is long. Errors in side chain packing and position also increase with decreasing identity, and variations in these packing. Like other methods of structure prediction, current practice in homology modelling is assessed in a biannual large-scale experiment known as the Critical Assessment of Techniques for Protein Structure Prediction or CASP.

Because it is difficult and time-consuming to obtain experimental structures from methods such as X-ray crystallography and protein NMR for every protein of interest, homology modelling can provide useful structural models for generating hypothesis about a protein's function and directing further experimental work.

The simplest method of template identification relies on serial pairwise sequence alignments aided by database search techniques such as FASTA and BLAST. More sensitive methods based on multiple sequence alignment - of which PSI-BLAST is the most common example. Protein threading, also known as fold recognition or 3D-1D alignment, can also be employed as a search technique for identifying templates to be used in traditional homology modelling methods.

Assessment of homology models without reference to the true target structure is usually performed with two methods: statistical potentials or physics-based energy calculations. Both methods produce an estimate of the energy (or an energy-like analogue) for the model or models being assessed.

Statistical potentials are empirical methods based on observed residue-residue contact frequencies among proteins of known structure in the PDB. They assign a probability or energy score to each possible pairwise interaction between amino acids and combine these pairwise interaction scores into a single score for the entire model. Examples of popular statistical potentials include Prosa and DOPE. Statistical potentials are more computationally efficient than energy calculations.

Physics-based energy calculations aim to capture the interatomic interactions that are physically responsible for protein stability in solution, especially Van der Waals and electrostatic interactions. These calculations are performed using a molecular mechanics force field. A force field specifically constructed for model assessment is known as the Effective Force Field (EFF) and is based on atomic parameters from CHARMM.

The most common method of comparing two protein structures uses the Root-Mean-Square Deviation (RMSD) metric to measure the mean distance between the corresponding atoms in the two structures after they have been superimposed. However, RMSD does underestimate the accuracy of models in which the core is essentially correctly modelled, but some flexible loop regions are inaccurate.

Uses of the structural models include protein-protein interaction prediction, protein-protein docking, molecular docking, and functional annotation of genes identified in an organism's genome. Even low-accuracy homology models can be useful for these purposes, because their inaccuracies tend to be located in the loops on the protein surface, which are normally more variable even between closely related proteins. The functional regions of the protein, especially its active site, tend to be more highly conserved and thus more accurately modelled.

[i] Idealization of bond geometry and removal of unfavourable nonbonded contacts are automatically performed by energy minimization with CHARMM (Brooks et al., 1983), using the PARAM22 parameter set and a cutoff distance for interactions of 8 A°.

[ii] The Swiss-prot database (Bairoch and Boeckmann, 1992) contains more than 43.00 sequences, whereas the Brookhaven Protein Data Bank (PDB) [Bernstein et al., 1977] contains 3000 entries, approximately 1000 of which are distinct proteins.

[iii] Multiconformer databases attempt to represent the flexibility of a molecule with a few, selected conformations. For example, a conformational search might yield thousands of candidate conformations, of which a few hundred might be selected for energy minimzation, detailed solvation calculations, or graphic analysis.

Comparative model building consists of the extrapolation of the structure for a new (target) sequence from the known 3D-structure of related family members (templates). One compares the target sequence with a database of sequences derived from the Brookhaven Protein Data Bank (PDB), using programs such as Fast A and BLAST.

A homologous protein is a protein that belongs to the same family, has the same function and shares more than thirty per cent similarity with the protein of interest. The side-chain is generated automatically using a build-in rotamer explorer module. Homology has precise difinition : having a common evolutionary origin.

9.4 GENERAL PROCEDURES

The steps to create a homology model are as follows :

- Identify homologous proteins and determine the extent of their sequence similarity with one another and the unknown.
- Align the sequences.
- Identify structurally conserved and structurally variable regions.
- Generate coordinates for core (structurally conserved) residues of the unknown structure from those of the known structure(s).
- Generate conformations for the loops (structurally variable) in the unknown structure.
- Build the side-chain conformations.
- Refine and evaluate the unknown structure.

In most cases of homology modelling, we have the sequence of a protein for which we want to model the three dimensional structure (the unknown). We then apply sequence search methods to identify proteins with which the unknown has some degree of sequence similarity and for which the three - dimensional structures are available.

Ideally, one will have several homologues to develop a homology model, but modelling can be done with only one known structure.

Although less common, some cases do arise in which the three-dimensional structure of a protein is known and one wants to identify homologues. In these cases, searches of three dimensional databases are performed. An example of a program that provides this type of database searching is Dali. Four general types of scoring have been applied for sequence alignment :

(1) Identity : Considers only identical residues.

(2) Genetic Code : Considers the number of base changes in DNA or RNA to interconvert the codons for the amino acids.

(3) Chemical Similarity : Considers the physico-chemical properties (e.g., polarity, size, charge) with greater weightage given to alignment of similar properties.

(4) Observed Substitutions : Considers substitution frequencies observed in alignment of sequences.

After the known structures are aligned, they are examined to identify the structurally conserved regions (SCRs) from which an average structure or framework, can be constructed for these regions of the proteins. Variable regions (VRs), in which each of the known structures may differ in conformation, also must be identified. Databases are now available that contain large numbers of protein structures that have been obtained by comparative (homology) modelling. Two of these databases are listed here :

- ModBase
- 3Dcrunch.

Programs that provide structure analysis include PROCHECK and 3D-Profiler. PROCHECK is based on an analysis of (phi,psi) angles, peptide bond planarity, bond lengths, bond angles, hydrogen-bond geometry and side-chain conformations of known protein structures as a function of atomic resolution.

3D-profile is based on the statistical preferences of each of the 2 amino acids for particular environments within the protein. Each residue position in a 3D model can be characterized by environment. Preferred environments for amino acids are derived from known three-dimensional structures and are defined by three parameters: (1) the area of each residue that is buried, (2) the fraction of side-chain area that is covered by polar atoms (i.e., O and N), and (3) the local secondary structure.

Several methods are being developed for the classification of proteins based on their structural and functional features.

- SCOP (Structural Classification of Proteins)
- CATH (Class, Architecture, Topology, and Homology)
- HOMSTRAD (Homologous Structure Alignment Database)

Proprotein three-dimensional structures are best determined by experimental methods such as X-ray crystallography and Nuclear Magnetic Resonance (NMR) spectroscopy. Despite significant advances in these techniques, many protein sequences are not easily accessible to structure determination by experiment. Over the last two years, the number of sequences in the comprehensive public sequence databases, such as Swiss Port/TEMBL and GenPept increased by a factor of 2.3. In contrast, despite structural genomics, the number of experimentally determined structures deposited in the Protein Data Bank (PDB) increased by only a factor of 1.4 over the same period. Thus, the gap between the numbers of known sequences and structures continues to grow.

The various optimization approaches include a Monte Carlo simulation, simulated annealing, a combination of Monte Carlo and simulated annealing, the dead-end elimination theorem, genetic algorithms, neural network with simulated annealing, mean field optimization, and combinatorial searches.

A homology modelling routine needs three items of input :

1. The sequence of the protein with unknown 3D structure, the **"target sequence"**.

2. A 3D template is chosen by virtue of having the highest sequence identity with the target sequence. The 3D structure of the template must be determined by reliable empirical methods such as crystallography or NMR, and is typically a published atomic co-ordinate "PDB" file from the Protein Data Bank.

3. An **alignme** between the target sequence and the template sequence.

The homology modelling routine arranges the backbone identically to that of the template. This means that not only the positions of alpha carbons, but also the phi and psi angles and secondary structure, are made identical to the template. Next, the more sophisticated homology modelling packages adjust side chain positions to minimize collisions, and may offer further energy minimization or molecular dynamics in an attempt to improve the model.

Overall differences in protein backbone structures are correlated with the root mean square deviation of the positions of alpha carbons or **rmsd.** Proteins are functional molecules in cells and are the major targets for drug action. To design a rational drug, we must firstly find out which proteins can be the drug targets in pathogenesis. Proteomics has great promise in identification of protein targets and biochemical pathways involved in disease processes. Proteomics as a whole increasingly plays an important role in the multi-step drug development process. The process includes target identification and validation, lead selection, small molecular screening and optimization, and toxicity testing. Furthermore, sub-disciplines such as computational proteomics, chemical proteomics, structural proteomics and topological proteomics offer significant contributions especially in computer-aided drug design.

During the early 1980s, structural biologists began to design rational drugs based on protein structures. The first projects were underway in the mid-1980s, and the first successful story, computer-aided rational design of peptide-based HIV-proteinase inhibitors, was published by the early 1990s.

3D structure of a target protein or nucleic acid is determined by X-ray crystallography or NMR. Using recently constructed protein and nucleic acid databases, new computational methods use the 3D structural information of the unliganded target to design entirely new lead compounds de novo. In this way, large virtual combinatorial libraries of compounds can then be screened computationally before going to the effort and expense of actual synthesis and biological studies. The ability to rapidly and accurately dock large numbers of candidate molecules into the binding site of a target macromolecule is a key component of lead generation.

Table 9.1 : Useful Websites in Computer-Aided Drug Design and Proteomics

Sr. No.	Database Description	UTL
1.	Ontario Center for Structural Proteomics.	http://www.uhnres.utoronto.ca/proteomics/
2.	Network service for comparing protein structures in 3D.	http://www.ebi.ac.uk/dali/
3.	Databases and Tools for 3D Protein Structure Comparison and Alignment.	http://cl.sdsc.edu/cc.html
4.	Integrated Sequence-Structure Database.	http://www.protein.bio.msu.su/issd/
5.	PROCAT 3D enzyme active site templates.	http://www.biochem.ucl.ac.uk/bsm/PROCAT/PROCAT.html
6.	Structural Classification of Proteins.	http://scop.mrc.lmb.cam.ac.uk/scop/
7.	Topology of Protein Structure.	http://www.tops.leeds.ac.uk/
8.	Biomolecular Interaction Network database.	http://www.blueprint,org/bind/bind.php
9.	TopNet for Topological Proteomics.	http://network.gersteinlab.org/genome
10.	Protein Data Bank.	http://www.rcsb.org/pdb/
11.	Protein sequence analysis and structure prediction.	http://www.embl-heidelberg.de/predictprotein/predictprotein.html

The major resources for computational proteomics are currently available protein and nucleic acid structures, the 3DGENOMICS (http://www.sbg.bio.ic.au uk/3dgenomics/) and PDB (http://www.rcsb.org/pdb/). When directly calculating and predicting a three-dimensional structure, the availability of a high quality, closely related template is essential to the success of the modelling process. Generally for a homology, model to be useful, adequate sequence identity (> 30%) should exist between target and template protein.

A homology model is generally constructed by extracting structural information from a template protein and applying this in the generation of a target protein's three-dimensional structure according to their mutual sequence similarity. Several algorithms are available to generate a homology model including the programs Modeller (Sali and Blundell, 1993), SYBYL Composer (Blundell et al., 1988), Insightll Homology (Greer, 1990), IGM (MolSoft, San Diego, CA). There are also several internet-based services available such as the Swiss-Model website and server (Schwede et al., 2003), the WHAT IF server (Vriend, 1990) and the 3D-Jigsaw Comparative Modelling Server (Bates et al., 2001; Contreras-Moreira and Bates, 2002). Generally, all modelling approaches follow the same four steps : (1) template identification; (2) sequence alignment; (3) model generation; and (4) model optimization and validation.

In the template identification step, a database of known sturures, usually retrieved from the RCSB protein data bank (Deshpande et al., 2005), is queried using sequence similarity search algorithms such as BLAST (Altschul et al., 1990) or PSI-BLAST (Altschul et al., 1997), or fold recognition algorithms (Godzik, 2003).

The second step, sequence alignment, is the most critical step to any successful homology modelling project. All homology modelling programs provide commands or modules for the automatic sequence alignment of two or multiple proteins. However, these machine-generated alignments frequently contain errors mainly due to the absence of knowledge regarding conserved sequences within a protein family and the functional role of individual amino acid residues. As emphasized in every homology modelling experiment, manual adjustment of machine-generated sequence alignment is essential for generating a successful model. When adjusting the alignment, care should be taken to align conserved sequences and to move gaps to the more variable extra membranous loop regions.

The third step, model generation, has been well established in each modelling tool and does not usually require human intervention.

Validation is an essential process to ensure accuracy of the generated model and there are two types of approaches available. Theoretical validation, where independent structural stereochemistry check programs are used to verify the quality of the model, and experimental validation where the model is tested against biological results.

PROCHECK (Laskowski 1997; Luthy et al., 1992), and WHAT IF (Vriend, 1990) are commonly used tools for external evaluation of the correctness of homology models. Generally, these programs develop rules and parameters extracted from available crystal structures and apply these to the model structure. The fitness that is presented by a 'fit score' indicates the compatibility of the model to the available crystal structures.

The majority of homology modelling studies also tests the model against available experimental data, including site-directed mutagenesis, cross-linking data, and low-resolution electron microsocopy studies.

Three automated programs are widely used for pharmacophore generation, distance comparisons (DISCO) (Martin et al., 1993), GASP (Jones et al., 1995) and Catalyst HIPHOP (Clement and Mehl, 2000). All programs attempt to determine common molecular features based on the superposition of active compounds.

Catalyst/hypoGen analysis requires a full range of test compounds from active to inactive along with their measured activities derived from experimental data. The result extends the usual pharmacophore. It not only identifies a query compound as active or inactive like in the tradition of a pharmacophore model, but also predicts the activity based on the regression of the training dataset.

Genetic Algorithm Similarity Program (GASP) is a genetic algorithm, developed for the superimposition of sets of flexible molecules (Jones et al., 1995).

With the input of a full range of training set compounds ranging from inactive to active, the HypoGen algorithm can generate hypothesis with features common amongst active molecules and missing from the inactive molecules (Li et al., 2000). This is accomplished in three steps, a constructive step, a subtractive step and an optimization step. Hypothesis common amongst the active compounds are identified in the constructive step, which is very similar to the regular pharmacophore perception procedure. Hypothesis common among inactive compounds are removed from the previous result in the subtractive step. The resultant hypothesis is then optimized using simulated annealing to further finetune the model parameters, thereby improving model quality.

Printed in the USA
CPSIA information can be obtained
at www.ICGtesting.com
LVHW050846260923
759107LV00009B/122